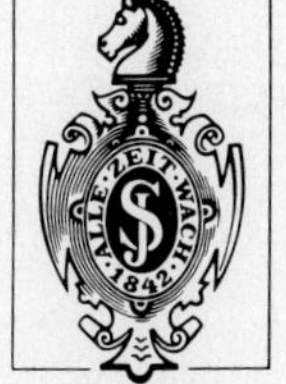

Marwali Harahap (Ed.)

Complications of Dermatologic Surgery

Prevention and Treatment

With 10 tables and 87 illustrations

Springer-Verlag
Berlin Heidelberg New York
London Paris Tokyo
Hong Kong Barcelona
Budapest

Harahap, Marwali, M.D.
Department of Dermatology
University of North Sumatra Medical School
Rumah Sakit Umun Pusat
H. ADAM MALIK
Jalan Bunga Lau No. 17
Medan 20136, Indonesia

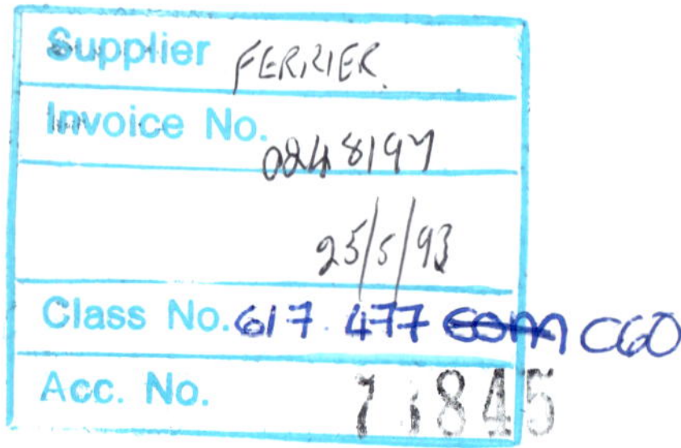

ISBN 3-540-55 337-1 Springer-Verlag Berlin Heidelberg New York
ISBN 0-387-55 337-1 Springer-Verlag New York Berlin Heidelberg

Printed: Druckhaus Beltz, 6944 Hemsbach
Bookbinding: J. Schäffer, 6718 Grünstadt
27/3145/5 4 3 2 1 0 – Printed on acid-free paper

Preface

The scope of dermatologic surgery is so wide that inevitably a large number and variety of complications arise. Of course the majority of complications can be prevented by careful preoperative preparation, meticulous surgical technique, and proper postoperative care, but when they do occur, they can be recognized and managed with skill and competence.

This book provides a valuable source of reference for the prevention, recognition, and management of complications in dermatologic surgery. Avoiding problems is at least as important as dealing with them, and so all the chapters in this book deal with both prevention and management.

This book addresses dermatologic surgeons in practice or in training and to surgeons in other specialties who may be required to undertake repair of skin defects.

Many of the authors accepted the responsibility of contributing to this work in addition to their many other obligations. For this, I am extremely grateful to them.

MARWALI HARAHAP

Contents

List of Authors

Philip L. Bailin, M. D., F. A. C. P.
  Department of Dermatology, Cleveland Clinic Foundation, Cleveland, OH,
  USA

Robert L. Baran, M. D.
  Unité de Dermatologie, Hôpital Général de Cannes, 06400 Cannes, France

Eugene L. Bodian, M. D., F. A. C. P.
  New York Hospital – Cornell Medical Center, 525 East 68th Street,
  New York, NY 10021 and New York University Medical Center, NYU-Skin
  and Cancer Unit, 560 First Avenue, New York, NY 10016, USA

Brian B. Burkey, M. D.
  Department of Otolaryngology – Head and Neck Surgery,
  Vanderbilt University Medical Center, S-2100 Medical Center North,
  Nashville, TN 37232, USA

Roger I. Ceilley, M. D.
  Department of Dermatology, University of Iowa, 600 University Ave.,
  Suite 450, West Des Moines, IA 50265, USA

William P. Coleman, III, M. D.
  Department of Dermatology, Tulane University School of Medicine,
  New Orleans, LA, USA, and The Coleman Clinic, 4425 Conlin Street,
  Metairie, LA 70006, USA

Paul S. Collins, M. D.
  Department of Dermatology, Stanford University Medical School,
  Stanford, CA, USA

Daniel W. Collison, M. D.
  Section of Dermatology, Dartmouth-Hitchcock Medical Center,
  One Medical Center Drive, Lebanon, NH 03756, USA

Rodney P. R. Dawber, MA, MB, CH. B, FRCP
  Department of Dermatology, The Slade Hospital, Headington,
  Oxford OX3 7JH, UK

Melvin L. Elson, M. D.
  The Dermatology Center, Inc., 4535 Harding Rd., Ste. 300, Nashville,
  TN 37205–2120, USA

Harvey Finkelstein, MDCM, FRCPC
  Department of Dermatology, University of Ottawa, 451 Smyth, Ottawa,
  Ontario, Canada K1N 8M5 and Ottawa Regional Cancer Center,
  Civic Division, 190 Melrose, Ottawa, Ontario, Canada K1Y 4K7

James E. Fulton, Jr., M. D.
  Acne Research Institute, 1617 Westcliff Drive, Suite 100, Newport Beach,
  CA 92660, USA

Ann F. Haas, M. D.
  Department of Dermatology, University of California at Davis,
  1700 Stockton Blvd., Sacramento, CA 95816, USA

Eckart Haneke, Prof. Dr. med.
  Department of Dermatology, Ferdinand-Sauerbruch-Klinikum Elberfeld,
  Arrenbergerstraße 20–56, 5600 Wuppertal 1, FRG

Marwali Harahap, Prof. Dr.
  Department of Dermatology, University of North Sumatra Medical School
  and Academic Hospital, Rumah Sakit Umum Pusat, H. ADAM MALIK,
  Jalan Bunga Lau 17, Tuntungan, Medan 20136, Indonesia

Robert Jackson, MDCM, FRCPC
  Department of Dermatology, University of Ottawa, 451 Smyth, Ottawa,
  Ontario, Canada K1N 8M5 and Department of Dermatology, Ottawa Civic
  Hospital, 1053 Carling, Ottawa, Ontario, Canada K1Y 4E9

Pearon G. Lang, Jr., M. D.
  Departments of Dermatology, Otolaryngology, and Communicative
  Sciences, Medical University of South Carolina, 171 Ashley Avenue,
  Charleston, SC 29425, USA

S. Teri McGillis, M. D.
  Department of Dermatology, Cleveland Clinic Foundation, Cleveland, OH,
  USA

Deborah Moritz, M. D.
  University of California Los Angeles, Department of Dermatology,
  Cleveland Clinic Foundation, Cleveland, OH, USA

Ronald L. Moy, M. D.
  Dermatology Center, Mohs Micrographic Surgery, 200 UCLA Medical Plaza,
  Los Angeles, CA 90024-6957, USA

Michael J. Sullivan, M. D.
   Department of Otolaryngology – Head and Neck Surgery, The Ohio State
   University, 456 West 10th Avenue, Room 4123, Columbus, OH 43210, USA

Nicholas R. Telfer, MD, MRCP
   Dermatology Center, Mohs Micrographic Surgery, 200 UCLA Medical Plaza,
   Los Angeles, CA 90024–6957, USA

Anna Tong, BS
   Dermatology Center, Mohs Micrographic Surgery, 200 UCLA Medical Plaza,
   Los Angeles, CA 90024–6957, USA

Walter P. Unger, MD, FRCPC, FACP
   Department of Dermatology, University of Toronto, Toronto, Ontario,
   Canada

Allison T. Vidimos, R. Ph., M. D.
   Department of Dermatology, Cleveland Clinic Foundation, Cleveland, OH,
   USA

Ronald G. Wheeland, M. D., F. A. C. P.
   Department of Dermatology, University of California at Davis,
   1700 Stockton Blvd., Sacramento, CA 95816, USA

George B. Winton, M. D.
   Department of Dermatology, James E. Quillen School of Medicine,
   East Tennessee State University, Johnson City, TN 37604, USA

Local Anesthesia and Regional Anesthesia

George B. Winton

Introduction

The use of local and regional anesthesia in surgical practice is considered to be safe, certainly much safer than the use of general anesthesia. For example, a 1955 survey of local anesthesia used for dental procedures found only two deaths in an estimated 90 million cases over a span of 10 years [1]. Such a statistic can lull one into an inappropriate sense of security. Significant complications other than death can and do occur with the use of local anesthetics which can cause considerable difficulty for patients [2]. The incidence of adverse reactions to regional blocks in a hospital setting is approximately 0.2% [3] while the incidence of adverse responses to dental local anesthesia may be as high as 2.5% [4]. The latter figure includes a substantial number of psychological reactions. It is imperative that any physician utilizing local and regional anesthesia understand the potential risks and be prepared to manage complications. This chapter covers local and systemic adverse reactions including allergy, drug interactions, and reactions peculiar to certain drugs, and also reviews precautions that one should take to prevent difficulties.

Complications Related to Use of Vasoconstrictors

Vasoconstrictors such as epinephrine are added to local anesthetic solutions to prolong anesthesia, control bleeding, and reduce systemic toxicity by reducing the rate of anesthetic absorption into the general circulation [5–7]. Toxic reactions include tachycardia, elevation of blood pressure, tremors, anxiety, diaphoresis, tachypnea, palpitations, headache, weakness, arrythmias, including ventricular fibrillation, cerebral hemorrhage, and cardiac arrest [5, 8, 9]. All of these effects can also be precipitated by excessive endogenous adrenalin which may result from an adverse psychological response to the injection or to surgery. The high rate of adverse reactions to dental procedures has been attributed largely to psychological effects because they do not seem to be dose related and may occur even when no vasoconstrictor is utilized [10]. It should also be noted that many of the listed effects of vasoconstrictor toxicity can also be produced by overdosage of the anesthetic agent and some can even be seen during an anaphylactic allergic reaction. To determine whether excessive vasoconstrictor is causing a particular constellation of signs and symptoms requires careful monitoring of blood pressure. In both anesthetic toxicity and anaphylaxis, blood pressure falls fairly rapidly, while excessive catecholamines cause it to rise [9].

Because the amount of subcutaneous epinephrine necessary to cause a systemic pressor effect is about 0.5 mg, which corresponds to 50 ml of a 1 : 100 000 solution, it is unlikely that adverse reactions would be encountered in most dermatologic surgery unless an intravascular injection is made. Even in cardiac patients 0.2 mg is considered safe [11, 12]. If injection has been made slowly, only a small amount of vasoconstrictor enters the circulation, and symptoms of toxicity passes quickly with no specific treatment [2]. Any patient who experiences angina should receive oxygen and sublingual nitroglycerin [12]. In the unlikely event that symptoms of anxiety are prolonged, 20–40 mg secobarbital given intramuscularly or intravenously is beneficial [2]. For the rare patient in whom a dangerous blood pressure elevation persists, treatment with a short-acting vasodilator such as nitroprusside [12] or small incremental doses of chlorpromazine [9] has been recommended. Cautious management is mandatory to prevent hypotension secondary to the treatment as vasoconstrictor is cleared from the circulation. Such serious circumstances are far more likely to appear during spinal or epidural anesthesia than during dermatologic surgery.

Contraindications to the use of vasoconstrictors include pheochromocytoma and hyperthyroidism. Relative contraindications include hypertension or cardiac disease, emotional disturbance, narrow angle glaucoma, peripheral vascular disease, concomitant use of general anesthesia, use of phenothiazines and tricyclic antidepressants, anesthesia in acral areas, use of beta blockers, and presence of early or late pregnancy [5, 7, 8, 13–16]. The relative contraindications which relate to drug interactions are discussed in a later section.

The use of vasoconstrictors, or any drug for that matter, during early pregnancy may affect organogenesis. Epinephrine in high doses can cause uterine artery spasm leading to diminished placental perfusion [17]. In late pregnancy epinephrine may delay labor [7, 16]. However, neither local anesthetics nor epinephrine is considered teratogenic, and it is unlikely that small doses utilized in dermatologic surgery would be detrimental. Therefore a total proscription of vasoconstrictor use in pregnancy is probably unwise although appropriate caution should be observed [18]. Prilocaine should be avoided during any stage of pregnancy because it may cross the placental barrier to produce fetal methemoglobinemia [19].

There has been a general precaution against the use of vasoconstrictors in acral areas such as the penis, digits, and earlobes [5, 7, 13, 16]. While this contraindication is only relative, certain situations require particular concern. The presence of diabetic angiopathy, Raynaud's phenomenon, cardiovascular disease, or impaired peripheral circulation rule against the use of vasoconstrictors [8]. Likewise, any circumferential injection of anesthesia into an appendage, especially when the fluid pressure of the agent would itself cause some vasoconstriction, should be done without epinephrine [20].

The ability of the vasoconstrictor to control local bleeding and reduce systemic absorption and toxicity from the anesthetic itself must be weighed against the unlikelihood of an adverse reaction in a robust patient. Many anesthetics are vasodilators, and epinephrine is quite useful in countering this effect. Dermatologists have found that small quantities of epinephrine can be safely infiltrated into localized areas of the ears, nose, penis, and even the tips of the digits in healthy patients [16].

A similar line of reasoning should be applied to the cardiac patient who is to have cutaneous surgery at any site. Patients who have had a myocardial infarction within the previous 6 months may have on unstable myocardium susceptible to life-threatening arrhythmias. If possible, surgery should be postponed until the scar and conduction tissue are stable. When surgery is performed, the relative advantages and disadvantages of vasoconstrictor use must be weighed for each patient. It may be safer to use modest quantities of lidocaine and epinephrine than to use a less reliable agent. The rise in heart rate and blood pressure due to inadequate pain control has been shown to produce more significant ECG changes than the injection of lidocaine with vasoconstrictor for dental procedures [19].

In 1983 Foster and Aston [14] reported an unusual interaction of epinephrine and propranolol in patients receiving local anesthesia. In this reaction, malignant hypertension, stroke and even cardiac arrest occurred after the injection of a local anesthetic containing epinephrine into patients taking propranolol. Theoretically, propranolol blocks both beta-1 cardiac receptors and beta-2 vascular bed receptors. The beta-2 receptors normally function to dilate vascular smooth muscle. When beta-2 receptors are blocked by propranolol and alpha receptors, which serve to constrict vasculature, are stimulated by epinephrine, the vasoconstrictive effects are unopposed and therefore exaggerated. Blood pressure rises precipitously, and a vagal response then slows the heart rate [16].

Following this report, Dzubow [15] prospectively studied ten patients undergoing cutaneous surgery and was unable to reproduce the reaction. He noted that patients receiving plain lidocaine experienced a significant fall in blood pressure following injection while those receiving lidocaine with epinephrine showed no change. The catastrophic reactions reported earlier may represent dose related or idiosyncratic responses or may be unrelated to this combination of drugs.

The prevention of the epinephrine-propranolol interaction can be achieved in several ways. A pure beta-1 blocker should theoretically be safe and can be substituted for propranolol under the supervision of an internist or cardiologist. A lower concentration of epinephrine (e. g., 1 : 500 000) may be equally effective in some cutaneous surgery [21–23]. The anesthetic can be injected slowly over a longer period of time with blood pressure monitoring. This choice seems easiest in view of Dzubow's data [15]. Finally, a longer acting anesthetic without epinephrine can be used. The slow absorption and lack of vasodilatory effect make prilocaine a good candidate, although its tendency to produce methemoglobinemia should be considered [16].

Treatment for the epinephrine-propronolol reaction includes intravenous administration of chlorpromazine in 1-mg increments with careful monitoring. No more than 5 mg is usually necessary. A hydralazine drip, 20 mg in 250 cm^3 saline, also administered with monitoring, is equally effective. If bradycardia persists after control of hypertension, atropine can be given [14].

Local Complications

General

The vast majority of local complications are due to poor technique although inappropriate use of epinephrine and the effect of certain drug combinations also produce an occasional adverse reaction.

Pain on Injection

A certain amount of discomfort is unavoidable when injecting local anesthetics. Pain can be minimized by using a good injection technique, which includes pinching the skin, inserting the needle slowly through a hair follicle to inject the first wheal, slowly injecting an initial wheal at the dermal-subcutaneous junction, and extending anesthesia by making subsequent injections through previously anesthetized areas [24]. The pain of the initial needle stick can further be minimized by first applying a topical aerosol refrigerant to skin surfaces [25] or viscous lidocaine to mucosal surfaces [2].

Much of the discomfort of anesthetic injections has been related to the presence of citric acid, which stabilizes epinephrine and gives the solutions a pH of approximately 4.0 [26–28]. Less painful injections can be achieved by first neutralizing the agent with sodium bicarbonate. An appropriately neutralized solution can be made by adding 5.0 ml 7.5% sodium bicarbonate solution to a 50 ml vial of 1% lidocaine with epinephrine. The neutralized solution should remain stable for 1 week [28]. The safety of this technique is not fully established [26], and its use should probably be restricted to local injection and not applied to regional blocks.

An alternative is to mix plain anesthetic with fresh epinephrine just prior to use. If 0.3 ml 1 : 1000 epinephrine is added to 30 ml anesthetic, a 1 : 100 000 concentration results having a pH higher than commercially mixed solutions [26].

Hematoma

A hematoma may result from puncture of blood vessels, injection into highly vascular areas, or injection of a patient with faulty coagulation. In most cases application of direct pressure is an adequate remedy. Should faulty coagulation seem to be present, consideration should be given to postponing surgery until an evaluation can be accomplished. Hematomas can form during trigeminal nerve blocks and are best prevented by aspirating before injection and avoiding injections into foramina [2]. Should a nerve block result in hematoma, the patient must be monitored carefully for evidence of infection at 48-h intervals [2].

Edema, Inflammation, Abscess

These complications all relate to the injection of foreign materials. Edema has been observed in dental practice and is believed to be caused by metallic ions (copper, zinc, nickel) in the anesthetic solution [29]. By avoiding metal syringes and bowls this complication is prevented. Inflammatory and infective complications can be prevented by use of proper sterile technique.

Necrosis

Persistent pain following the use of local anesthesia may be the first sign of necrosis of tissue. It may result from multiple injections into a small area, use of epinephrine concentrations higher than 1 : 100 000 or from high-pressure injections into thin, firmly adherent tissue such as the hard palate [2], nasal mucosa, or external auditory canal.

Nerve Injury

Penetration of the needle into a nerve sheath can cause injury leading to persistent anesthesia or paresthesia following nerve block. Contaminants such as alcohol can cause similar problems [2]. There have also been reports of prolonged anesthesia following nerve blocks using chloroprocaine solutions containing sodium bisulfite at pH 3.0. Follow-up in vitro testing has shown that the combination of low pH and presence of sodium bisulfite in the anesthetic solution can produce irreversible conduction blockade [30]. Should such complications occur, there is no treatment to be given. In most cases regeneration of the nerve occurs over a period of several months [2].

Needle Breakage

Needle breakage tends to occur when the needle is redirected within tissue without withdrawing it far enough to allow a pivot. Breakage generally occurs at the hub [2, 12]. A needle tip lost within a body orifice such as the mouth, nose, or ear may require radiographic localization before retrieval is attempted. To avoid this problem, use an anesthetic needle long enough so that it does not have to be inserted completely into tissues.

Inadvertent Motor Blockade

Because of the spreading ability of anesthetic solutions, inadvertent blockade of facial nerve branches can occur during facial surgery. Femoral nerve block has also been reported after hernia repair under local anesthesia [31]. The initial difficulty is ascertaining whether a motor nerve has been severed during the procedure. If the facial nerve is anesthetized, the patient may not be able to close an eye completely. Therefore, the eye should be patched until function returns [2].

Blindness and Double Vision

Injection of too much anesthetic under high pressure when performing an infraorbital nerve block can cause diffusion of agent into the orbit, producing temporary blindness [2]. Hematoma within the orbit can also be produced by an improperly placed block. If anesthesia reaches one or more extraocular muscles, double vision can occur [2, 32]. Permanent blindness has also been reported [33] following injection of a large volume of lidocaine with vasoconstrictor into the nasal septal mucosa. It was suspected that spasm of the ophthalmic artery had occurred due to retrograde flow from nasal vessels with subsequent thrombus formation. To prevent this rare complication, injections should be limited to 5–10 cm^3, all air should be removed from the syringe, and injection into the highly vascular turbinates should be avoided. Injection of oily substances, collagen, or crystal liquids should be done only with extreme caution.

Systemic Reactions to Anesthetics

Vasovagal Reaction

The most common systemic reaction is a vasovagal episode in an anxious patient. Here pallor, tachypnea, hypotension, diaphoresis, bradycardia and syncope are seen and can usually be reversed by elevation of the legs (Table 1) [5]. In severe cases, oxygen and aromatic spirits of ammonia should be administered. If these measures fail, one should look for a more serious medical cause of the syncope [2]. Differentiation from vasoconstrictor overdosage is usually possible because of the low blood pressure observed. Differentiation from anaphylaxis should be possible because of the lack of respiratory distress. Because vagovagal episodes commonly occur just as anesthesia is being administered, the possibility of anesthetic overdose can usually be dismissed especially if there have been no premonitory signs of CNS excitability (e. g. twitching, seizures). Vasovagal episodes can be prevented by placing the patient in a supine position preoperatively.

Table 1. Management outline for acute local anesthetic toxicity [2, 6, 9, 36, 39, 42, 53]

Symptoms	Diagnosis	Therapy
Pallor, sweating, nausea, bradycardia, hypotension	vasovagal episode	Supine position (lateral position in obstetrics); O_2, ephedrine, atropine if needed.
Apprehension, cold sweat, tachycardia, arrhythmia, elevated blood pressure	Reaction to vasopressor	Observe for recovery if due to small intravascular injection. Otherwise may use O_2, SL NTG, secobarbital, nitroprusside, or chlorpromazine as needed.
Tremors, twitching, excitation, nervousness	Moderate anesthetic toxicity	O_2, head-down position, hyperventilation, diazepam or thiopental. (Do not overtreat.)
Convulsions	Moderate to severe anesthetic toxicity	Maintain respiration, protect patient from injury; diazepam or thiopental.
Apnea	Severe anesthetic toxicity	Artificial ventilation, intubate if possible to avoid aspiration; maintain blood pressure.
Apnea and cardio-vascular collapse	Severe anesthetic toxicity	As above, with closed chest cardiac massage, adrenaline.
Skin rash, hypotension, tachycardia, bronchospasm, abdominal pain, strider, shock	Allergy to anesthetic	Epinephrine, antihistamine, corticosteroid, O_2 by mask, IV fluids, CPR if necessary.

Systemic Toxicity

General

Direct systemic toxicity to a local anesthetic can result from exceeding the recommended maximum dose or from making an accidental intravascular injection. High blood levels of anesthetic may also result from delayed clearance of anesthetic from the body secondary to a preexisting disease or to a drug interaction.

The maximum recommended doses of commonly used anesthetics are listed in Table 2. These doses are applicable to both local infiltration anesthesia and nerve blocks. It is rare that larger quantities would be necessary in most dermatologic surgery. If a large volume of agent is required, the concentration can be reduced by adding normal saline. Because toxicity of local anesthetics is related to serum levels rather than to the quantity of agent present in the tissue, it is sometimes possible to exceed the recommended dosage in poorly vasularized

Table 2. Maximum doses of local anesthetics [5, 6, 13, 16, 25]
Adult doses are listed. Consult *Physicians' Desk Reference* for pediatric doses.

Anesthetic	Maximum single dose (no epi./epi.)
Cocaine	150 mg
Procaine	500 mg/600 mg
Lidocaine	300 mg/500 mg
Mepivacaine	300 mg/500 mg
Bupivacaine	175 mg/250 mg
Prilocaine	400 mg/600 mg
Etidocaine	300 mg/400 mg

sites. It is possible to exceed these amounts in liposuction surgery, for example, because the agent is absorbed into the circulation quite slowly and may not reach a peak until 12 h after injection [34].

Intravascular injection is a more common cause of systemic toxicity for dermatologists. A high pressure injection into a named artery on the face may reach the cerebral circulation causing an immediate seizure. The twin precautions of aspirating before injecting nerve blocks and injecting slowly prevents a catastrophe. Should toxicity nevertheless occur, this is short lived. Aspirating before local infiltration is inconvenient and possibly less important because large vessels are not likely to be encountered. Difficulties can be avoided by simply keeping the needle tip in motion while injecting locally. Again, this technique prevents any large amount of agent from reaching a vessel should one be penetrated.

Anesthetics containing an ester linkage (e. g., cocaine, procaine, tetracaine) are metabolized in the tissues or in the local circulation by pseudocholinesterase. Patients with an inherited deficiency of this enzyme are susceptible to toxicity from these drugs [13]. The amide anesthetics (e. g., lidocaine, bupivacaine) are metabolized in the liver, and preexisting liver disease may delay elimination from the body. Both esters and amides are excreted by the kidney, and renal malfunction can therefore lead to toxic accumulation of anesthetics or their metabolic by-products [2].

There are several drug interactions that affect local anesthetic use. These are discussed in a separate section.

Symptoms

The symptoms of anesthetic toxicity are immediate if they result from intravascular injection or delayed 5–30 min if they are caused by the gradual build-up of high blood levels [9, 35]. The latter circumstance leads to a slowly accelerating constellation of symptoms which facilitates early recognition and effective intervention. The former circumstance is not a serious problem if small amounts of drug are involved. If large amounts are involved, death may result from cardiovascular collapse before treatment can be instituted [9].

At low blood levels the toxicity of local anesthetics is manifested by CNS excitability, possibly associated with a transient increase in blood pressure and pulse [9]. As blood levels rise, signs of cardiovascular and respiratory depression appear and CNS excitability gives way to CNS depression [9].

Initially, low blood levels of 1–5 mg/ml (lidocaine) produce excitatory symptoms of lightheadedness, euphoria, tingling of the lips, ringing of the ears, a bitter taste in the mouth, and a general chill. This blood level is achieved when lidocaine is used as an antiarrhythmic drug [36] and has been observed during routine hair transplantation procedures [37]. At moderate blood levels of 8–12 mg/ml (lidocaine), an anesthetic seizure can occur. Sometimes a prodrome of slow speech, jerky tremors, and hallucinations is seen [36]. At high blood levels of 20–25 mg/ml (lidocaine) the cardiac effects are noted, and a general CNS depression occurs. Shallow respirations give way to apnea and cardiovascular collapse [36].

Prevention

To prevent toxic overdoses several rules should be followed [6, 36]:
a) use the minimum effective dose of anesthetic, especially on the head and neck,
b) aspirate before injecting,
c) use divided doses when injecting large areas,
d) use nerve blocks with minimal local infiltration whenever possible,
e) allow sufficient time for the anesthetic to work before reinjecting,
f) avoid injecting inflammed tissues (anesthetic is less effective),
g) use a vasoconstrictor when indicated,
h) consider preoperative sedation with diazepam to increase the seizure threshold when large amounts of anesthetic must be used.

The last recommendation must be approached with caution because high doses of minor tranquilizers may suppress early CNS symptoms of anesthetic overdose so that abrupt cardiovascular depression is the first sign of trouble [38].

Treatment

The treatment of anesthetic overdose depends on the relative blood levels present and the signs and symptoms observed. At low blood levels, manifested by lightheadedness or dizziness, place the patient in a head-down position with legs elevated and administer oxygen. If blood pressure is low, ephedrine 50 mg may be given intramuscularly or 10–25 mg intravenously (adjust dosage for children and debilitated patients) [6].

Moderate blood levels may produce signs of impending convulsions such as tremors, twitching, and excitation. A seizure can sometimes be prevented by placing the patient in a recumbent position, administering oxygen, and encouraging hyperventilation. Diazepam 10 mg intramuscularly or 3–10 mg intravenously provides further protection [6, 39]. Should a seizure occur, it normally lasts less than 60 s [39]. The most important immediate actions are to protect the patient from physical injury and to insure adequate ventilation. If the patient becomes unresponsive, manual ventilation or mouth-to-mouth respiration should be administered. Diazepam, as described above, or thiopental 50–100 mg intravenously can be used to arrest seizure activity; however, in any case overtreatment should be avoided. Both drugs can cause CNS depression which can delay the return of the patient to full consciousness [39] and may cause apnea [9], especially when combined with high blood levels of anesthetic.

At high blood levels cardiovascular collapse can occur requiring full cardiopulmonary resuscitation. In most cases respiratory depression precedes circulatory collapse [9]. Cardiovascular collapse does not usually occur if respirations become inadequate; sufficient oxygen is supplied to the patient by artificial means. Artificial ventilation is then continued until spontaneous respiration returns [9]. If blood pressure is falling and respirations are shallow and rapid, vasopressors and artificial ventilation should be begun at once [36].

Allergic Reactions

Allergic reactions to local anesthetics are quite rare, probably accounting for only 1% of adverse effects due to these agents [40]. Allergy to ester-linked agents is far more common than allergy to the newer amides. Para-aminobenzoic acid liberated by the hydrolysis of ester-linked anesthetics is believed to be responsible for the allergic reactions. There is a theoretical possibility that allergy to the esters could be cross-reactive with methylparaben, used as a preservative in multiuse vials of amide anesthetics [35]. Therefore paraben sensitivity must be ruled out whenever allergy to an amide is suspected. There appear to be few documented accounts of true allergic reactions to an amide-linked anesthetic itself, and there appears to be little or no cross-reactivity between the two groups [5, 41]. However, patients who are allergic to one ester may be allergic to the whole group while those allergic to an amide may be able to use an alternative amide successfully [12]. Many patients who believe that they are allergic to local anesthetics have instead suffered at one time a vasovagal reaction or an adverse response to epinephrine or lidocaine due to intravascular injection. Nonetheless, the presence of allergy should be ruled out prior to rechallenge.

A full range of allergic manifestations is possible, including both immediate and delayed hypersensitivity syndromes. More than 80% of reactions are cell-mediated, resulting in contact dermatitis [42]. The remainder are caused by circulating antibodies producing urticaria, angioedema, dyspnea, hypotension, or cardiovascular collapse.

The proper method of evaluating patients with suspected allergy is complicated by a high incidence of false-positive reactions on intradermal testing [42], not all of which can be attributed to preservatives. Furthermore, a patient sensitized to IgE antibodies may suffer acute, fatal anaphylaxis upon exposure to a minute test dose. It has also been shown that there is poor correlation between patch test and prick and intradermal test results, meaning that type I and type IV hypersensitivity can occur independently [43]. Nonetheless, there is now substantial opinion that skin testing can be useful if it documents that a tested drug is safe even if allergy to some other specific agent cannot be determined with certainty [5, 44, 45]. Testing should be done in a facility equipped to handle anaphylaxis or other emergencies, and it should be supplemented with progressive subcutaneous challenge of larger test doses [45, 46].

The initial treatment of an immediate hypersensitivity reaction consists of the subcutaneous injection of 0.5 ml (0.1–0.3 ml in children) 1 : 1000 epinephrine [2]. Massage of the injection site increases the rate of absorption. Ventilation should be maintained with oxygen by mask or by mouth-to-mouth resuscitation if needed. Epinephrine injection can be repeated at 5 to 15-min intervals as long as symptoms persist [42]. Hypotension should be treated with fluids and vasopressors such as phenylephrine or methoxamine [42]. In cases of severe, persistent bronchospasm, 250–500 mg aminophylline can be administered intravenously. Corticosteroids and antihistamines are not antianaphylactic and are useful only as adjuncts to epinephrine in the treatment of anaphylaxis [42]. They may be useful in preventing a recurrence of symptoms and in avoiding the use of additional epinephrine [2].

If allergy is manifested only as an urticarial skin rash, a single injection of epinephrine followed by a course of an antihistamine such as diphenhydramine, 50 mg orally four times daily, should be effective. Medication should be taken for several days.

Idiosyncratic Reactions

Occasionally patients develop an adverse reaction to a normal amount of anesthetic which has been properly administered. The signs and symptoms are variable and unpredictable but tend to resemble toxic reactions to the anesthetic agent. While some of the more bizarre symptoms are probably psychogenic, there may exist a few individuals who have a low threshold for the toxic effects of these drugs. When skin-tested for allergy, these patients may be normal, and they may not react to anesthetic administered with epinephrine. When plain anesthetic is given in even low doses, however, toxicity occurs [2, 47]. The most important aspects of treatment are maintenance of an airway and support of respiration and circulation [2].

Adverse Reactions Specific to Certain Drugs

Adverse effects on the myocardium due to abuse of cocaine are well known. Recently, myocardial infarction has been reported following clinical use of cocaine for anesthesia of the nasal mucosa [48]. In this case topical cocaine had been used in conjunction with lidocaine and epinephrine. It was believed that cocaine interferred with the reuptake of epinephrine at adrenergic nerve terminals leading to an exaggerated sympathetic stimulation. To avert myocardial infarction in this situation, nitroglycerin should be administered at the first sign of a hypertensive crisis. Alpha and beta blocking agents are good adjunctive treatments [49, 50].

Prilocaine causes methemoglobinemia in a dose-related fashion. It is therefore relatively contraindicated in a patient with compromised oxygen-carrying capacity. Such patients might include children with cyanotic heart disease or individuals with chronic renal or pulmonary disease [13]. It should also be avoided in pregnant women [19]. Methemoglobinemia can be reversed with methylene blue.

Bupivacaine has been associated with cardiac arrest that was resistant to resuscitation following anesthetic overdosage. This anesthetic has a prolonged effect on the cardiac conduction system compared to lidocaine and causes arrhythmias at serum concentrations just slightly above the seizure threshold. Resuscitation is not impossible but requires rapid oxygenation, higher than normal epinephrine doses to treat electromechanical dissociation, and the use of bretylium rather than lidocaine to treat reentrant arrhythmias [35].

Persistent nerve block following use of chloroprocaine with epinephrine is discussed above (see "Local Complications").

Drug Interactions

The simultaneous administration of propranolol or cimetidine may slow hepatic clearance of amide anesthetics. A deficiency of plasma pseudocholinesterase or administration of drugs which compete for this enzyme impedes metabolism of ester anesthetics [35, 38]. Interestingly, amide anesthetics are potent inhibitors of plasma cholinesterase, and therefore the administration of an ester to someone who has recently received an amide might cause unexpected toxicity [38].

Tricyclic antidepressants inhibit the uptake of catecholamines. There is a theoretical risk that exogenously administered epinephrine in an anesthetic agent could cause excessive accumulation, precipitating a hypertensive crisis. In the amounts used in dentistry, no rise in blood pressure is seen [19]. Indeed, the levels of catecholamines released in response to anxiety and exercise are much higher than those produced by local injections. It therefore seems reasonable to use epinephrine with anesthetic in these cases, observing appropriate caution [19].

Cardiovascular collapse has been seen following regional administration of bupivacaine in patients taking either verapamil or the beta blocker timolol. In both cases it is more likely that the drugs potentiated the regional block of sympathetic fibers rather than a systemic effect of bupivacaine [51].

The opioid-antiemetic combinations used to sedate children prior to office surgical procedures can reduce the seizure threshold and increase CNS depressant effects of local anesthetics. Deaths have been reported in the dental literature when overdoses of the sedative combinations were used. In these cases more than three times the recommended dose were administered [51].

Malignant Hyperthermia

Malignant hyperthermia (MH) is an inherited, sometimes lethal syndrome most commonly triggered by inhalational anesthetics such as halothane and the muscle relaxant succinylcholine. It occurs in 1 : 15 000 anesthetic administrations in children and in 1 : 50 000 administrations in adults [52]. There have been reports of MH following spinal and epidural anesthesia using amide anesthetics, and the safety of using such agents for local injections in patients with a history of MH has been questioned. It is generally agreed that ester anesthetics are safe in this regard.

In an extensive review of this problem, Shira [52] could find no cases of well-documented MH in patients given amide anesthetics for dental injections. He concluded that these agents could be safely administered for routine dental treatment to patients with a known susceptibility to MH. Their use for routine cutaneous surgery should also be safe.

Conclusion

In general, the dermatologic use of local and regional anesthesia is quite safe. Although the exceptional adverse reaction is rare, the physician must be able to recognize and manage it appropriately.

References

1. Seldin HM, Recant BS (1955) The safety of anesthesia in the dental office. J Oral Surg 13:199–208
2. Laskin DM (1984) Diagnosis and treatment of complications associated with local anesthesia. Int Dent J 34:232–237
3. Dhuner KG (1972) Frequency of general side reactions after regular anesthesia with mepivacaine with and without vasoconstrictor. Acta Anesthesiol Scand Suppl 48:23–52
4. Persson G (1969) General side effects of local dental anesthesia with special reference to catecholamines as vasoconstrictors and to the effect of some premedicaments. Acta Ondontol Scand Suppl 53:1–141
5. Thomas RM (1982) Local anesthetic agents and regional anesthesia of the face. J Assoc Milit Dermatol 8:28–33
6. Abadin A (1975) Capsule anesthesiology: use of local anesthetics in dermatology. J Dermatol Surg Oncol 1:65–70
7. Farber GA (1982) Anesthesia for skin surgery. In: Epstein E, Epstein E Jr (eds) Skin surgery, 5th edn. Thomas, Springfield, pp 54–64
8. Robinson JK (1979) Reply to letter to the editor. J Dermatol Surg Oncol 5:945
9. Moore DC (1981) Regional block, a handbook for use in the clinical practice of medicine and surgery. Thomas, Springfield, pp 19–43
10. Milgram P, Fiset L (1986) Local anaesthetic adverse effects and other emergency problems in general dental practice. Int Dent J 36:71–76
11. Buckley JA, Ciancio SG, McMullen JA (1984) Efficacy of epinephrine concentration in local anesthesia during periodontal surgery. J Periodontol 5:653–657

12. Henderson JJ, Nimmo WS (1983) Practical regional anesthesia. Blackwell, Oxford, pp 96–102
13. Baker JD, Blackman BB (1985) Local anesthesia. Clin Plast Surg 12:25–31
14. Foster CA, Aston SI (1983) Propranolol-epinephrine interaction, a potential disaster. Plast Reconstr Surg 72:74–78
15. Dzubow LM (1986) The interaction between propranolol and epinephrine as observed in patients undergoing Mohs surgery. J Am Acad Dermatol 15:71–75
16. Winton GB (1988) Anesthesia for dermatologic surgery. J Dermatol Surg Oncol 14:41–54
17. Ralston DH, Schnider SM (1968) The fetal and neonatal effects of regional anesthesia and obstetrics. Anesthesiology 48:34–64
18. Gormley DE (1990) Cutaneous surgery and the pregnant patient. J Am Acad Dermatol 23:269–279
19. Martin IC (1988) Medical problems with local analgesia. Dent Update Suppl 2:S15–S18
20. Ecker RI (1980) More on local anesthesia of the digits. J Dermatol Surg Oncol 6:165
21. Grabb WC (1979) A concentration of 1 : 500 000 epinephrine in a local anesthetic solution is sufficient to provide excellent hemostasis. Plast Reconstr Surg 63:834
22. Graham WP III (1983) Anesthesia in cosmetic surgery. Clin Plast Surg 10:285–287
23. Siegel RJ, Vistnes LM, Iverson RE (1973) Effective hemostasis with less epinephrine. Plast Reconstr Surg 51:129–133
24. Robinson JK (1979) Advantages and technique of inducing local anesthesia with a smallbore, angled needle. J Dermatol Surg Oncol 5:465–466
25. Stegman SJ, Tromovitch TA, Glogau RG (1982) Basics of dermatologic surgery. Yearbook Medical Publishers, Chicago, pp 23–31
26. Grekin RC, Auletta MJ (1988) Local anesthesia in dermatologic surgery. J Am Acad Dermatol 19:599–614
27. Stewart JH, Cole GW, Klein JA (1989) Neutralized lidocaine with epinephrine for local anesthesia. J Dermatol Surg Oncol 15:1081–1083
28. Stewart JH, Chinn SE, Cole GW, Klein JA (1990) Neutralized lidocaine with epinephrine for local anesthesia II. J Dermatol Surg Oncol 16:842–845
29. Gordh T (1979) Complications and their treatment. In: Eriksson E (ed) Illustrated handbook in local anesthesia. Lloyd-Luke, London, pp 16–19
30. Cousins MJ, Bridenbaugh PO (1988) Neural blockade in clinical anesthesia and management of pain. Lippincott, Philadelphia, pp 130–131
31. Chan Tyk, Davidson T (1990) Femoral nerve block after intra-operative subcutaneous bupivacaine injection. Anaesthesia 45:163–164
32. Stromberg BV (1985) Regional anesthesia in head and neck surgery. Clin Plast Surg 12:123–126
33. Rettinger G, Christ P (1989) Visual loss following intranasal injection. Rhinology Suppl 9:66–72
34. Bridenstein JA (1989) Lidocaine during liposuction. J Dermatol Surg Oncol 15:775–776
35. Mulroy MF (1989) Regional anesthesia: an illustrated procedural guide. Little Brown, Boston, pp 31–41
36. De Fazio CA (1981) Local anesthetics: action, metabolism, and toxicity. Otolaryngal Clin North Am 14:515–519
37. Maloney JM III, Lertora JJL, Yarborough J et al. (1982) Plasma concentrations of lidocaine during hair transplantation. J Dermatol Surg Oncol 8:950–954
38. Wildsmith JAW, Armitage EN (1987) Principles and practice of regional anaesthesia. Churchill Livingstone, Edinburgh, pp 28–29
39. De Jong RH (1977) Local anesthesia, 2nd edn. Thomas, Springfield, pp 112–114
40. Verill PJ (1975) Adverse reactions to local anesthetics and vasoconstrictor drugs. Practicioner 214:380
41. Fregert S, Tegner E, Thein I (1979) Contact allergy to lidocaine. Contact Dermatitis 5:185–188

42. Adriani J, Zepernick R (1981) Allergic reactions to local anesthetics. South Med J 74:694–699
43. Ruzicka T, Gerstmeier M, Przybilla B, Ring J (1987) Allergy to local anesthetics: comparison of patch test with prick and intradermal test results. J Am Acad Dermatol 16:1202–1208
44. Aldrete JA, Johnson DA (1969) Allergy to local anesthetics. JAMA 207:356–357
45. DeShazo RD, Nelson HS (1979) An approach to the patient with a history of local anesthetic hypersensitivity: experience with 90 patients. J Allergy Clin Immunol 63:387–394
46. Incaudo G, Schatz M, Patterson R, Rosenberg M et al. (1978) Administration of local anesthetics to patients with a history of prior adverse reaction. J Allergy Clin Immunol 61:339–345
47. Levy SM, Baker KA (1986) Considerations in differential diagnosis of adverse reactions to local anesthetic: report of a case. J Am Dent Assoc 113(2):271–273
48. Chin YC, Brecht K, Das Gupta DS, Mhoon E (1986) Myocardial infarction with topical cocaine anesthesia for nasal surgery. Arch Otolaryngol Head Neck Surg 112:988–990
49. Gordon BR (1987) Topical cocaine nasal anesthesia (Letter). Arch Otolaryngol Head Neck Surg 113:211
50. Das Gupta DS (1987) Topical cocaine nasal anesthesia (Reply). Arch Otolaryngol Head Neck Surg 113:211
51. Reynolds F (1987) Adverse effects of local anesthetics. Br J Anaesthesia 59:78–95
52. Shira RB (1988) The use of amide local anesthetics in patients susceptible to malignant hyperthermia. Oral Surg Oral Med Oral Pathol 66:405–415
53. Zenz M, Panhans C, Niesel HC, Kreuscher H (1988) Regional anesthesia. Year Book Medical Publishers, Boca Raton, pp 15–16

Electrodesiccation and Curettage

HARVEY FINKELSTEIN and ROBERT JACKSON

Definition and Description of Electrodesiccation

Electrosurgery in dermatologic practice involves the use of electricity in different physical ways and for different indications [1, 2]. Electrosurgery may include the modalities of electrodesiccation (electrofulguration), electrosection, electrocoagulation, electrocautery, and electrolysis (Table 1).

Table 1. Electrosurgical Modalities

	Active Electrodes	Type of current
Electrodesiccation (electrofulguration)	One	Highly damped
Electrocoagulation	Two, either both active or one active and one dispersive	Moderate damping
Electrosection	Two, one active and one dispersive	Slightly damped or continuous save

Electrocautery – not an electrode, hot platinum wire and thus no current through patient; electrolysis – two electrodes but low voltage and frequency, uses direct current.

Electrodesiccation is the method used with curettage in the treatment of benign or malignant diseased tissue; it aids in tumor destruction and provides hemostasis. Electrodesiccation uses one active electrode. The spark gap apparatus produces a high-frequency (500–1000 kHz) alternating current of high voltage (2000 V or more) and low amperage (100–1000 A). Damped oscillations are produced so that in effect with each oscillation the voltage diminishes until there is no voltage and hence a gap. This cycle repeats itself. In electrodesiccation, the electrode contacts the tissue. Electrofulguration is identical except that the electrode is held just above the tissue to create a sparking. The two terms are now considered synonymous. The alternating current is of sufficiently high frequency to avoid causing nervous or muscular response yet still produces heat. The heat results from the living tissues' resistance to the passage of current, and the electrode warms up secondarily from the tissue heat. The pathologic results of electrodesiccation are shrunken and shriveled cells with condensed and elongated nuclei giving rise to an appearance of streaming. Blood vessels are thrombosed [3].

The lesions treatable by electrodesiccation and curettage include:

basal cell carcinomas (superficial, multicentric, and papular variety but not morpheaform), actinic keratoses, squamous cell carcinomas (small), Squamous cell carcinoma in situ (including Bowen's disease), seborrheic keratoses, verruca vulgares, and pyogenic granulomas.

It is not the purpose of this paper to describe in great detail the indications and contraindications of the use of electrodesiccation: these have been discussed elsewhere [4, 5]. Many of the complications which we describe can be attributed to the improper selection of cases to be treated by the method. Where appropriate, this is pointed out in the discussion of the complications.

Technique of Electrodesiccation and Curretage

The technique of electrodesiccation and curettage has been well described [6–8]. Good technique is crucial in helping to avoid complications. Once an appropriate lesion has been selected for removal, an adequate shave or wedge biopsy should be taken in every case where the possibility of a cancer exists. Use of the curette to supply the biopsy material should be discouraged because the specimen is often inadequate due to crushing fragmentation, small size, and lack of orientation. A punch biopsy can leave a deep scar and interfere with curettage [4].

The following technique description is appropriate and relevant to the removal of basal cell carcinomas. Once the surgical site has been anesthetized and a biopsy properly taken, curettage is begun to remove the remainder of the diseased tissue. Cure of the malignant tumor by good technique is the first priority. Minimizing normal tissue destruction and hence the resulting scar is an important consideration but should never take precedence over removal of a cancerous growth. Scars can always be revised later. For malignant lesions, curettage followed by electrodesiccation is usually performed three times or until no discernible tumor is left. Less than three curettages or reluctance to surgically remove at least 2 mm beyond the normal appearing border increases the risk of tumor recurrence from peripheral pseudopods of cancer cells. The skill of the operator has been shown to influence cure rates [9]. Choice of the size and shape of curette should be guided by the shape and location of the cancer. Proper selection of curettes helps to spare normal tissue while allowing good destruction and removal of diseased tissue. The last curettage should be done with a smaller instrument to facilitate removal of small finger projections or pockets of cancer.

Curettage works best with untreated tumors where no previous surgical or biopsy scarring confuses the feel of the cancer. The gelatinous tissue feel of a basal cell carcinoma is absent in a morpheaform basal cell carcinoma or in sequestrated tumor islands in scarred tissue. The firm gritty tissue of a squamous cell carcinoma is identifiable by the curette from normal tissue at the edges and base of the tumor.

Bleeding control is aided by stretching the surgical site between two or three fingers depending on the technique [8]. Stabilization by stretching of the tissue also allows for more effective curettage.

Practical considerations with the use of the electrosurgical machine arise which have bearing on the surgical result. Power settings on the spark gap apparatus should not be excessively high to prevent an inordinate amount of tissue destruction with resultant scarring. The longer the active electrode is applied to the tissue, the more tissue is destroyed. A ball electrode tip as compared to a needle gives rise to more destruction because of the greater contact area.

Effective hemostasis is achieved only if the surgical field is almost free of blood. Current and heat is diffused too quickly by excess blood, and hence good technique in the mechanical control of bleeding is important.

If the cancer is clearly much larger and more invasive than one anticipated, or if one penetrates into fat (the acrid odor of burning fat is usually the first clue), one should obtain hemostasis and stop. Further treatment can be planned after the biopsy results are available.

We have divided the complications from electrodesiccation and curettage into three groups (see Table 2): acute (up to 3 weeks), subacute (up to 3 months), and chronic/late (over 3 months). These time allotments are quite arbitrary, and there may be some overlaps particularly between the subacute and chronic.

Acute Complications

Pain

Pain arises due to inadequate anesthesia or from the injection of the anesthetic itself. The methods of anesthesia, whether regional, local, field block, or nerve block, and the pharmacology and selection of anesthetic agents and their complications are reviewed elsewhere in this volume. The value of preoperative medication with drugs such as benzodiazepine (diazepam 5 mg) or antihistamines (diphenhydramine HCl 25–50 mg) should not be underestimated for procedures involving children or very anxious adults. Postoperative pain is not a problem. Its presence strongly suggests a secondary coccal infection.

Table 2. Complications of electrodesiccation and curettage

Acute	Chronic/late
Pain	Scarring
Cardiac arrest	Early, fresh
Anaphylaxis	Linear
Vasovagal fainting	Contractures
Fire and burns	Facial scars
Excessive bleeding	Scars in young
	Scars in sun-damaged
Subacute	Hypertrophic
Infection	Keloids
Eczema	Tumor recurrence
Excess granulation tissue	Transmission of infection
Nonhealing wound	
Damage to underlying structures	

Cardiac Arrest

Fortunately, cardiac arrest is a very rare event. Clinical settings in which this is more likely include
a) patients with unstable cardiovascular disease,
b) pacemaker patients, and
c) anaphylactic allergic reactions to an anesthetic.

Appropriate history must include questions related to allergic reactions and cardiac status prior to beginning any procedure. Removal of tumors where electrodesiccation and curettage is the treatment of choice should not present much risk even with a strong history of ischemic heart disease. Usually the procedure is short and blood loss minimal. However, longer procedures in the elderly or high-risk patient, in whom electrosurgery may be used as part of larger excision, graft, or flap techniques, should be done in the hospital setting. Dermatologists and office staff should be well versed in basic cardiopulmonary resuscitation technique. Insufflation bags and apparatus to secure an airway may be considered part of basic equipment in the office for those skilled in their use.

Pacemaker patients may present a problem when electrosurgical technique involves high-frequency modalities such as electrodesiccation, electrocoagulation, and electrosection. By contrast, electrolysis and electrocautery are not problems. Electrolysis involves very low electrical exposure. Electrocautery involves no electricity transfer at all. The risk involved even with high-frequency electrosurgery is negligible with contemporary well-shielded pacemakers. Nevertheless, it is prudent to understand the potential interactions between different pacemaker types and the high-freqency electrosurgical device.

Two types of pacemakers exist. The older, rarely used variety has a fixed rate with no sensing device and is very resistant to electromagnetic interference. There are two versions of the newer demand synchronous pacemaker. There is a ventricular inhibited type which fires only when the heart rate drops below a certain level. Bradycardia or asystole may result if electrical output by the electro-surgical device is sensed as a heartbeat. There is also a ventricular trigger device which fires with each spontaneous beat or at a preset rate when no spontaneous beat occurs. Extra systole, tachycardia or fibrillation may result from electrical interference when this is sensed as a heartbeat.

Sebben [10] reviewed precautions which should be taken with the use of electrosurgery on pacemaker patients. He points out that "simple electrodesiccation of small lesions on relatively healthy pacemaker patients poses neglible risks."

If there are unusual circumstances, Sebben suggests the following. Heart monitoring can be done by checking the peripheral pulse. An AM radio tuned to 5400 kH$_z$ can monitor the pacemaker rate if held near the chest. Electrosection which involves higher energy and larger bursts is best performed in hospital. One should avoid working directly on a lesion over or near the site of the implanted pacemaker. Patients with external pacemakers should not receive electrodesiccation. The length of electrical bursts should be kept as short as possible, preferably less than 5 s. Patients should be grounded and at a site far away from the heart and pacemaker. The electrosurgical procedures should be avoided or postponed if the medical condition of the patient is such that other factors, including anoxia and electrolyte imbalances, put them at greater risk for arrythmia if interference occurs.

Anaphylaxis, which may progress to cardiac arrest, can arise as a complication to an anesthetic agent. The older ester (e. g., procaine) aminoacyl anesthetics presented more of a problem than the more common amide (e. g., xylocaine) type now in wider use. Methods of alternative anesthesia and appropriate medical therapy for acute life-threatening allergic reactions is reviewed in the chapter in this volume on anesthesia. Injectable adrenaline and antihistamine must be readily available in the surgical setting, whether office, clinic or inpatient.

Vasovagal fainting can be prevented by always having the patient lying down. If the patient feels faint during the procedure, keep him lying down until he feels better. Then allow the patient to sit up slowly and stay sitting for a few minutes with someone beside him in case he faints again. If the patient seems that he may be very upset by the procedure, preoperative medication can help considerably. Be wary of having patient's relatives or friends in the same room, as they are not accustomed to the procedure. We have seen more problems with relatives or friends fainting than with patients themselves fainting. Keep the patient who has felt faint in the office until he feels comfortable, even if this takes an hour or so. While this may be awkward, it is better than having the patient faint in elevators or going down stairs.

Fire and Burns

Electrosurgery must be carried out in the absence of flammable or explosive cleansing and sterilizing or anesthetic agents. Care should be taken to remove any pools of alcohol or alcohol mixtures in a skinfold or natural crevice such as the ear. Soaked drapes or cotton swabs should be removed before a procedure begins. The skin and hair, in particular, should be completely dry and free of alcohol. The patient using portable oxygen in the office setting or oxygen in the operating room may present an explosive hazard. The flammability of methane from flatus in the perianal area makes this an area where great caution should be taken when carrying out electrosurgery. Fire extinguishers appropriate for electrical fires, using a nontoxic gas as the retardant, should also be available.

Ground plates are not normally used in most simple electrodesiccation procedures. When a ground plate is used, because of pacemaker risk or because electrosection or electrocoagulation modalities are also being used for other surgical removals, care must be taken in its placement, for superficial or deep burns from tissue cooking may result from unwanted groundings. The site of the plate and its manner of application are important [11, 12]. The plate should be applied where soft tissue allows a large area of contact. It must also be placed as close as possible to the operative site so that resistance to current is lower, and less power is required. The further the current must travel to the plate, the more likely are unwanted groundings and hence subsequent skin burns. One must beware of other electrical equipment in contact with the patient. The thigh or buttock, which may offer good placement for surgery between the feet and chest, may be too far removed when operating on the head and neck. Great care must also be taken that the plate establishes good contact with the patient and does not become displaced during the procedure. Finally, remember that the active electrode presents a hazard if there is accidental activation, and hence it should never be rested on the patient when not in use.

Excessive Bleeding

During the operation excessive bleeding may occur because of poor technique, inappropriate selection of tumor (too large, too deep, etc.) or coagulopathies. The importance of tissue stabilization and the application of pressure with the digits stretching the operative site wound to control bleeding on the performance of electrodesiccation and curettage has already been mentioned. Direct pressure or squeezing beneath the wound also controls bleeding on genitalia, digits, nose, lips and external ears. Remember that a "dry field" is necessary for effective coagulation with the monoterminal electrode. The character of the bleeding does change with removal of the tumor from diffuse pooling to pinpoint bleeding, which is easier to control. Using local anesthetic with adrenaline has vasoconstrictive benefits during the curettage and electrodesiccation.

Electrodesiccation and curettage of a lesion on a digit rarely requires a tourniquet. If one is used, a clamp or hemostat should be left on the compressing band so that one does not inadvertently leave the tourniquet on after the procedure. If a tourniquet is used on a digit, electrodesiccation becomes much more potentially damaging to vital underlying structures including nerve, tendon, and bone. The virtual lack of blood flow does not allow for the usual dissipation of heat that one might be more accustomed to when using the electrodesiccating needle in other locations. Lower settings of voltage and shorter bursts are indicated.

Bleeding that does occur is a function of the size and number of blood vessels cut. Presumably, larger tumors which have sufficient depth to be adjacent to larger veins and arteries will have been selected for surgical procedures other than electrodesiccation and curettage. The surgeon must know the anatomy so as to avoid larger arteries which may be lacerated inadvertently during the biopsy or actual curettage. The application of the spark from the apparatus or continuous pressure is usually sufficient to control bleeding from small dermal and subdermal venules and arterioles, but hemostats and sutures should be available for use if larger vessels are nicked and result in free venous flow or arteriolar or arterial spurting.

Whether due to a drug or a patient's endogenous coagulopathy, good history taking is paramount in predicting bleeding problems. History of excessive bleeding from the nose, gums, or even minor cuts may indicate the need to check the platelet count, bleeding time, prothrombin time, and blood smear.

Some patients in the senior age group, who are most frequently those presenting for solar-induced malignancy, are on drugs that make surgery more difficult. Acetylsalicylic acid (ASA) is widely used in this age group for patients with atherosclerosis. This drug is also found in many over-the-counter medications for respiratory symptoms or stomach upset. The patient often neglects to mention these. The ASA affects platelet function for 7–10 days even after it is discontinued and increases slightly the risk for bleeding during the procedure and postoperatively. Other drugs which may affect clotting include dipyridamole and ibuprofen [13]. These drugs are very minor contraindications to routine electrodesiccation and curettage surgery; in general, most cases in which curettage is the treatment need not be postponed. This contrasts with the patient on heparin received during dialysis or those on coumarin-type drugs. Surgery in these patients is best postponed, if possible, until the effect of the drug has been reversed. Even if adequate hemostasis seems to be achieved in the office, much bleeding may occur later. Consultation with the patient's family physician or internist is indicated before these drugs are discontinued or their action reversed with vitamin K or plasma factor concentrates. When curettage and electrodesiccation is undertaken in patients in whom anticoagulant-types of medications cannot be stopped, meticulous care needs to be taken to make sure that good hemostasis has been achieved before the patient leaves the office. The patient should wait in the office for at least 1 h after surgery to verify that there has been complete control of bleeding. A pressure dressing is helpful. The patient should be instructed on the appropriate use of pressure to a bleeding wound if problems arise at home and to limit physical activity for 24 h following surgery. The patient should be reassured and be prepared for some bleeding that might occur when the initial crusted electrocoagulum separates.

Bleeding may occur, usually from some minor trauma, any time up to 2–3 weeks. It is particularly common on the red lip about 7–10 days after the initial procedure. Control is usually possible by pressure, repeat electrodesiccation, or suturing. The latter two procedures require local anesthesia. Late bleeding may also be a sign of secondary coccal infection.

It is useful to have the patient placed with his feet and legs down for a few minutes after performing a procedure on lesions in these areas. One can thus discover and recoagulate vessels that are oozing before the patient leaves the office.

Subacute Complications

Infection

Wounds following electrodesiccation and curettage surgery infrequently become infected simply because they are dry and sterile after the procedure. Personal preference by the dermatologist may influence postoperative wound care. Many dermatologists prefer to have the patient keep the wound dry for 24 h after surgery and only then begin application of alcohol or hydrogen peroxide twice daily for cleansing until healed. This results in a thick dry crust. Others suggest the regular use of an antibiotic ointment under occlusion (for example, mupirocin, fusidic acid) to help prevent possible infection and to keep the crust soft and thin. There is some evidence that keeping the wound moist promotes epithelialization and speeds complete healing. Remember that sensitivities to topical antibiotics are not uncommon. Infection may rarely occur and present with pain, swelling, and erythema surrounding the wound with purulent discharge at the edges below the crust. This can be easily shown by gentle squeezing of the crusted lesion. Tender regional lymphadenitis may also be present. The usual organisms are *Staphylococcus aureus* and *Streptococcus pyogenes*. Infection is more common where there is persistent moisture (as in intertriginous areas), or when the patient of his own volition keeps the wound consistently occluded by an occlusive dressing. Wound infections should be treated promptly with systemic antibiotics.

A rare problem in the external ears of diabetics is the development of a chondritis and life-threatening infection due to *Pseudomonas aeruginosa*.

Eczema

Eczema of the skin surrounding the wound may be seen as a primary irritant or contact allergic reaction. It occurs from a topical application to the wound site, usually an antibiotic. Reactions to adhesive tape or Band-Aids are linear. Treatment of the eczema consists of stopping the offending agent, tap water compresses, and moderately potent topical corticosteroids. Rarely an infected weeping wound may give rise to an infectious eczematoid dermatitis.

Excessive Granulation Tissue

Proud flesh (excess granulation tissue) may develop on occasion in the site of electrodesiccation and curettage. Reepithelialization does not occur, and the patient returns with the wound weeping, bleeding, and forming excessive crusts.

Areas which are especially liable to develop proud flesh are on the forehead, temples, and bald scalp where there is evidence of severe solar dystrophy. Patients should be informed when they can expect the final crust to fall off their wound. It is often useful to see the patient 4 weeks after surgery.

When excess granulation tissue does occur, the weekly application of a 75% silver nitrate stick destroys the heaped-up tissue. Clobetasol 17-propionate ointment can be used on the granulation tissue and should be applied three or four times daily. If the granulation tissue does not disappear, and the wound does not heal, removal by electrodesiccation and curettage can be done with a biopsy to exclude recurrent or residual tumor.

Nonhealing Wound

Five causes of a nonhealing wound are infection, eczema, excess granulation tissue, very slow healing in an area with a relatively poor blood supply such as the shin, and recurrent tumor. Wounds on the legs, where dependency with or without venous disease may slow healing, benefit from compression dressings. The problem of recurrent tumor is dealt with below.

Damage to Underlying Structures

Both the physical damage of curettage and electrical damage of electrodesiccation may put important structures at risk. Careful selection of tumors should eliminate consideration of this therapy for deep, large, and long-standing carcinomas which may be close to important anatomical structures such as nerves (e. g., on sides of fingers) arteries (e. g., temporal artery) or ducts (e. g., nasolacrimal).

When electrodesiccation is done on the dorsal hand or digits where nerves and tendons run close to the surface, care should be taken to avoid damage to these structures.

Chronic/Late Complications

Scarring

The scarring which occurs after electrodesiccation and curettage may present a problem to the patient because of symptoms or cosmetic outcome. Postoperative advice should include care of the wound, reassurance about expected purpura, edema, weeping, and crusting and the type of scar that might be expected for the particular surgical site and size of tumor. It is useful to mark the probable size of the wound with ink and show the patient the eventual size of the wound. Most patients underestimate the size of their cancer, especially when on the face. The patient can be reassured about the natural history of scars when follow-up for carcinoma recurrence is normally done.

Healing occurs by secondary intention after curettage. Wounds usually heal in 4–6 weeks, but when the wound is large, and where the blood supply is poor and subcutaneous tissue lacking, such as on the ear and on the shin, additional time may be required. When the last crust falls off, and final epithelialization has been completed, the patient can expect erythema. Usually, with time, the erythema also fades and leaves hypopigmentation, atrophy, and occasionally telangiectasia (Fig. 1). The hypopigmentation is less obvious in fair-skinned as compared to darker skinned individuals but is more obvious in skin severely damaged by the sun. Hyperpigmentation may also occur. In general, the cosmetic result improves with maturation of the scar so that by 10–15 years after the procedure over 80% of surgical scars are judged to be excellent to good cosmetic results. This contrasts with 47% after 1 year and 78% after 3 [9]. In light of these statistics, cosmetic repair of scars should not be hurried, but postponed for 2–3 years. Good technique, with appropriate use of electrosurgical power settings and application of the electrode discharges, helps to minimize tissue destruction and subsequent inordinate hypertrophic or atrophic scarring. To minimize scarring after curettage of benign lesions, such as seborrheic keratoses, electrodesiccation is best avoided and replaced by other coagulation methods such as the application of Drysol (aluminum chloride hexahydrate 20%) or a modified Monsel's solution (3.8 molar solution of ferric chloride) [14].

Fresh scars after electrodesiccation and curettage may be raised and somewhat sensitive. This can be confused with recurrence of the tumor. A raised scar, which may first resemble a recurrence, will often flatten, soften, and shrink over 6 months, obviating the need for biopsy [15].

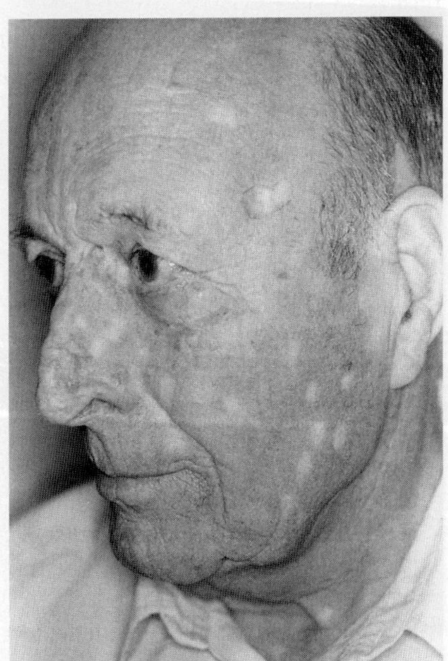

Fig. 1. Multiple atrophic hypopigmented scars after electrodesiccation and curettage

The mild hypertrophy of a scar which occurs early and quickly improves should be distinguished from a more persistent hypertrophic scar or keloid. Keloids, unlike hypertrophic scars, involve the wound site and creep beyond the treatment borders and do not improve with time. History and examination of previous wounds may allow recognition of patients at risk for keloid formation.

Scars take on a linear appearance when subjected to marked underlying muscle pull (e. g., scapular area, side of neck; Fig. 2). Scar contractures may result in unwanted deformation of anatomy and function, particularly in the periorbital or perioral regions, especially when the wound is over 2 cm. The red lip/skin junction, canthi, and eyelids close to the margins are examples of tumor sites where electrodesiccation and curettage are best avoided.

Flattening, softening, and lightening of scars can be expected after curettage and electrodesiccation. Concave surfaces on the face hide scars and result in better cosmetic results when compared to scars on convex surfaces [16]. The convex surface of the nose and chin, in particular, often give rise to depressed, stellate scars. Unfortunately, excisional surgery is not possible on the nose. In general, cosmetic repair of defects caused by electrodesiccation and curettage should be postponed for 2–3 years for two reasons. First, to be sure that a recurrence is not hidden under the graft or flap; second, many electrodesiccation and curettage

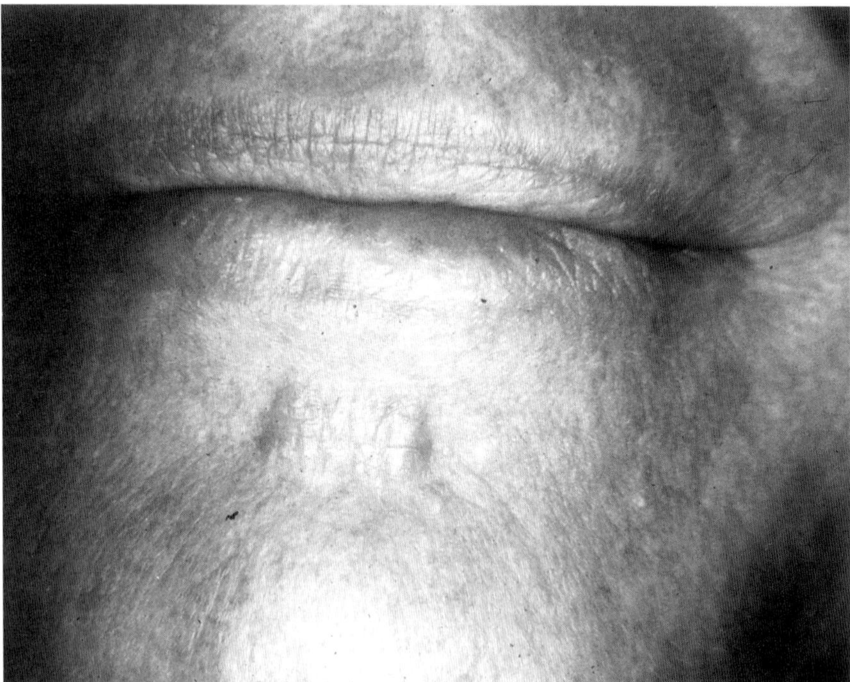

Fig. 2. Linear hypertrophic scar in center chin

scars improve with time. The Mohs' micrographic technique might be substituted as the primary therapy if grafting is desired at the time of initial surgery. In certain wounds on the face a combination of primary closure and secondary intention healing may give a better cosmetic result.

The round atrophic scar of electrodesiccation and curettage does not blend well in younger patients (under 40 years) who lack the lines and imperfections of aging and sun damage. Alternative therapies should be considered for these cases. In the extensive solar-induced poikilodermatous skin the white atrophy of the slightly thickened scar can stand out against the background of yellow elastosis, red telangiectasia, and brown hyperpigmentation.

Hypertrophic scars are estimated to occur in 10%–15% of cases after removal of basal cell carcinomas by electrodesiccation and curettage. Keloids are much rarer, in approximately 1% of cases [9, 17]. Hypertrophic scars occur most often on the upper chest and lateral arms, but the face, back, and abdomen can also be affected (Figs. 3, 4). When itchy or irritable and cosmetically distressing, they can be improved by methods which include (a) intralesional triamcinolone 10–40 mg/cm^3, with or without prior cryotherapy with liquid nitrogen; and (b) clobetasol 17-propionate, with or without occlusion, or flurandrenolide-impregnated tape. Radiation treatment for hypertrophic scars is never required. Surgical revision with perioperative steroid injection has a great risk of creating a new

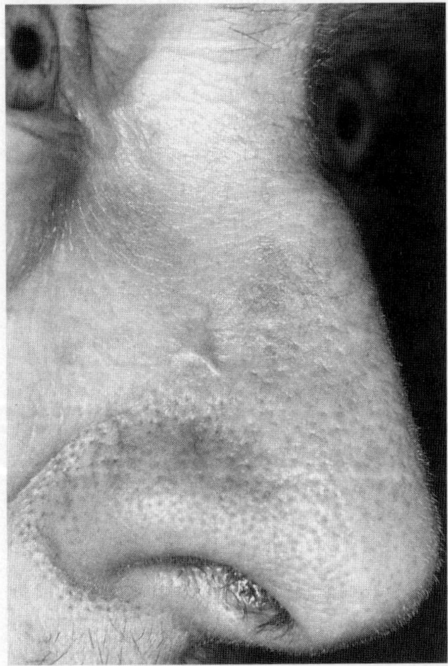

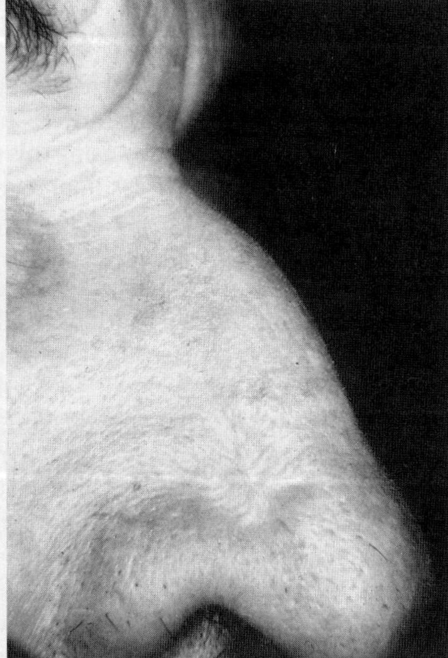

Fig. 3. Stellate hypertrophic scar at junction of cheek and nose skin

Fig. 4. Cross-hatched scar superior to ala

hypertrophic scar. In general, hypertrophic scars become less obvious and less tender in 1–2 years.

Keloids are rare following electrodesiccation and curettage. They are managed in the same way as keloids from other causes. Electrodesiccation and curettage should not be used on weight-bearing areas of the plantar surfaces. Painful scars or keloids on these areas are very disabling and virtually untreatable.

Concern for surgical cosmesis should not override the importance of eliminating a skin cancer.

Tumor Recurrences

Recurrences of malignant tumors treated with electrodesiccation and curettage can occur months to years after the procedure. They may arise for various reasons, especially inappropriate choice of tumor or poor technique. Malignant lesions for which electrodesiccation and curettage should be avoided because of the high likelihood of recurrence include:
a) basal cell or squamous cell carcinomas over 2 cm,
b) morpheaform basal cell carcinoma,
c) lesions occurring in embryonal planes of the face (those located in the nasal labial fold, oral commissures, external auditory canal, inner canthi of the eye and scalp) are all higher risk tumors; for a contrary view, see [18],
d) lesions deeply invasive and extending into subcutaneous tissue, and
e) recurrent tumors where scar formation makes identification of tumor by curettage difficult.

This is true for recurrences whether after cryotherapy, radiation, excisional surgery, or previous curettage or Mohs' surgery. With the proper selection of tumor and skilled surgery, cure rates using this modality have been shown to be well over 90%. This is despite the occasional demonstration of residual intact tumor cells after the procedure. The postsurgical inflammation and the host's immunological response perhaps help to eliminate residual basal cell carcinomas.

Recurrences of malignancies which do occur after electrodesiccation and curettage can be managed by various modalities. Where Mohs' micrographic surgery is available, this gives the best cure rate [19]. The Mohs' surgeon must consider operating not only in the obvious area of clinical recurrence but also on the entire previously treated scarred area of skin so as not to miss rests of tumor cells [20]. Radiotherapy and surgical excision provide a good second choice but both lack exact pathologic control of margins. Also, unlike Mohs' operation, tissue sparing is not achieved as easily with excision or radiotherapy. Preservation of vital structures and achieving a good cosmetic surgical result, particularly in the central facial area, are particular advantages of the Mohs' technique. Repeat electrodesiccation and curettage should usually be avoided for recurrent malignant tumors because of the difficulty that the prior scarring creates for the curettage. There are, however, some cases in which it may be considered, for example, in recurrences of superficial tumors such as superficial multicentric basal cell carcinomas.

Transmission of Infection

The electrodes used in electrosurgery may pose no less an infectious risk than improperly sterilized surgical instruments such as the curette [21]. The smoke created may also carry microorganisms. Finally, fluid droplets from tissue during electrosurgery may be sprayed over a distance of up to 29 cm [22].

The heat generated by the tip does not necessarily destroy micro-organisms. It is not self-sterilizing. It has now been shown experimentally that *Staphylococcus aureus* can be transferred from inoculated tissue to sterile tips and from innoculated electrode tips to sterile tissue [23]. This may have a bearing on postoperative wound infection. Herpesvirus and hepatitis B virus have also been shown to survive electrical discharge [24, 25].

There have as yet been no documented cases of patient-to-patient or patient-to-surgeon transmission of these organisms or human immunodeficiency virus with electrosurgical techniques, but the possible risks indicate the importance of appropriate precautions. The surgeon should wear gloves, and both mask and goggles should be considered because of spray effect. Electrodes should be sterilized between patients or disposable electrodes used. All dermatologic surgeons should consider immunization with hepatitis B vaccines. When treating viral warts with electrodesiccation, evacuating the smoke plume via appropriate apparatus to avoid inhalation of intact papillomavirus is also good practice.

Conclusion

Electrodesiccation and curettage is an important part of dermatologic surgical practice. Its application, limitations, and complications are reviewed here. Expert technique with a sound understanding of the basic principles of electrodesiccation and curettage and its role in the management of skin tumors must be acquired. Many of the problems arising from electrodesiccation and curettage are due to the inappropriate choice of lesion to be treated – not the treatment modality.

In these litigious times it is prudent to make sure that the patient understands the technique and the possible sequelae. Alternative therapies should also be discussed in difficult or problem cases. Particular attention should be paid to obtaining consent from parents, in the case of children, and guardians or trustees in the case of the infirm elderly or the mentally incompetent.

References

1. Jackson R (1970) Basic principles of electrosurgery: a review. Can J Surg 13:354–361
2. Boughton RS, Spencer SK (1987) Electrosurgical fundamentals. J Am Acad Dermatol 16:862–867
3. Clark WL, Morgan JD, Asnis EJ (1924) Electrothermic methods in treatment of neoplasms and other lesions with clinical and histological observations. Radiology 2:233
4. Jackson R, Laughlin S (1988) Electrodesiccation and curettage. In: Schwartz Robert A (ed) Skin cancer – recognition and management. Springer, Berlin Heidelberg New York

5. Jackson R (1984) Treatment of epitheliomas: electrodesiccation and curettage. In: Epstein E (ed) Controversies in dermatology. Saunders, Philadelphia, pp 112–114
6. Williamson GS, Jackson R (1964) The treatment of basal cell carcinoma by electrodesiccation and curettage. Can Med Assoc J 90:409–418
7. Jackson R, Laughlin S (1984) Electrosurgery. Dermatol Clin 2(2):233–244
8. Adam John E (1986) The technic of curettage surgery. J Am Acad Dermatol 15:697–702
9. Kopf AW, Bart RS, Shrager D et al. (1977) Curettage-electrodesiccation treatment of basal cell carcinoma. Arch Dermatol 113:439–443
10. Sebben JE (1983) Electrosurgery and cardiac pacemakers. J Am Acad Dermatol 9:457–463
11. Taylor KW, Desmond J (1970) Electrical hazards in the operation room, with special reference to electrosurgery. Can J Surg 13:362–374
12. Sebben JE (1987) Hazards of electrosurgery. J Am Acad Dermatol 16:869–872
13. Salasche SJ (1986) Acute surgical complications: cause, prevention and treatment. J Am Acad Dermatol 15:1163–1185
14. Epstein E, Maibach HJ (1964) Monsel's solution. Arch Dermatol 90:226–228
15. Epstein E (1970) Curettage and electrodesiccation. In: Epstein E (ed) Skin surgery, 3rd edn. Thomas, Springfield, p 265
16. Zitelli JA (1983) Wound healing by secondary intention – a cosmetic appraisal. J Am Acad Dermatol 9:407–415
17. Baer RI, Kopf AW (1964–1965) Complications of electrodesiccation and curettage. In: Baer RI, Kopf AW (eds) The year book of dermatology. Year Book Medical Publishers, Chicago, pp 14–16
18. Wentzell JM, Robinson JK (1990) Embryologic fusion planes and the spread of cutaneous carcinoma: a review and reassessment. J Dermatol Surg Oncol 16:1000–1005
19. Rowe DE, Carroll RJ, Day CL (1989) Mohs' surgery is the treatment of choice for recurrent (previously treated) basal cell carcinoma. J Dermatol Surg Oncol 15:414-431
20. Wagner RF Jr, Cottel WI (1987) Multifocal recurrent basal cell carcinoma following primary treatment by electrodesiccation and curettage. J Am Acad Dermatol 17:1047–1049
21. Sebben JE (1990) Contamination risks associated with electrosurgery. Arch Dermatol 126:805–808
22. Berberian BJ, Burnett JW (1986) The potential role of common dermatologic practice technique in transmitting disease. J Am Acad Dermatol 15:1057–1058
23. Bennett RG, Kraffert CA (1990) Bacterial transferance during electrodesiccation and electrocoagulation. Arch Dermatol 126:751–755
24. Colver GB, Peutherer JF (1987) Herpes simplex virus dispersal by hyfercator electrodes. Br J Dermatol 117:627–629
25. Sheretz EF, Davis GL et al. (1986) Transfer of hepatitis B virus by contaminated reusable needle electrodes after electrodesiccation in simulated use. J Am Acad Dermatol 15:1057–1058

Dermabrasion

JAMES E. FULTON, JR.

Introduction

Postdermabrasion complications may develop under the best of circumstances. These complications may include keloids, hypertrophic scars, hyper-or hypopigmentation, blocked pores, milia formations, the appearance of enlarged pores, the loss of the natural skin texture, or acne flare-ups.

The incidence of these complications can be reduced by presurgery screening, using good surgical techniques, and providing the optimum in wound management [1]. Methods can also be employed to accelerate the resolution of certain complications [2]. The procedures used before, during, and after surgery are presented in this chapter.

Avoiding Dermabrasion Complications

Presurgery Screening

The most important first step is presurgery evaluation. What is the mental status of this individual? Is this person capable of understanding directions and capable of following them for the 10 days after surgery? If patients speak a foreign language, even though they are somewhat fluent in the language used, communication can degenerate during the anxiety of surgery and wound healing. Cultural differences may also come into play after surgery. Patients should be checked for their ability to communicate and follow instructions and also examined for their current mental status. Patients with previous hospitalization for mental disorders may have a flare-up of their underlying condition during the postoperative period. It is often helpful to do a small test spot dermabrasion or chemical peel-up under the side burn or a full-face Jessner peel to study the mental and physical aspects of the patient. This allows more time to become acquainted with the patient.

The next step is to obtain a complete informed consent. The patients must understand exactly what is to be done and how they may help in wound healing. They must wear a masklike dressing for several days following surgery, and their eyes may be swollen shut. This knowledge before surgery makes them better patients after surgery.

Their physical status must be reviewed. They should have no underlying skin conditions that are active. It is best to have their acne under complete control and the red erythematous residual acne lesions completely faded. This gives the operator a much better surface to plane.

Their history is equally important. If they have been involved in drug abuse, they require substantially more anesthesia during the procedure, and they tend to be less compliant patients, often suffering with a low pain threshold. If they have had repeated episodes of herpes simplex of the lip, this may be a problem during surgery and may require prophylactic acyclovir to prevent a flare-up of the herpes and a spread onto the abraded areas [3]. Their dietary history is important. Vegetarians, especially those who are not scientific and have an unbalanced vegetarian diet, may show slow wound healing.

In addition to physical examination and history, we perform routine laboratory work including a CBC, a panel of chemistries, a hepatitis surface antigen screen, and an HIV determination. We also do a nasal culture by swabbing the anterior nares. We have found that patients with a normal nasal flora have less chance for a surface wound infection compared to those that culture out virulent gram-positive or unusual gram-negative bacteria. If we find an unusual bacteria or an unusual antibiotic resistance pattern, we may change the postoperative antibiotic.

Pretreatment with topical vitamin A acid (tretinoin) speeds wound healing and reduces the incidence of postoperative milia formation [4]. We normally prefer to start the patient a month in advance, with tretinoin 0.25%, increased to .05% if needed, to produce a slight peeling indicating a therapeutic level of tretinoin exposure.

Surgical Techniques

The most important aspect of dermabrasion is to perform a complete anatomical segment. This usually means a full-face dermabrasion that travels 1/8 in. into the hairline and a 1/2 in. below the jawline, including the whole face, the upper and lowers lips, and the lower eyelids. Often, we combine the dermabrasion with a chemical peel, especially around the eyes [5]. We normally perform a full-face dermabrasion. However, one can perform an upper-face dermabrasion or a lower-face dermabrasion and feather the edge into the temple area; one may also carry out a nose dermabrasion and feather it off into the cheeks, or a perioral dermabrasion and feather it off into the nasolabial fold. However, all things being equal, we prefer the full-face dermabrasion to obtain a uniform pink color throughout the facial area. When combined with the simultaneous chemical peel around the eyes and onto the neck area, this results in a uniform pigmentation. This is especially important on more darkly pigmented individuals. If we do end up with slight hypo-or hyperpigmentation, the only line of dermabrasion is below the jawline. This minimizes complications.

Anesthesia is important, as we do not want the patient to feel uncomfortable and to move during the procedure. This may cause a complication of a broken tooth, a skin laceration, or catching the rapid rotating wheel in the hair. Our usual anesthesia is intravenous sedation by a registered nurse anesthetist, combined with a regional nerve block of the nerves of the face [6].

Although most physicians still freeze the skin before dermabrasions, our results suggest that freezing results in frostbite. This additional damage leads to an increased incidence of complications [7]. Currently, we freeze only in selected areas. The dermabrasion is usually started with the Bell Hand Engine equipped with the large dome fraise (Robin's Instruments, Chatham, NJ, USA). We begin with a light abrasion over the right cheek area. We no longer use the postage-stamp method of dermabrasion because it takes too long. We do the whole cheek, and then go to the other cheek, and then the forehead, finishing up with the chin and nose area. We proceed very lightly at first, and then return for the second or third time. This repetition allows tissue edema to build up, allowing us to plane much more vigorously without catching the rapid rotating wheel in the soft tissue. Without the benefits of the freeze, the operator must be especially aware of the direction of fraise rotation. If the unit is rotating away from the orifice or away from the hair, the fraise may catch the tissue or hair.

We are very careful around the teeth, eyes, and hair. We make sure the unit is rotating into the orifice, into the hair, or into the eyelid area, so that we do not catch loose skin, hair, or teeth. If there is a particular offensive line, wrinkle, or acne scar, we freeze selected areas with fluroethyl spray before the dermabrasion to allow a little deeper penetration in selected areas such as the central cheek area or glabellar area. We attempt to carry out the procedure without freezing in the jawline area, which is the danger area for keloid formation.

Once the planing is completed, and a uniform, smooth, rosy facial anatomy is evident, the patient is bandaged in a semiocclusive dressing (Omiderm, D.R. Labs, San Rafael, CA, USA). This plastic dressing begins to adhere immediately to the moist abraded skin. It is additionally held in place with a Webril 6 netting. This holds the dressing in place for the 1st day or so until it becomes fixed. Since we have usually performed a chemical peel on the periorbital area, the patient is allowed to recover from anesthesia with an ice pack over the eye area.

The patient is sent home with the home care kit that includes:

> tube net (four pieces), 4 x 4 gauze pads, cleanser (Cetaphil), thermometer, drinking straws, eucerin ointment (4-oz jar), aloe vera solution and spray, antibiotic tablets, acyclovir (Zovirax) capsules (if needed for fever blisters), pain tablets, sleeping tablets, and an ice bag for the eyes.

The home care kit is designed to get patients through the next 10 days of recovery. It includes a thermometer so they can take their temperature twice daily, and report any elevations over 101° F. It also includes acyclovir to avoid a herpes flare-up. We originally used this only in selected cases, but because of many patients' poor history, we now use acyclovir five times daily for the initial 5 days after surgery in every case.

Postoperative Considerations

One of the greatest advances in dermabrasion care has been the use of an occlusive bandage after the dermabrasion procedure. Our current favorite is a plastic film from Israel. This dressing immediately adheres to the skin and is useful to protect the wound for the first 4–5 days postoperatively. It prevents oxygen in the air from drying out the wound but has a porosity that allows fluid to transpire through the plastic. This dressing is held in place with Webril netting. The netting can be changed daily if a patient so desires. We spray the wound with an aloe vera gel to take advantage of the aloe vera stimulated wound healing [8].

It is important for the next few days that the patient be up and moving around. While resting he must keep his head upon several pillows. This keeps the edema and swelling down. Excessive edema may delay the wound healing and permit bacterial infections or pigmentary changes. At about 4–5 days, the wound dressing method is altered. The patient begins to apply a petrolatum-based ointment (Eutra, Swiss-American Products, Dallas, TX, USA). The petrolatum dressing is applied over the plastic, and as it begins to soften the edges, the plastic dressing is gradually cut off. It usually takes a day or so for the dressing to come off gradually. The patient must avoid pulling the dressing off, as it may pull the new tissue with it. Basically, the home care program is a gentle debridement with frequent showers. We wash the dressing and the ointment with a cleanser (Cetaphil, Owens Lab, Fort Worth, TX, USA) and then reapply the ointment until the wound debris softens again before the next shower in 4–6 h. This is repeated until the dressing and debris are eliminated.

The secret to rapid wound healing and complication avoidance is preventing the formation of crust. This is best accomplished by gently cleansing the area with Cetaphil and the palms of the hands about every 6 h. Between showers the area is kept greased with Eutra. As the wound changes from red to pink, which signifies a new epithelial cover, we change the dressing to a bland cream (Eucerin, Beiersdorf, Norwalk, CN, USA). This dressing is used for 3–4 days. After this, a day treatment lotion, containing sunscreen, can continue as the skin moisturizer. We change the dressing about every 4 days to avoid an allergic reaction from a preservative. If a persistent crust develops, we switch to an antibiotic ointment (Polysporin, Burroughs-Wellcome, Research Triangle Park, NC, USA) or a silver-sulfadiazine ointment (Silvadene, Marion Labs, Kansas City, MO, USA). We do not suggest that the patient use hydrogen peroxide cleansing as we have seen delayed wound healing from too aggressive peroxide cleansing. After 15 days ur so, we often suggest that the patient begin using a bleaching lotion to prevent hyperpigmentation.

In summary, it is important to analyze the surgical steps. Divide them into pre-, peri-, and postoperative periods. Use steps to optimize wound healing and prevent infections. Any delay in wound healing may precipitate one of the feared complications.

The goal is to obtain rapid wound healing in 8 days. One must deal with an informed patient, soliciting his help in wound management to achieve mutual goals. With this extensive patient education program and postoperative management we have essentially eliminated infection as a postoperative complication.

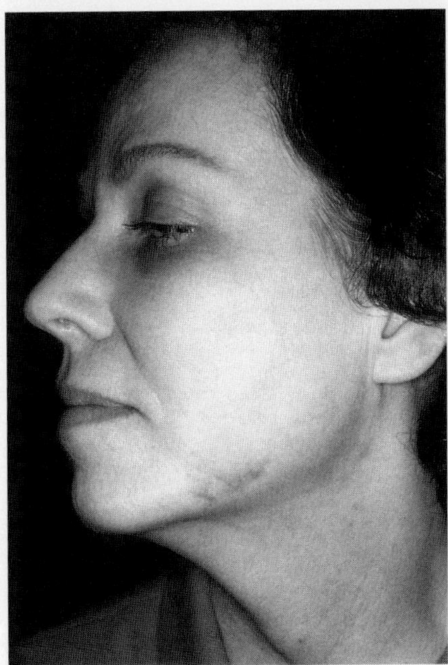

Fig. 1. Persistent red streak signifying pending keloid or hypertrophic scar

Managing Complications

Persistent Red Streak

The most feared complication from chemical peeling or facial dermabrasion is keloid or hypertrophic scar. These occur most often along bony prominences such as a jawline and are usually the result of genetic predisposition, combined with delayed wound healing induced by freezing. Freezing along the jawline can produce a deeper wound and delay wound healing. This delayed wound may evolve into a persistent red streak, and if this begins to itch, it is a sure sign of an oncoming hypertrophic scar or keloid (Fig. 1). Immediately, we begin therapy with a silicone sheet (Sylastic, Dow-Corning-Wright, Memphis, TN, USA). Preferably, the silicone dressing is worn 24 h a day for 2–3 weeks or until the persistent streak has healed. It can be worn less, but the minimum appears to be 12 h a day [9].

The silicone sheet has been a great life-saver in treating these early signs of keloid formations. It is also useful in a keloid that has developed. In addition, intralesional steroids and a steroid cream or ointment can be used when the silicone sheet is not in place.

Hyperpigmentation

The management of hyperpigmentation is relatively easy. If darkly pigmented individuals are informed that they may react with postinflammatory hyperpigmentation after the surgery, they understand that it will fade in a month or so.

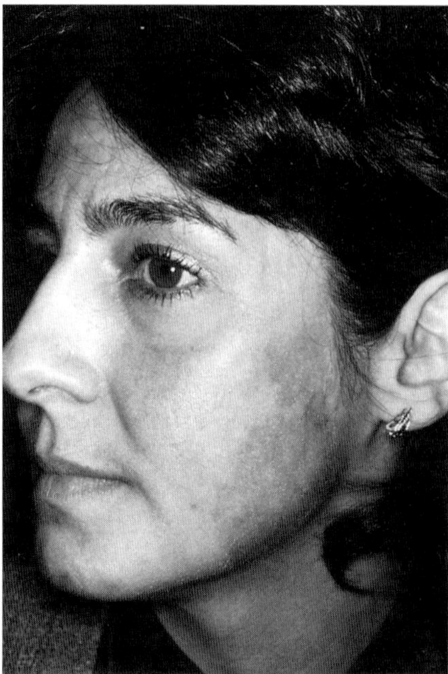

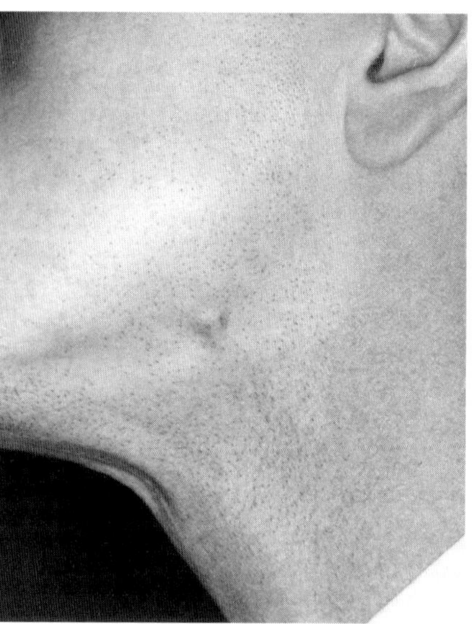

Fig. 2. Postinflammatory hyperpigmentation following dermabrasion. This resolves over the next 3 weeks

Fig. 3. Hypopigmentation of the jawline. This can usually be blended with several 20% TCA peels

However, the hyperpigmentation may also develop in a light-skinned individual, even with blue eyes (Fig. 2). In the United States these patients are quite often part American Indian. In any case, the use of tretinoin in the evening and bleaching lotion with sunscreen during the day fades these lesions more rapidly. They usually disappear within 3 months. Again, the educated, forewarned patient is much more understanding.

Hypopigmentation

Hypopigmentation is a much more serious problem. The loss of melancytes is usually permanent. The melanocytes do not divide very effectively, and there are always fewer melanocytes after a dermabrasion or chemical peel. This may be clinically visible especially at lines of demarcation, such as the lower jawline (Fig. 3). This is why it is so important to mask the potential color change by a full-face dermabrasion. To avoid a demarcation below the jawline area it is quite common to perform a light chemical peel (20% TCA) on the neck area before the dermabrasion starts. Do not perform the chemical peel after the dermabrasion, as the raw dermabraded skin receives a deeper peel.

Milia

During the wound healing process, the large pores dump new skin cells onto the surface to repave the area rapidly. The smaller pores are quite often sealed over by these advancing skin cells. After 3-4 weeks, these small sealed pores begin to build up dead skin cells and oil just below this new epidermis. These develop into a millet-seed-like lesion called a milia. These are not really a complication but are better called a sequela of a dermabrasion procedure. They occur quite often and are simply a normal occurrence after surgery (Fig. 4). Mandy [4] has felt that this incidence of milia is reduced by pretreatment with tretinoin. However, confirming studies have not been conducted. Usually, these milia go through a life cycle over 2–3 months and disappear. Again, advance education of the patient reduces his anxiety about these millet-seed lesions. They can be extracted simply with a needle puncture and a Schamberg extractor.

Enlarged Pores

Unfortunately, many acne sufferers have large pores and oily skin. When the dermabrasion planes acne scars, it may leave the appearance of enlarged pores (Fig. 5). Quite often the pore size is larger under the surface, near the area of the sebaceous ducts. This larger opening may be evident after the dermabrasion. Unfortunately, these enlargements are permanent and only worsen with subsequent procedures. Obagi (personal communication) feels that the pore size can be reduced by pretreatment for 1 month with isotretinoin (Accutane, Hoffman-LaRoche, Nutley, NJ, USA). However, this has not been confirmed.

Acne Flare-Ups

Quite often after the dermabrasion procedure, the predisposing acne problem may flare up. This may be because we have stirred up the metabolism of the skin pores or because we have used heavy occlusive ointments during the wound healing. It is quite common for a mild acne flare-up to develop after the dermabrasion procedure. Usually in 3 weeks, topical treatment can again be instituted with a benzoyl peroxide wash, followed by topical erythromycin solution. These two treatments plus a reduction in skin moisturizing agents are usually effective in bringing the flare-up under control. However, some cases become more persistent and may require the addition of systemic antibiotics such as tetracycline or instituting isotretinoin therapy.

Conclusion

The most important aspect of dermabrasion surgery is to avoid complications. As we have discussed, this can be done by working with an informed patient, preparing the skin ahead of time with tretinoin treatment, and performing an in-

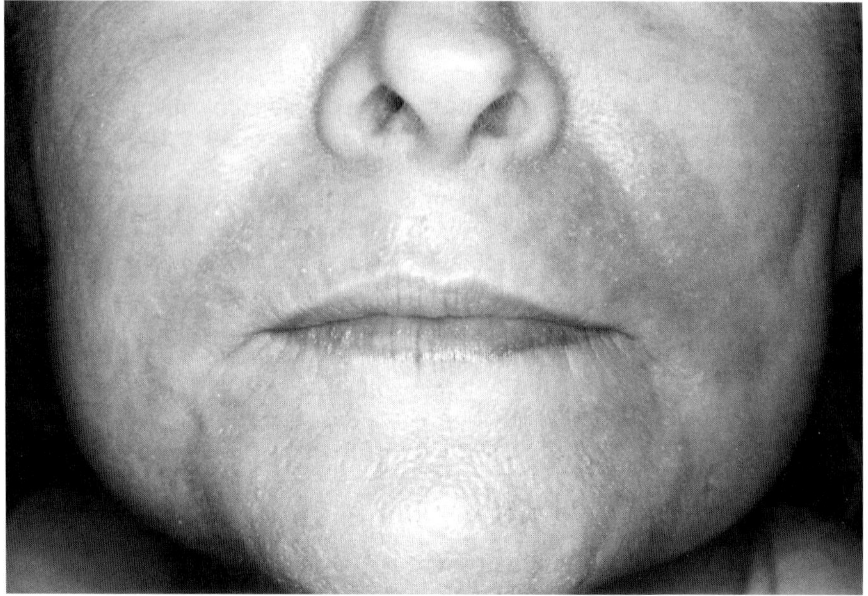

Fig. 4. Multiple milia formations after dermabrasion

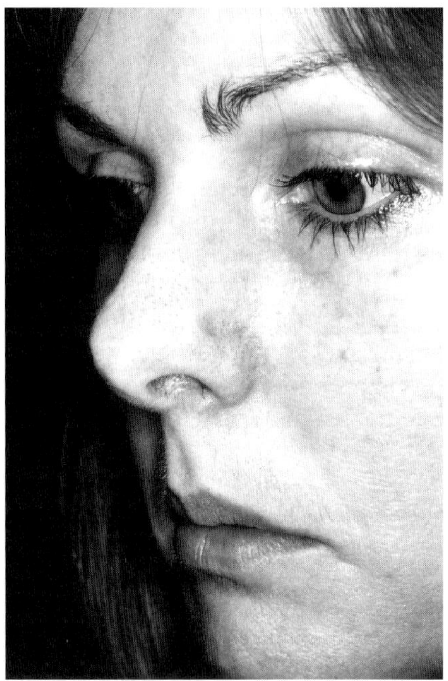

Fig. 5. Enlarged pores following a dermabrasion. These changes are permanent

depth history and physical examination. The best surgery technique appears to be full-face dermabrasion, done without freezing. Freezing selected areas can be performed when more damage is needed over a wrinkle or acne scarred area. After the procedure a semiocclusive wound dressing is helpful for the first 5 days of surgery. This is followed by an ointment dressing for 5 days and then a cream moisturizer. This allows rapid wound healing, and the wound is closed in 8–10 days. This minimizes the complications of dermabrasion surgery. The management of a persistent red streak, pigmentation change, or milia can usually be accomplished easily with an informed patient.

References

1. Fulton JE (1987) Modern dermabrasion techniques: a personal appraisal. J Dermatol Surg Oncol 13:780–789
2. Fulton JE (1991) The prevention and management of postdermabrasion complications. J Dermatol Surg Oncol 17:431–437
3. Fulton JE (1991) Management of herpes simplex flare-ups following dermabrasion or chemical peel procedures. AJ Cosmet Surg 8:11–13
4. Mandy SH (1986) Tretinoin in the pre and post operative management of dermabrasion. J Am Acad Dermatol 15:878–882
5. Fulton JE (1990) Step-by-step skin rejuvenation. Am J Cosmet Surg 7:199–205
6. Fulton JE (1990) Modern dermabrasion techniques. Am J Cosmet Surg 6:19–24
7. Fulton JE (1991) Delayed wound healing induced by spray refrigerants during full-face dermabrasions. Am J Cosmet Surg 8:65–69
8. Fulton JE (1990) Stimulation of postdermabrasion wound healing with aloe vera gel-polyethelene oxide dressing. J Dermatol Surg Oncol 16:460–467
9. Quinn KJ (1987) Silicone gel in scar treatment. Burns 13:33–40

Cryosurgery

Rodney P. R. Dawber

Many of the effects of the freezing methods employed in clinical practice produce inflammatory changes that are probably important for successful treatment; therefore morbidity, side effects and complications cannot always be treated as separate entities in cryosurgery, as is seen with many of the changes described below. Specific complications depend largely on the regime employed and on the site, pathology and size of the lesion to be treated.

Table 1 shows a list of the more well-known complications. We will consider some of the commoner effects listed since anyone new to cryosurgery should have detailed knowledge of these in order to explain to patients the most likely events prior to healing. It is important to note that many of these complications may under some circumstances be advantageous, for example, the altered

Table 1. Some complications of cryosurgery (Modified from Zacarian) [I]

Immediate	Delayed
Pain	Postoperative infection and febrile reaction
Headache affecting forehead, temples and scalp	Haemorrhage
Insufflation of subcutaneous tissue	Granulation tissue formation
Haemorrhage	Pseudoepitheliomatous hyperplasia
Oedema	Hyperpigmentation (Fig. 6)
Syncope	Milia
Blister formation (Fig. 1)	Hypertrophic scars (Fig. 3)
	Nerve/nerve ending damage
	Bone necrosis and arthralgia, mainly terminal phalanx or interphalangeal joints
	Digital extensor tendon rupture
	Hypopigmentation (Fig. 8)
	Ectropion and notching of eyelids
	Notching and atrophy of tumors overlying cartilage (Fig. 4)
	Tenting or notching of the vermilion border of the lip
	Atrophy
	Hair and hair follicle loss

sensation, making pain relatively mild in relation to the often severe inflammation produced.

Pain

All patients will feel some degree of discomfort when local anaesthesia is not used. The subjectivity of pain means that this varies from patient to patient; even multiple, prolonged freeze-thaw cycle methods cause but little pain in some individuals. However, a few generalisations are possible: Even the shortest, cotton-wool bud freeze gives a perceptible sensation of "hot" or "burning". Tissue-penetrating regimes and those methods giving rapid lowering of temperature and ice formation often give discomfort within seconds of their commencement, for instance, liquid nitrogen spray techniques – probably due to the pre-anaesthetic effects of freezing on cutaneous nerve endings. Pain during the thaw phase, particularly after "tumor dose" methods, may last for many minutes and be profound and quite intense. Certain anatomical sites are more likely to produce pain – particularly fingers, pulp and periungual area, helix and concha of the ear, lips temples and scalp [1, 2]. Necessarily aggressive cryosurgery, such as for malignancy, when carried out to skin immediately over bone, may rarely lead to "bone pain" lasting several days. Even though pain of the above type is usually transient, a throbbing sensation after digital freezing may persist for 1–2 h. These factors make the choice of whether to use local anaesthetic or not sometimes difficult. In general, single-freeze schedules used for benign or preneoplastic skin lesions do not require local anaesthesia; this may also be the case with superficial malignant lesions.

Headache, often migraine-like, is not uncommon with freezing of lesions on the forehead, temples and scalp. This is usually transient but occasionally lasts for many hours; headache is not always directly related to the site of freezing [1].

Nitrogen Gas Tissue Insufflation

This is extremely rare and is most likely to occur with open spray liquid nitrogen techniques carried out immediately after biopsy, particularly around the orbit [3]. It can be avoided by starting with only gentle spraying directed at an angle or by using pressure rings or cones. In 22 years of cryosurgery practice, the author has never personally seen this complication.

Oedema

This occurs to some degree with every patient – a product of the acute inflammation and "leaky" capillaries, the amount of oedema relating directly to the severity of the regime carried out. Pronounced idiosyncratic oedema occasionally occurs even from short-freeze schedules. The severest oedema is typically seen

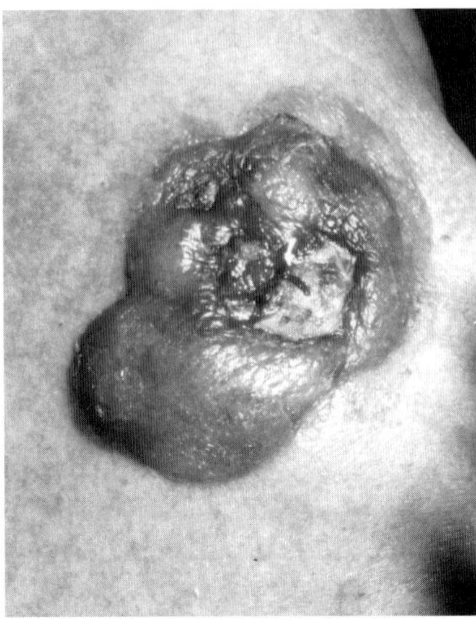

Fig. 1. Blister formation at the site of a treated basal cell carcinoma; no anti-inflammatory treatment was used in this case

in lax skin sites, such as eyelides, lips, labia minora (less common with labia majora), and foreskin.

Whilst oedema equates with subcutaneous swelling, blister formation relates to the dermoepidermal split produced by the freeze schedules most commonly used in clincial practice (Fig. 1). Associated epidermal cell death may lead to "weeping" erosions for several days. If sufficient capillary and venular damage occurs then haemorrhagic bullae may develop within 12–24 h (Fig. 1). Such blisters are often painless, presumably because of the temporary peripheral nerve ending damage [4]; also, they heal rapidly without scarring [5] (Fig. 4), but any associated hypopigmentation may be permanent.

Haemorrhage and Vascular Necrosis

Within 4–7 days of aggressive cryosurgery, mainly tumor schedules, it is not uncommon for the treated field to become cyanosed, with subsequent necrosis ("venous gangrene") and sloughing of the dead tissue. This is probably due to delayed thrombosis of capillaries and venules and may be an important and necessary part of tumor death and high cure rates, reminding one that initial ice formations and temperature decrease are not the sole factor in cancer therapy.

Haemorrhage, sometimes excessive, may occur with cryosurgery by several mechanisms. If a pedunculated or prominently papular lesion is manipulated during its solid ice phase, any ice cracks that appear may be associated with bleeding during the thaw; this is usually capillary/venous bleeding and is transient. If cryosurgery is preceded by biopsy or curettage, for example, to "debulk" tumors, post-freezing bleeding may last many minutes; it is easily controlled by application of 70% aluminium chloride solution, rarely needing electrocoagulation [2]. The rarest and most dramatic form of haemorrhage is the delayed type, up to 14 days after treatment. This may relate to the delayed necrotic phase after treatment of a tumor which had already invaded large arterioles or a larger artery. Arterial bleeding of this type may be profuse and dangerous and requires immediate pressure to minimise blood loss and early tying off of the affected vessel. The author has experience of one patient who bled from a deep vulval artery 11 days after a single, liquid nitrogen spray, freeze/thaw cycle treatment for multicentric pigmented Bowen's disease [6]; she required the transfusion of 4 pints of blood.

Inhibition of Inflammatory Complications

Most of the complications described above are the results of various components of the acute or chronic inflammatory reaction caused by freezing. Many attempts have been made to minimise or abort these effects without compromising cure rates. Zacarian [1] recommends cyproheptadine (Periactin) three times daily for a day before and several days after cryosurgery to minimize oedema; swelling and blister formation may be lessened by using topical clobetasol proprionate [7] or oral or parenteral steroids [8, 9] (bolus dose or short-term use). The topical steroid may usefully be applied 2 h before treatment and for 3–4 days afterwards (twice daily) to minimise inflammatory symptoms and signs.

Sensory Impairment

Some degree of paraesthesia or, less commonly, anaesthesia, is common after freezing [4]; indeed, the fact that cold can produce numbness has been known for many centuries [10].

The analgesic effect of cryosurgery has proved effective in the palliative management of various inoperable tumors by direct application to the tumor, while others have used a cryoprobe to produce analgesia in patients with intractable pain by blocking peripheral nerve function. These studies have also shown that, although all transmission is blocked in the frozen nerve, full recovery occurs after a variable period. This supports previous work directly freezing the sciatic nerve of nine rabbits with liquid nitrogen. In all cases nerve conduction was completely interrupted, but within 100 days rheobase and chronaxy measurements confirmed full restoration of normal function. Thus, if a nerve trunk underlying a treated skin lesion is inadvertently damaged, complete recovery of distal sensory or motor function can be expected; the return of sensation after freeze injury is sooner than after nerve section because the connective tissue nerve sheath is usually not destroyed.

When skin rather than peripheral nerves is frozen, it is well recognised that retreatment of the frozen area several days, or weeks, later will be relatively painless, and that pain after cryosurgery is minimal. Although the studies of Lloyd et al. [11] in Oxford have provided figures for the duration of pain relief after cryosurgery to various peripheral nerves, there was until recently little information on the duration of sensory loss after cutaneous cryosurgery. Patients, however, require this information particularly when a sensitive area such as the fingertip is to be rendered anaesthetic by freezing.

Subsequent work in 1985 [4] showed that appreciation of all three modalities of sensation tested – touch, pain and cold – were initially reduced in all subjects studied. The recovery took up to 1.5 years for the longest freeze. Compared with control skin, all treated areas sampled within the first few weeks of cryosurgery were found to have an absence of axons in the upper dermis and a noticeable reduction in the deeper dermis. The longer the freeze time, the more pronounced were these changes. Even with the longest freeze time, however, Schwann's cell and connective tissue pathways were present in normal numbers at all levels, with areas of Schwann's cell proliferation. Apart from mild lymphocytic infiltration around a few of the neurovascular bundles, there was little evidence of inflammation and minimal fibroblastic activity. Dilatation of occasional superficial blood vessels was the only vascular change detected. Biopsy specimens taken at later stages contained increasing numbers of axons at all levels.

Faber et al. [12] carried out sensory testing by means of a graded bristle technique following treatment of 183 skin lesions in 169 patients; mild transient sensory loss was detected in 28% of treated lesions. They noted that this did not appear to be influenced by the freezing technique used or the type of wound healing but was site dependent, for example, the trunk and neck showing more prolonged impairment that the face; on the eyelid, however, sensory loss was not detected at all. It is, of course, these effects that may be the basis of the successful use of cryosurgery for pruritus vulvae and ani [13], the symptoms of lichen sclerosus et atrophicus, prurigo nodularis and lichen simplex (neurodermatitis).

Scarring

Hypertrophic or contractile scars [1, 2] are rare after therapeutic doses of cryosurgery. If the former occurs, it requires similar treatment to similar lesions produced by other modalities of treatment. It is generally stated that freezing does not induce scarring. The work of Shepherd and Dawber [14] has shown that cryosurgical regimes which involve severe and prolonged freezing of the skin are quite capable of producing obvious scarring (Figs. 2, 3) [5]. Preservation of the fibrous network is the rule after treatment schedules used in clinical practice; this acts as a network around which cellular components regenerate. This process often gives an excellent cosmetic result, although dermal thinning may be a feature in the long term. Fibroblasts appear to be less susceptible to damage by freezing than epidermal cells. The possible protective nature of the blistering which accompanies healing deserves further in vivo study.

Paradoxically, early keloids, for example, after ear piercing, may be treatable by liquid nitrogen spray [14]. Cartilage necrosis is extremely rare after freezing; therefore, ear, eyelid and nasal lesions give good cosmetic results after cryosurgery [15]. It should be remembered that the only consistent exception to this

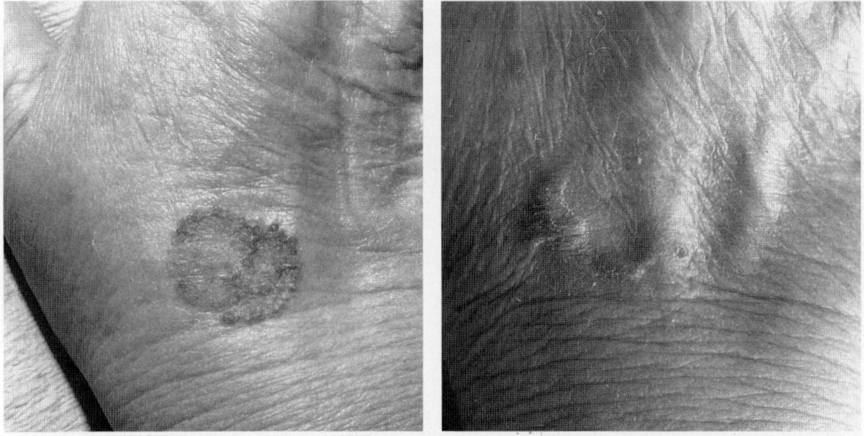

Fig. 2 a, b. Carcinoma-in-situ of the dorsum of the hand successfully treated with liquid nitrogen-spray – one FTC. The hypertrophic healing **(b)** occurred with 3 weeks; biopsy showed only dense elastic fibres which flattened spontaneously 16 weeks after treatment

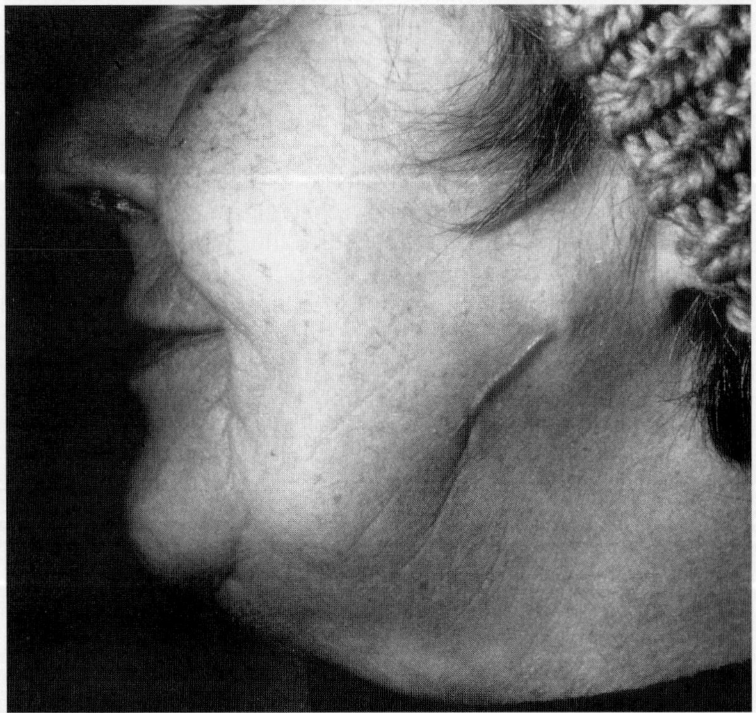

Fig. 3. Linear hypertrophic scar 6 weeks after two-FTC therapy for basal cell carcinoma; the pathophysiological basis for this linear lesion after a circle of destruction is not exactly known

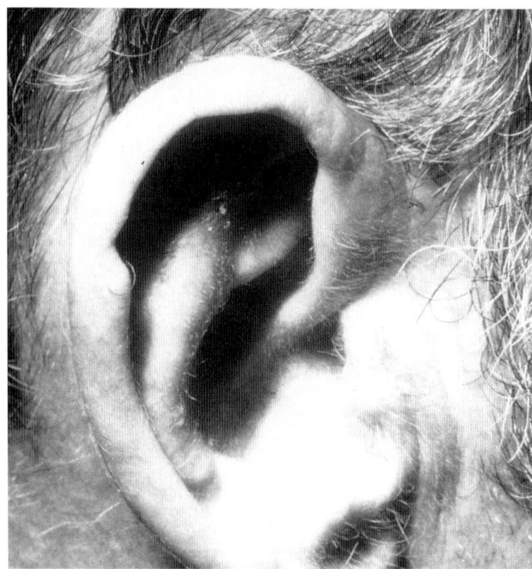

Fig. 4. Ear "notching" following the treatment of a squamous carcinoma (two FTCs)

dogma is cartilage already invaded by tumor. Even if tumor cure is achieved, a cartilage defect may occur; this is more likely to occur with squamous carcinoma than basal cell carcinoma (Fig. 4).

Scarring in the general sense of permanent visual alteration in the skin appearance after treatment must include the effects on adventitious glands of the skin and hair follicles. Follow-up histology after tumor treatments consistently reveals loss of sweat, sebaceous and apocrine gland structures; indeed this information has led to cryosurgery being used in some centres to treat hidradenitis suppurativa, various components of acne vulgaris, and axillary hyperhidrosis. Loss of the larger, normal, sebaceous pores after nasal and centrifacial skin treatments significantly alters the appearance of the skin and contributes greatly to the difficulty of cosmetically masking such blemishes (Fig. 5). Hair follicle damage after other than the shortest freeze times is so consistent that cryosurgery is generally only considered on sites such as the scalp and beard area for the treatment of small lesions. Burge and Dawber [16] have recently presented evidence to suggest that short freeze times may sometimes cause "resorption" and permanent loss of follicles without surrounding scarring, whilst "tumor regimes" lead to overall dermal damage with associated follicular scarring. The permanence of this loss suggeststhat the dermal papillae are irrevocably damaged by the freezing methods used in clinical practice.

Pigmentary Changes

Post-inflammatory hyperpigmentation, usually temporary, is common after short treatments for benign lesions, particularly on below knee skin; it may also develop in a halo distribution around a treated tumor site (Fig. 6). If hypopigmentation or

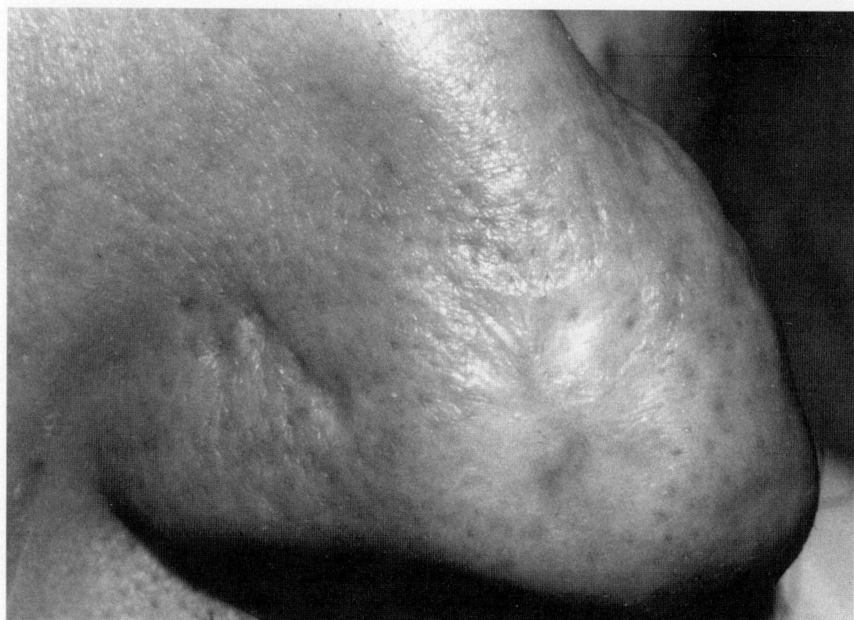

Fig. 5. Loss of pilosebaceous "pores" following treatment of basal cell carcinoma. This may be very obvious even in the absence of connective tissue scarring

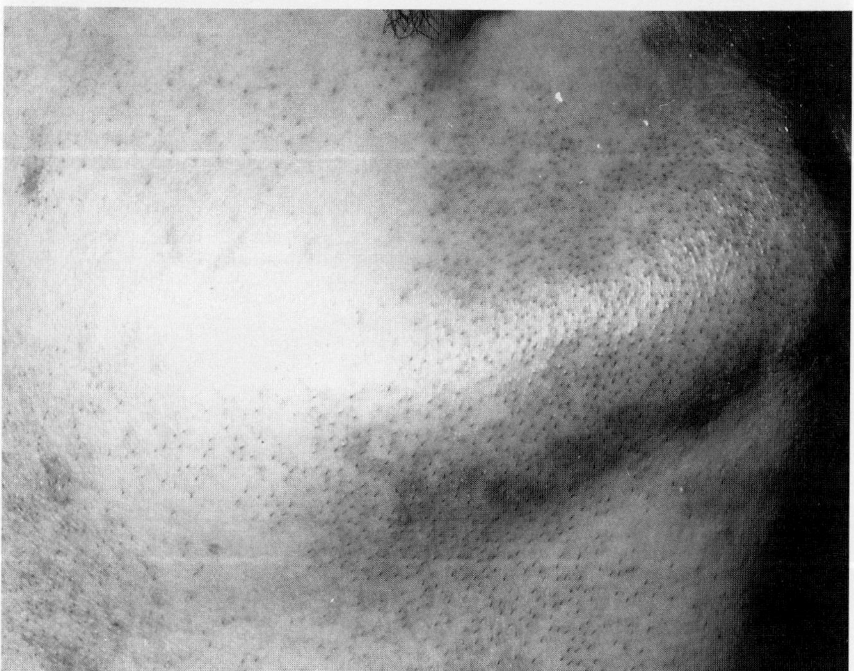

Fig. 6. Temporary patchy hyperpigmentation of the beard area following the treatment of multiple warts

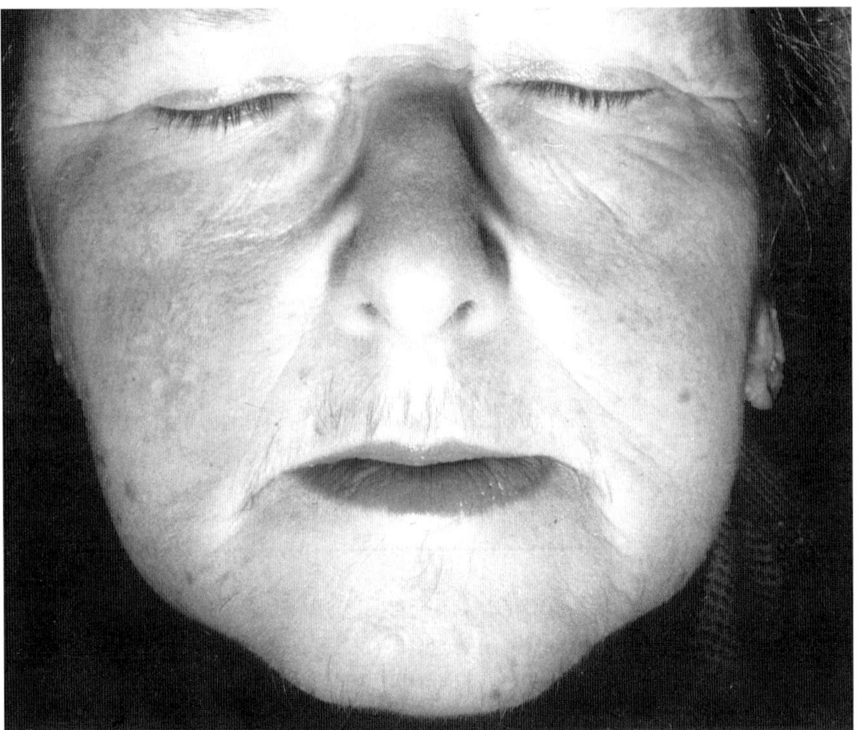

Fig. 7. Central hypopigmentation with a halo of hyperpigmentation 6 months after treatment of lentigo maligna

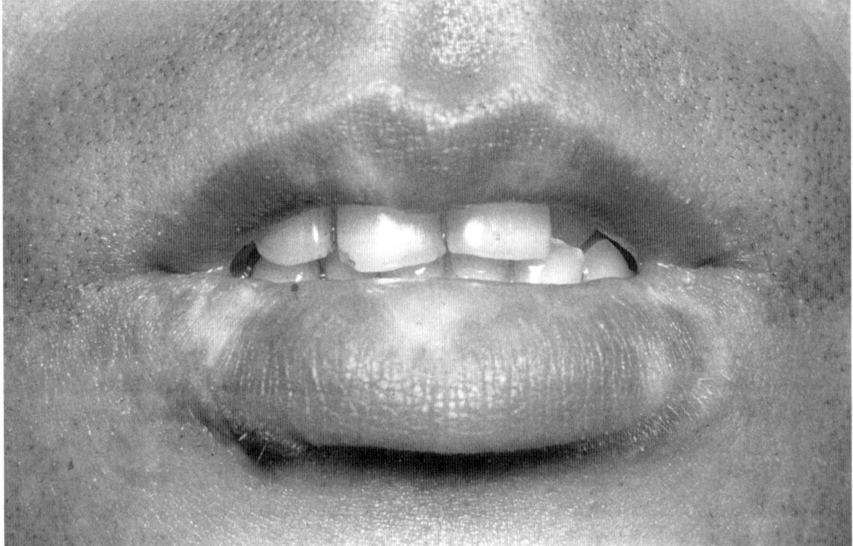

Fig. 8. Hypopigmentation – in this case temporary – in a negroid individual, following repeated Q-Tip liquid nitrogen application to digitate and filiform warts of the lips

depigmentation occur they are usually permanent, even though non-functioning melanocytes may recolour the white areas [10]. As a result, patients, particularly those with non-white skin, should be cautioned about potential pigmentary problems (Figs. 7, 8).

This description of the commoner complications, morbidity and side effects may be highly inhibitory to the budding cryosurgeon. Experience and increasing knowledge of which lesions *not* to treat, mean that in general it is quite possible to obtain good results from freezing with very little in the way of adverse effects.

Contra-indications

Known complications make it possible to suggest certain contra-indications, although there are no absolute contra-indications to cryosurgery. Indeed, many of those listed in cryosurgical and dermatological surgery books simply imply that for many skin lesions better cure rates can be obtained with other modes of treatment, for instance, morphoeic basal cell carcinoma. Also, certain sites and skin types lessen the usefulness of cryosurgery, mainly for cosmetic reasons, such as scalp and beard areas, negroid skin [10].

Many concurrent diseases may adversely affect the success rates and healing after cryosurgery. The author entirely agrees with Zacarian [1] that the following diseases should in general preclude the use of cryosurgery:
- Intolerance to cold
- Cryoglobulinaemia [17]
- Cryofibrinogenaemia [17]
- Raynaud's disease
- Cold urticaria
- Pyoderma gangrenosum
- Collagen and autoimmune disease
- Concurrent treatment with renal dialysis
- Concurrent treatment with immunosuppressive drugs
- Platelet deficiency disease
- Blood dyscrasies of unknown origin
- Multiple myeloma
- Agammaglobulinemia

One of the most important contra-indications is the absence of an accurate diagnosis. This is not to denigrate clinical judgement, however, which generally are adequate. Apart from the commonest types of basal cell carcinoma, *no* skin tumors should be treated without histological confirmation of diagnosis. This therefore means that destructive cryosurgery equipment that is easy to use must not be put in the hands of inexperienced physicians without adequate supervision and training.

References

1. Zacarian SA (1985) Cryosurgery for skin cancer and cutaneous disorders. Mosby, St. Louis, pp 283–297
2. Torre D (1986) Cryosurgery of basal cell carcinoma. J Am Acad Dermatol 15:917–929
3. Elton RF (1983) Complications of cutaneous cryosurgery. J Am Acad Dermatol 8:513–516
4. Sonnex TS, Jones RL, Weddell AG, Dawber RPR (1985) Long-term effects of cryosurgery on cutaneous sensation. Br J Dermatol 290:188–190
5. Shepherd JP, Dawber RPR (1984) Wound healing and scarring after cryosurgery. Cryobiology 21:157–169
6. Mortimer PS, Sonnex TS, Dawber RPR (1982) Cryotherapy for multicentric pigmented Bowen's disease. Clin Exp Dermatol 8:319–322
7. Hindson TC, Spiro J, Scott LV (1985) Clobetasol proprionate ointment reduces inflammation after cryotherapy. Br J Dermatol 112:599–602
8. Kuflik EG (1983) An attempt to reduce periorbital oedema in cryosurgery of eyelid tumors. Skin Allergy News 14:5–6
9. Kuflik EG, Webb W (1985) Effects of systemic corticosteroids on post-cryosurgical edema and other manifestations of the inflammatory response. J Dermatol Surg Oncol 11:464–468
10. Dawber RPR (1988) Cold kills. Clin Exp Dermatol 13:137–150
11. Lloyd JW, Barnard JDW, Glynn CJ (1976) Aryoanalgesia – a new approach to pain relief. Lancet 2:932–934
12. Faber WR, Naafs B, Sillevis Smitt JH (1987) Sensory loss following cryosurgery of skin lesions. Br J Dermatol 119:343–347
13. Detrano SJ (1984) Cryotherapy for chronic non-specific pruritis ani. J Dermatol Surg Oncol 10:483–484
14. Shepherd JP, Dawber RPR (1982) The response of hypertrophic and keloid scars to cryotherapy. Plast Reconstr Surg 70:677–682
15. Burge SM, Shepherd JP, Dawber RPR (1984) Effect of freezing the helix and rim or edge of the human and pig ear. J Dermatol Surg Oncol 10:816–819
16. Burge SM, Dawber RPR (1990) Hair follicle destruction and regeneration in guinea pig skin after cutaneous freeze injury. Cryobiology 27:153–163
17. Stewart RG, Graham GF (1978) A complication of cryosurgery in a patient with cryofibrinogenaemia. J Dermatol Surg Oncol 14:43–45

Cutaneous Laser Surgery

Deborah Moritz, S. Teri McGillis, Allison T. Vidimos
and Philip L. Bailin

Introduction

Medical laser technology began in the early 1960s with the skin being one of the first target organ systems to be approached [1]. In the past decade, significant advances have been made in the use of lasers for the treatment of a variety of cutaneous disorders.

The word laser is an acronym for light amplification by the stimulated emission of radiation. While not emitting ionizing radiation in most cases, laser light energy exerts its effects on tissue by being absorbed and converted to heat, which subsequently results in tissue modification and/or destruction. Three factors influence the effects of laser light on cutaneous tissue: selective wavelength absorption, duration of contact and power density (i. e., irradiance). Selective wavelength absorption refers to the fact that specific wavelengths of light are preferentially absorbed by atoms and molecules in the skin, such as melanin and hemoglobin. These are known as chromophores. The absorption of light is therefore determined not only by the wavelength of light emitted but also by the absorbing chromophore in the tissue. Without specific chromophores incident light is not selectively absorbed but is reflected and scattered into surrounding tissue, which can result in nonspecific tissue injury. The rate of heating and therefore the degree of destruction is determined by the power density (irradiance) and the duration of exposure, which together define the energy fluence delivered to the target tissue. Heat which is generated in a nonspecific manner leads to most of the side effects that are encountered during laser surgery.

Laser light is uniquely monochromatic (all of one wavelength), and the preferential peak of absorption of several cutaneous chromophores is now known to be maximal at certain energy wavelengths. Selective heating of tissue is achieved by matching a laser system that emits a certain wavelength to the specific target chromophore in the tissue to be treated. This in effect maximizes the therapeutic results and minimizes side effects and complications.

Duration of contact is the length of time a chromophore or tissue is exposed to an energy source. Prolonged contact generates heat which dissipates to surrounding tissue and therefore can lead to tissue necrosis.

Power density, or irradiance, of the laser exposure refers to the intensity of energy which impacts the target area of tissue. This is expressed as watts per square centimeter. The power density determines whether a vaporizational, cutting, coagulative, or necrotic tissue response results.

Many laser systems are commercially available; however, the lasers most commonly used in dermatology include the carbon dioxide, argon, dye, copper vapor, and ruby lasers.

Carbon Dioxide Lasers

The carbon dioxide laser emits light in the far infrared portion of the electromagnetic spectrum with a wavelength of 10 600 nm. The carbon dioxide laser can be used to treat a large number and variety of unrelated cutaneous tumors (listed in Table 1) [2]. The wide variety of lesions amenable to treatment with the carbon dioxide laser is due in part to the fact that the light energy emitted from the laser is absorbed by water rather than by specific chromophores. Because all living soft tissues are composed of 80%–90% water, the carbon dioxide laser energy is absorbed superficially within 0.1–0.2 mm of living tissue. This serves to minimize heat conduction and thermal damage to adjacent uninvolved tissue.

The carbon dioxide laser is very versatile in that it can be used to cut, coagulate, or vaporize tissue. In addition, it can be used in either a continuous or a superpulsed mode. In a continuous mode the laser energy is emitted at a constant power output. This stream of light can be interrupted or "gated" (by means of shuttering devices) at various intervals determined by the laser operator. In the superpulsed mode energy is emitted in very high power pulses of very short duration, which delivers bursts of energy to the tissue. This modality is said to have the benefit of offering a cooling phase to the target and therefore may lead to less nonspecific tissue destruction [3].

Side Effects and Complications

Side effects of carbon dioxide laser therapy can often be predicted, and true complications are fortunately rare. Side effects can be thought of as common cutaneous reactions that in most cases are anticipated. These include such things as "normal" scarring, which results when wounds heal by secondary intention, and postinflammatory pigmentary alterations. Hypopigmentation, for instance, occurs commonly and is secondary to thermal damage to nearby melanocytes. This complication is often unavoidable because many of the conditions treated with the carbon dioxide laser involve the dermis and can affect overlying and nearby melanocytes. Hyperpigmentation also occurs, especially in darker skinned individuals, but this is often temporary. A small percentage of patients may have persistent hyperpigmentation. This side effect can often last for several months but can be minimized with use of UV protection and avoidance of topical irritants. If it does occur, a trial of hydroquinone compounds may enhance resolution. Because side effects are often anticipated,

Table 1. Clinical application of the carbon dioxide laser (Modified from [2])

Cutting Tool

Patients with
  Bleeding disorders
  Epinephrine contraindication
  Pacemakers or monitoring devices

Lesions
  Keloids
  Acne keloidalis nuchae
  Burns (débridement)
  Decubitus ulcers

Procedures
  Moh's micrographic (microscopically controlled) surgery
  Bone perforation for stimulation of granulation tissue

Vaporizing Tool

Warts

Vascular lesions
  Nodular portwine stains
  Lymphangioma circumscriptum
  Pyogenic granulomas
  Adenoma sebaceum
  Angiokeratomas
  Angiosarcomas
  Venous lakes

Epidermal or mucosal disorders
  Epidermal nevus
  Erythroplasia of Queyrat
  Oral florid papillomatosis
  Actinic cheilitis
  Balantis xerotica obliterans
  Lichen sclerosus et atrophicus
  Bowenoid papulosis
  Bowen's disease
  Nail ablation
  Darier's disease
  Hailey-Hailey disease

Dermal processes
  Syringomas
  Trichoepitheliomas
  Neurofibromas
  Myxoid cysts
  Xanthelasma
  Tattoos

Cutting and Vaporizing Tool

Rhinophyma

Giant condylma acuminatum

---

these potential results can be discussed with the patient well in advance of the surgery.

Complications, on the other hand, are results that are not anticipated and often leave permanent, undesirable sequelae. Complications such as hypertrophic scarring and keloids can occur in anatomic areas with a known risk for these reactions. These include the neck, chest, mandibular ridge, back and upper arms. This complication can be anticipated in such regions, and intralesional corticosteroids can be initiated in the immediate post-operative period. In patients without a history of keloids, the side effect is not frequent enough to warrant routine prophylactic administration of intralesional corticosteroids. These unfortunate occurrences need to be addressed on an individual basis. Pressure dressings or burn garments worn over high-risk sites while healing and for several months afterwards may prevent hypertrophic scars and keloids from developing further. Hypertrophic scars are by far a more common result of laser surgery, and are confined to the boundaries of the wound treated. For the most part, these flatten spontaneously during the course of healing or with small amounts of intralesional corticosteroids. Keloids, on the other hand, outgrow the boundaries of the treated area and require much more aggressive care. Careful management of such patients is required.

Less common complications include postoperative bleeding, infection, and hypergranulation of the wound. Although the CO_2 laser seals blood vessels during treatment, vessels can reopen postoperatively and result in postoperative hemorrhage. This occurs more often in areas with a rich vascular supply or in deeper wounds where larger vessels are encountered. In addition, the neovascularization associated with wound healing can result in postoperative bleeding. Firm pressure is usually all that is needed to stop the bleeding. However, patients should be aware that excessive bleeding requires medical attention, and that they may require cautery or ligation of vessels which persistently bleed. Infection is an infrequent event with the laser since it produces sterile wounds (Fig. 1). Local antibiotic care generally suffices. Hypergranulation can occur during the healing phase of any wound which is allowed to heal by second intention (Fig. 2). Hypergranulation retards reepithelialization and therefore should be treated. Cautery, silver nitrate, or vaporization with the CO_2 laser can be used to treat the hypergranulation. The patient should be reevaluated in 2–3 weeks and retreated, if necessary.

Failure of the initial pathologic condition to respond to laser therapy can be considered a complication and is seen when treating recalcitrant warts, active cutaneous disease, and chronic cutaneous diseases which involve deep follicular epithelium (i.e., syringomas, trichoepitheliomas, Hailey-Hailey disease, Darier's disease). For the most part, the laser offers some temporary relief for many of these conditions. In many cases it is difficult to determine whether there is actually recurrence of disease or in fact a new primary lesion. For instance, when treating condyloma, it is not unusual to notice the development of new lesions along the periphery of the treated area several months following treatment. In the authors' practice it is generally accepted that a 6-month lesion-free period is necessary to effectively proclaim the treatment a "cure." The appearance of lesions prior to this

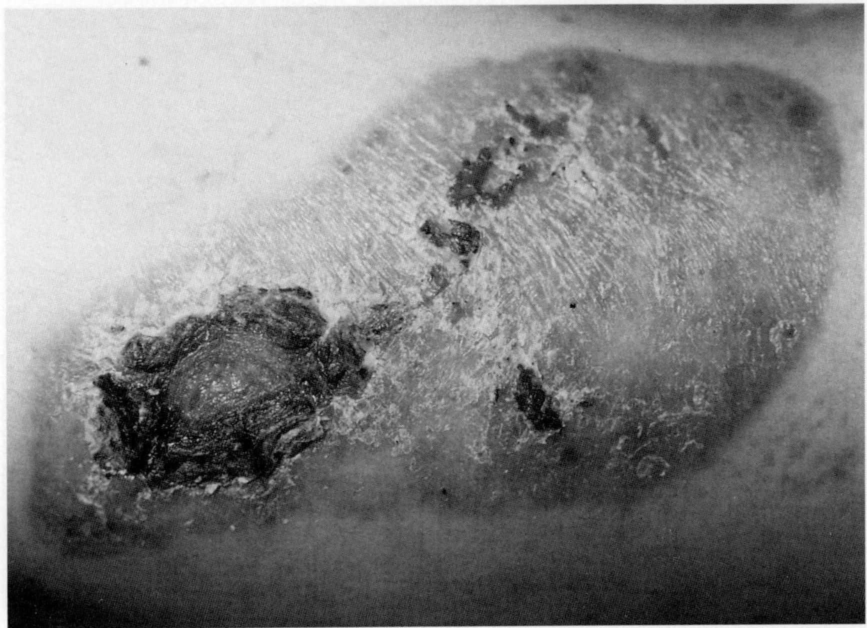

Fig. 1. Secondary infection of CO_2 laser wound

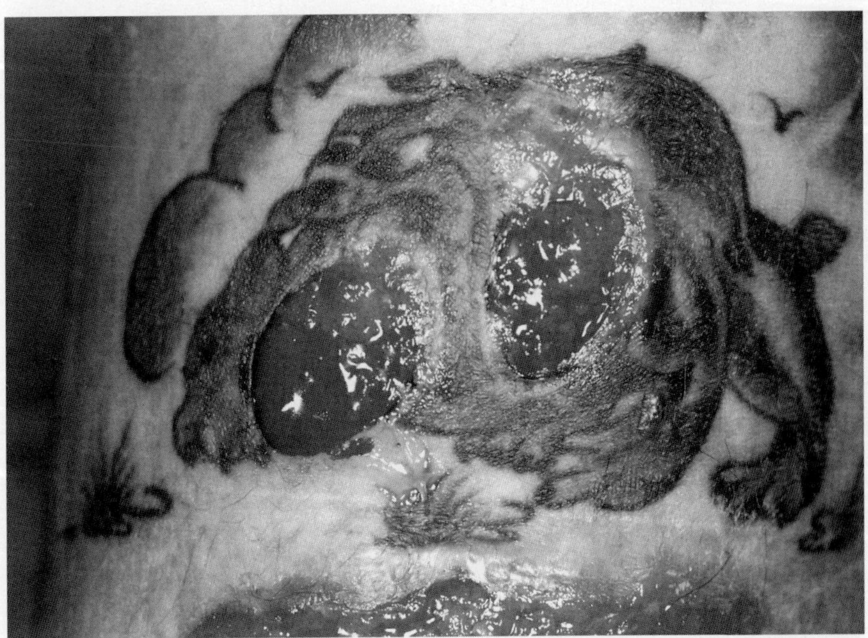

Fig. 2. Exuberant granulation tissue after CO_2 laser vaporization of tattoo

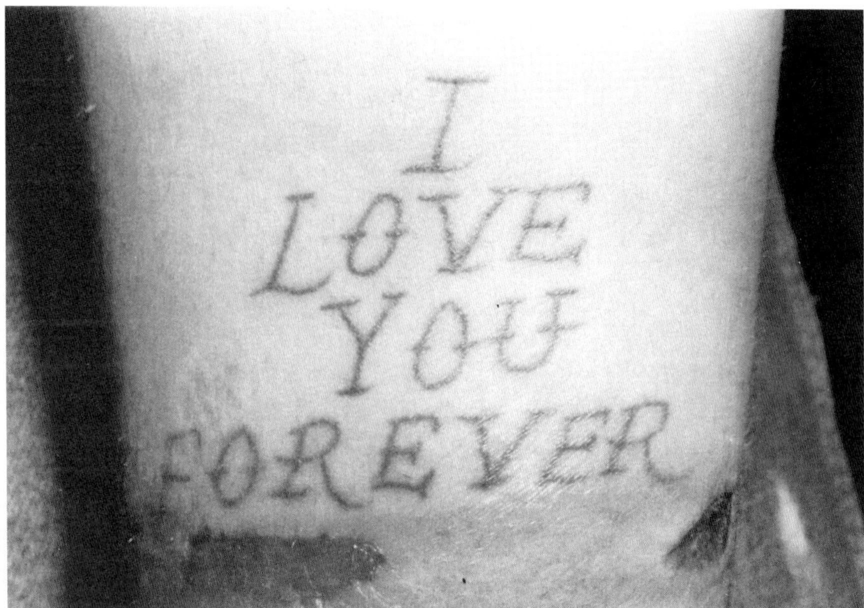

Fig. 3. Traumatic erosion overlying healed atrophic scar from CO_2 laser. (Courtesy of Robert Brodell, M.D., Warren, OH, USA)

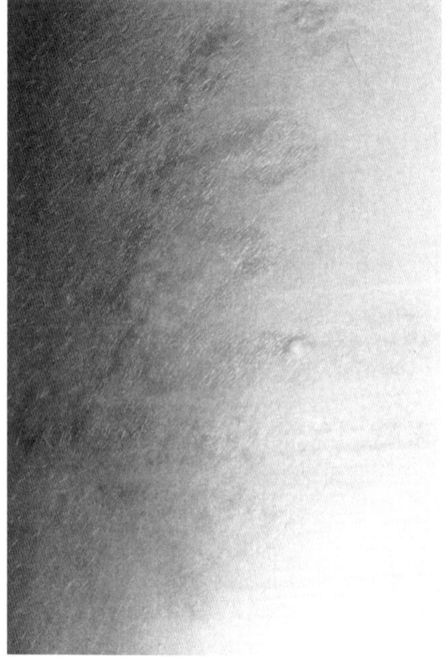

Fig. 4. Milia within the healed CO_2 laser wound. (Courtesy of Robert Brodell, M.D., Warren, OH, USA)

time often implies residual seeding of the virus. While not truly a complication, the patient, again, should be informed of this occasional occurrence.

When atrophic scarring occurs after healing, frictional stresses along the area can lead to superficial erosions (Fig. 3). If untreated, these can lead to local infection. Routine local preventative care is generally effective in averting these problems. Likewise, lymphatic bullae have also been reported in wounds allowed to heal by secondary intention [4]. Milia can also occur, which usually resolve spontaneously (Fig. 4). Compression dressings or garments overlying the newly healed epithelium can be used to prevent traumatic erosions and compress lymphatic channels and thus reduce this response. Contact reactions to dressings and ointments have also been observed but are not specifically related to the laser treatment.

General Carbon Dioxide Laser Wound Care

The carbon dioxide laser removes epidermis and dermis while treating cutaneous disease. Immediately postoperatively, wounds are dry and bloodless, displaying a surface of coagulated tissue proteins. These areas are cleansed with hydrogen peroxide and an antibacterial ointment is applied. The patient then continues this care beginning 24 h postoperatively on a twice-daily basis until full reepithelialization occurs. In areas that are potentially exposed to sun, trauma, or frictional stresses it is advised that the wounds be kept covered.

Nonwound Complications of Carbon Dioxide Laser

As with all laser systems, eye protection must be used by the laser operator, patient, and assistants since the eyes contain chromophores for all laser systems. The carbon dioxide laser vaporizes soft tissue water, and therefore any inadvertent eye exposure may result in a corneal ulceration or abrasion. This complication can be prevented by wearing appropriate eyewear, which includes plastic goggles or glasses [5–7]. When working around the patient's eye, a protective corneal shield should be placed to protect the ocular structures from the laser light. Placement of protective lenses may itself lead to corneal abrasions and conjunctivitis, which can be minimized by generously lubricating the shield with an antimicrobial ophthalmic ointment as well as by careful atraumatic placement [7]. The nontreated opposite eye must also be adequately protected with an eye patch during treatment. Following surgery, the patient's eye must be patched after removal of the shield until the topical anesthetic has worn off to prevent any inadvertent injury postoperatively.

Another issue that has surrounded use of the carbon dioxide laser is the possibility of infection from inhalation of vaporized viral particles in the laser plume. It is now known that a laser plume from infected individuals has been shown to contain infectious human papillomavirus particles [8, 9]. This has not yet been reported for hepatitis B or immunodeficiency virus; however, the theoretical risk for exposure exists. Plume exposure can be prevented with adequate evacuation of the smoke with a filtered vacuum device at the time of surgery. The operator and the patient, as well as anyone else in the room, should also wear high filtration surgical masks [8, 9].

Deflection of the laser beam off polished, shiny surgical instruments is a potential hazard that can be avoided by using Teflon-coated or anodized instruments [5]. Such deflection may cause inadvertent injury to nontarget areas of the patient or even injury to the laser operator and assistants. If protective drapes are impacted, ignition may occur. Wetting the drape surrounding the surgical field also helps to avoid accidental ignition. Nonflammable drapes are available.

Argon Lasers

The argon laser emits a continuous beam of six different wavelengths in the blue-green portion of the visible spectrum. Its active medium is argon gas. Of the emission, 80% is in the 488–514 nm range. Its chromophores are melanin and hemoglobin, and therefore it penetrates skin approximately 1–2 mm in depth before being totally absorbed.

The argon laser is commonly used for vascular lesions such as portwine stains, hemangiomas, telangiectasias, angiofibromas, and benign pigmented lesions [2] (see Table 2). Upon absorption by the target chromophore, which is hemoglobin, the energy is converted into heat which leads to the thermal damage. As the vessel being treated undergoes repair, microscopic fibrosis occurs which produces gradual improvement of the vascular lesion. Because there is some production of heat, which can be uncomfortable to the patient, local anesthesia may be required for treatment.

Table 2. Clinical application of the argon laser (Modified from [2])

Vascular	*Pigmented*
Portwine stain	Tattoos
Telangiectasias	Decorative
Rosacea	Traumatic
Cherry angiomas	
Angiokeratomas	Melanocytic
Venous lakes	Cafe-au-lait
Glomus tumors	Lentigines
Blue rubber bleb nevi	Blue nevi (Ota and Ito)
Adenoma sebaceum	
Pyogenic granulomas	
Cavernous hemangiomas	
Lymphemangiomas	
Kaposi's sarcoma	

Side Effects and Complications

Side effects and complications of argon laser surgery are relatively rare. The most common complications seen with the use of the argon laser are pigmentary alterations, textural change, hypertrophic scarring, and incomplete resolution of the lesions [10].

Since melanin is a chromophore that competes with hemoglobin, the most common side effect of argon treatment is a pigmentary change. Pigmentary alterations are usually temporary and should improve over time. However, 20% of patients experience persistent hypopigmentation in the area that has been treated [2]. Obviously, darker skinned patients have more competition from their natural melanin and are at slightly higher risk for this change (Figs. 5, 6). These areas do not tend to tan subsequently and may be further accentuated with sun exposure. Broad spectrum photoprotection is therefore recommended. Hyperpigmentation can be seen in dark-skinned individuals or those who fail to use adequate UV protection during the healing period. For the most part, the patient should be reassured that these areas will fade with time.

Benign melanocytic lesions can be treated with the argon wavelengths. While the continuous-wave argon laser can be used for eradicating pigment cells at a target site, there is a sublethal heating effect on the neighboring nontarget pigment cells. This can result in overproduction of pigment and therefore in a field of hyperpigmentation around or within the laser target area. However, this hyperpigmentation is usually transient. Adequate photoprotection (UVA/UVB) can minimize continued hyperpigmentation.

Textural changes are frequently seen in lesions in the process of being treated. These are identified by slight contour changes without evidence of true scarring. For the most part, these are the result of partial treatment of vasculature below. Areas that have complete resolution of vessels may be more depressed than those with remaining untreated vasculature. This is much akin to a sponge in which partial areas have been squeezed dry of water. This side effect often improves during the course of treatment, and patients should be reassured that this is not a permanent change.

Scarring is an unfortunate complication seen with argon laser. If excessive heat is generated in surrounding tissue, fibrosis occurs not only to the vessels but also to the support tissue which can ultimately lead to atrophic or hypertrophic scarring. Scarring after argon laser therapy has been reported at rates of 1.0%–4.5%. This scarring may be atrophic or hypertrophic (Fig. 7). Hypertrophic scarring is seen particularly in select high-risk areas such as the mandibular ridge, upper lip, and perialar regions. With careful testing and patient selection, these changes can be avoided [11]. Infants and young children are more prone to developing hypertrophic scars since they are in an active growth phase, and treatment with argon laser should be deferred until puberty unless absolutely indicated. As the argon laser may generate considerable heat, superficial bullae and/or crusts may form postoperatively. Should these areas become secondarily infected, there is an increased likelihood of forming scar tissue, and these

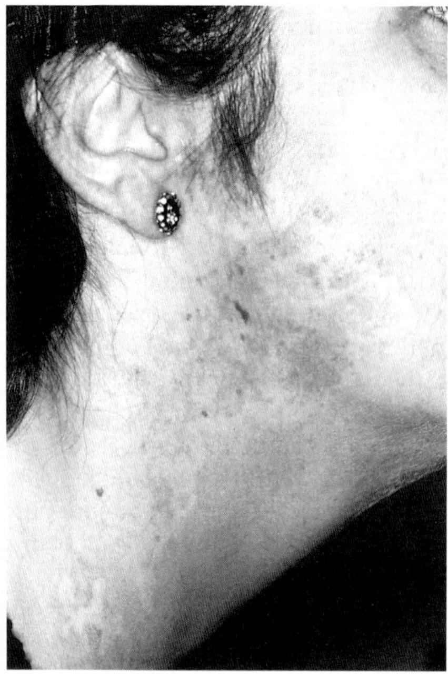

Fig. 5. Central hyperpigmentation and peripheral hypopigmentation in a port-wine stain treated with argon laser

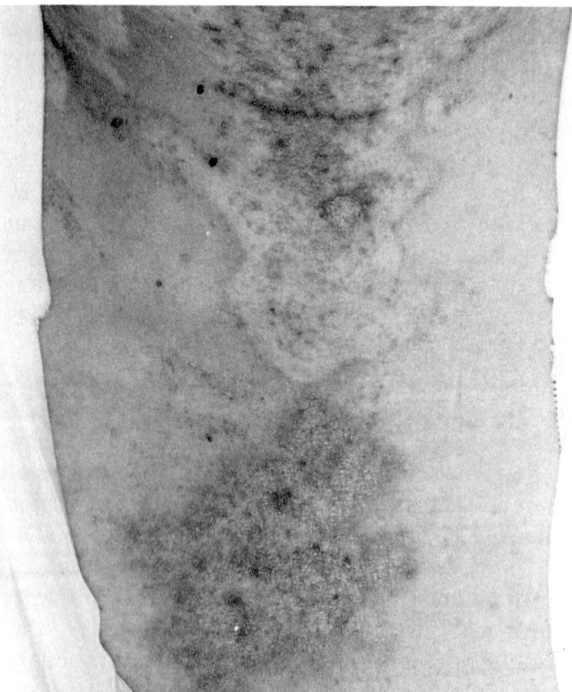

Fig. 6. Residual portwine stain with hypopigmentation and a rim of hyperpigmentation after argon laser

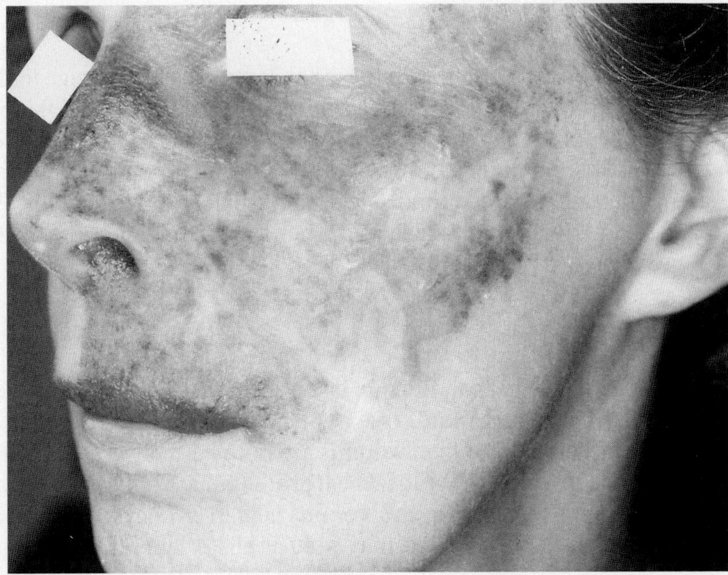

Fig. 7. Hypertrophic scarring and hypopigmentation over the cheek with residual portwine stain treated with argon laser

wounds should be managed with careful local antibiotic care. Atrophic scarring is fortunately rare and occurs from over-zealous treatment of the afflicted region. By using high-power settings and long exposure times much heat is generated, leading not only to obliteration of vasculature but also to surrounding dermis. This change is seen most often in thin or immature lesions, as well as those overlying bony prominences such as the malar eminence. Scarring has been dramatically reduced in the past few years because of a better understanding of the laser-tissue interactions and by lowering of exposure time. Modifications of the argon laser delivery systems have been achieved such that more evenly distributed energy can be delivered via a microprocessor system such as the Hexascan (Lihtan, Lyle, France) [12]. By testing small areas of the lesion with different settings, optimal treatment parameters can be established.

Incomplete Resolution of Lesions

Perhaps the most common "complication" of argon laser therapy is incomplete or partial resolution of the cutaneous condition being treated. Despite careful testing there are often regions within the lesion that are less responsive than others. This is due in part to the variable caliber and depth of the vasculature as well as to the differences in cutaneous textures. It is, however, preferable to retreat such an area with similar or lower energy fluence settings rather than attempt to eradicate the lesion completely by higher settings which may lead to adverse sequelae.

Nonwound Complication of Argon

Eye protection is required with the argon laser because damage to the retina may occur. The retina contains argon chromophores (both hemoglobin and melanin). This is in contrast to the type of injury occurring with the carbon dioxide laser, which affects the cornea. Goggles with appropriate optical densities to prevent laser penetration are required. These are usually orange in color. Protective eye shields should also be placed on the patient when treating periorbital lesions [6, 7].

Wound Care

In contrast to the carbon dioxide laser, which vaporizes epidermis and dermis leaving an exposed wound, the argon laser passes through the epidermis to reach its target below. Open wounds are not routinely created but occasionally small bullae result from the local heat production. Application of antibiotic ointment is generally effective, and wounds heal in 5–7 days. Postoperative application of ice packs for 12–24 h may reduce blister and crust formation.

Dye Lasers

Dye lasers utilize organic fluorescent compounds (dyes), each of which can emit wavelengths in the visible range. In dermatology, the most commonly used wavelengths are 577 nm (yellow) and 585 nm (orange). The main chromophore for these wavelengths is oxyhemoglobin. These wavelengths are felt to be more selective than those produced by the argon laser in that they are preferentially absorbed by oxyhemoglobin with much less competition from melanin chromophores. The dye lasers most commonly used in dermatology are of two types. These include the continuous-wave tunable dye lasers and the flashlamp dye laser systems. Continuous-wave dye lasers emit beams of relatively low energy at constant power. Since these lasers are truly "tunable" in that the operator has access to wavelengths anywhere from 480 to 630 nm. vascular and pigmented lesions can be treated (see Table 3). The spot sizes required to produce adequate power densities for meaningful tissue response with these laser systems are necessarily small (0.05–3.0 mm) so that treatment areas are also relatively small in size. The flashlamp dye lasers, on the other hand, emit streams of high power pulses of energy of very short duration, in the order of 450 microseconds. This short duration approximates the thermal relaxation time of the vessels. This term refers to the time interval for which a target tissue or structure must be heated in order for thermal transference to adjacent tissue to occur. Heating tissue for a period less than the thermal relaxation time results in minimal spread of heat energy to adjacent structures. The thermal relaxation time reflects the ability of the structure to retain heat within itself. This factor can be calculated for cutaneous blood vessels and is helpful for predicting how much time the laser should irradiate the tissue to effect selective blood vessel damage. The

Table 3. Clinical applications of the dye laser (Modified from [2])

Vascular (577/585 nm)

Portwine stains
Telangiectasias
Rosacea
Cherry angiomas
Angiokeratomas
Venous lakes
Glomus tumors
Blue rubber bleb nevi
Adenoma sebaceum
Pyogenic granulomas
Capillary hemangiomas

Pigmented (630 nm)

Cafe-au-lait
Lentigines
Junctional and small compound nevi
Dermal melanocytosis (nevus of Ota)

---

flashlamp pumped system has a short pulse duration which is well below the calculated 1–10 ms relaxation time of target vessels, and thus heat is said to be retained selectively within them. This delivery system is theoretically felt to minimize the risk of scarring. This system has the advantage of delivering energy with a fairly large spot size so that larger lesions may be treated in a single session.

The flashlamp dye laser system is now considered to be the treatment of choice for portwine stains in children [13, 14]. Likewise, it is especially amenable to treating immature or pale vascular lesions in adults. The continuous-wave tunable dye laser is effective in treating lesions that are darker or thicker.

Side Effects and Complications

Because of the more selective absorption of wavelengths in the 577–585 nm range, complications have been minimal for dye lasers. With both laser systems, multiple treatment sessions are required to achieve an 80%–90% lightening. Patients need to be informed of this well in advance.

Because the flashlamp dye laser system is used in children, there are many instances in which general anesthesia is required. The potential complications of general anesthesia perhaps remain greater than the complication of the laser itself, and a risk-benefit ratio must be determined on an individual basis. For many patients, however, either dye laser system can be used without any anesthesia or with local anesthesia, either topical or injected. Minor hyperpigmentation and skin texture alterations have been rarely reported with each laser system. The continuous-wave laser frequently leaves an orange-brown postinflammatory pigmentation which is temporary and fades with time. Purpura or bruising frequently follows pulsed dye laser therapy. A few isolated cases of atrophy and hypertrophic scarring have been reported with the flashlamp dys laser [14–16].

Nonwound Complications of Dye Lasers

Specialized eyewear is available for use with the tunable dye and flashlamp dye lasers. The operator needs to be aware of the wavelength which is being used so that appropriate specialized eyewear is selected. In cases in which the continuous-wave tunable dye laser is used, it is not uncommon to use wavelengths in the argon as well as the yellow and orange wavelengths. Tuning from one wavelength to another may require a change in eyewear.

The dye laser may require a dye change during the course of treatment. These organic dyes are highly toxic and need careful handling. It is imperative that all dyes be kept out of the treatment area, and it is suggested that they be locked away from other personnel. All dyes should be disposed of in a manner specified by the company.

Wound Care

The continuous-wave dye laser produces minimal epidermal changes. Should small bullae evolve, these can be easily treated with topical antibiotic care. Treated areas should not be exposed to direct ultraviolet exposure for several weeks following therapy.

The flashlamp dye laser produces purpura at the treatment site. This causes the treated area to look darker postoperatively. This fades in approximatlely 10 days, but patients should be advised of this outcome in advance. Because more extensive areas can be treated in a single session with this laser, tissue edema is not infrequent. This is seen especially when periorbital areas are treated. Ice packs applied immediately postoperatively provide some relief.

Neodymium-YAG Laser

The neodymium-YAG laser active medium is neodymium-yttrium-aluminum-garnet crystal doped with 1%–3% neodymium ions producing light in the near infrared spectrum at a wavelength of 1060 nm. There is no specific chromophore in skin. It has limited absorption and moderate scatter; therefore it results in deep penetration and moderate tissue injury. Because there is no specific chromophore, there is a much higher risk of target tissue injury accompanied by surrounding thermal damage. It is often used for the more nodular portwine stains and also mucosal or cavernous hemangiomas. It can also be used to coagulate recalcitrant warts and cutaneous carcinomas.

Side Effects and Complications

As with the other laser systems, the most common complications are related to the generation of heat to the surrounding tissue. There is a much higher incidence of all types of scarring including atrophic, hypertrophic, and keloidal scars. The target area most likely heals with some pigmentary abnormality, which is most commonly hypopigmentation. Because of the higher risk of scarring, this laser system is used primarily to treat destructive lesions, carcinomas, or in areas in which scarring can be hidden (such as the mucosa).

Copper Vapor Laser

The copper vapor laser emits 2 wavelengths of light, one of which is 578.2 nm and the other 510.5 nm. It produces a train of individual pulses in rapid succession. Its major chromophore is oxyhemoglobin. Indications and complications are similar to those of the dye laser.

Ruby Laser

The ruby laser has an active medium of a ruby crystal doped with chromium ions to emit a wavelength of 694 nm. This is a red visible light beam, and its chromophore is mainly melanin but can also be some forms of hemoglobin. The ruby laser has been found most recently to be useful in the treatment of blue-black tattoos on persons with fair (nonmelanized) complexions [17]. The tattoo pigment seems to absorb the wavelength of light, which results in gradual removal of the tattoo with minimal risk of scarring. Because of its limited indications, it is not presently widely available. Also, since many tattoos often contain more than one color, and the ruby laser can only be used on the blue-black portion of the tattoo, the remaining portion must to be treated with some other mechanism, such as surgical excision or CO_2 laser vaporization. It has been used (in the Orient) to treat large pigmented nevi and nevus of Ota or Ito. It may produce scarring from thermal transference.

Conclusion

Many of the complications listed under each laser system are all similar and are related to the heat generated by absorption of the laser energy by the specific chromophore (Table 4). Dissipation of the heat to surrounding tissue increases the risk of complications. All complications can be minimized by understanding laser systems fully and the cutaneous disease which is being treated. By increasing the selectivity of the chromophore, decreasing scatter, and decreasing the exposure time of the laser light, the complications can be minimized (Table 5).

Table 4. Complications of laser surgery

Laser system	Anticipated side effects	Complications
CO_2 laser	Scar (usually atrophic); hypopigmentation; hyperpigmentation	Hypertrophic scarring; keloids; bleeding; infection; failure of condition to respond; erosion of atrophic scar tissue; corneal ulcer/abrasion; lymphatic bullae (in second intention wounds)
Argon	Hypopigmentation; hyperpigmentation; inability of treated area to tan	Hypertrophic scarring; atrophic scarring; infection; failure of response
Dye	Pigmentary change; purpura	Failure of response

Table 5. Prevention and treatment of laser complications

Side Effect/Complication	Prevention	Treatment
Hypopigmentation		UVB, PUVA
Hyperpigmentation	UV protection; avoid topical irritants	Topical hydroquinones
Hypertrophic scarring	Pressure dressing; massage	Il corticosteriods; pressure
Keloids	Il corticosteroids in known keloid formers; pressure dressing; avoid high-risk areas	CO_2 laser excision; X-ray therapy; electron beam; pressure; Il corticosteroids
Bleeding (postoperative)	Avoid excessive trauma to wound bed; avoid air travel in first 24–48 h postoperatively	Pressure; cautery; ligation
Infection	Good wound care management; topical antibiotics	Systemic antibiotics
Failure of condition to respond	Patient selection	Trial of retreatment with different parameters; consider other form of therapy
Erosions over scar tissue	Avoid frictional stress	
Lymphatic bullae	Avoid second intention healing, if possible	Compression garments
Corneal abrasion or ulcer secondary to laser exposure	Protective goggles; protective contact lens when working near the eye	Antimicrobial ointment and patching until healed; opthalmologic evaluation
Corneal abrasion secondary to protective eyewear	Generous lubrication of lens prior to placement; irrigation of eye after removal of lens; patching of eye until topical anesthesia resolves	Antimicrobial ointment and patching until healed; ophtalmologic evalution

By understanding the laser systems fully, the most appropriate laser system can be chosen and used. Since all of the systems emit a wavelength which can be absorbed by components of the eye, protective eyewear is necessary for the patient and all operators. Since the CO_2 laser produces a plume, appropriate smoke evacuation is mandatory to prevent contamination of the air by infectious viral and/or bacterial particles. As newer laser systems are developed, selectivity will probably be increased; however there will probably be a narrowing of their usefulness. Since they are all very expensive, it is difficult for any one institution to have multiple laser systems, thus sometimes making availability to individual patients a problem.

References

1. Goldman L, Blaney DJ et al (1963) Effect of the laser beam on the skin. J Invest Dermatol 40:121
2. Dover JS, Arndt KA, Geronemus RG et al (1987) Illustrated cutaneous laser surgery: a practitioners guide. Appleton and Lange, East Norwalk
3. Hobbs ER; Bailin PL, Wheeland RG, Ratz JL (1987) Superpulsed lasers: minimizing thermal damage with short duration, high irradiance pulses. J Dermatol Surg Oncol 13:955–964
4. Moranz JF, Siegle RJ, Barret JL (1989) Lymphatic bullae arising as a complication of second intention healing. J Dermatol Surg Oncol 15:874–877
5. Friedman NR, Saleeby ER, Rubin MG, et al (1987) Safety parameters for avoiding acute ocular damage from the reflected CO_2 (10.6 µm) laser beam. J Am Acad Dermatol 17:815–818
6. Goldmann L, Rockwell J (1971) Lasers in medicine. Gordon and Breach, New York, pp 276–281
7. Wheeland RG, Bailin PL, Ratz JL, Schreffler DE (1987) Use of scleral eye shields for periorbital laser surgery. J Dermatol Surg Oncol 13:156–158
8. Sawchuk WS, Wever PJ, Lowy DR, Dzubow LM (1989) Infectious papillomavirus in the vapor of warts treated with carbon dioxide laser or electrocoagulation: detection and protection. J Am Acad Dermatol 21:41–49
9. Garden JM, O'Banion K, Shelnitz LS, et al (1988)Papillomavirus in the vapor of carbon dioxide laser-treated verrucae. JAMA 259:1199–1202
10. Ulbricht SM, Stern RS, Tang SV, et al (1987) Complications of cutaneous laser surgery. Arch Dermatol 123:345–349
11. Scheibner A, Wheeland RG (1989) Argon-pumped tunable dye laser therapy for facial port wine stain hemangiomas in adults – a new technique using small spot size and minimal power. J Dermatol Surg Oncol 15(3):277–282
12. Mc Daniel DH, Mordon S (1990) Hexascan: a new robotized scanning laser handpiece. Cutis 75:300–305
13. Reyes BA, Geronemus R (1990) Treatment of port-wine stains during childhood with the flashlamp-pumped pulsed dye laser. J Am Acad Dermatol 23:1142–1148
14. Tan OT, Sherwood K, Gilchrest BA (1989) Treatment of children with port-wine stains using the flashlamp-pulsed tunable laser. N Engl J Med 320:416–421
15. Glassberg E, Lask GP, Tan EML, et al (1988): The flashlamp-pumped 577 nm pulsed tunable dye laser: clinical efficacy and in vitro studies. J Dermatol Surg Oncol 14:1200–8.
16. Swinehart JM (1991): Hypertrophic scarring resulting from flashlamp-pumped pulsed dye laser surgery. J Amer Acad Dermatol 25:845-6.
17. Reid WH, McLeod PJ, Ritchie A, Ferguson-Pell M (1983) Q-switched ruby laser treatment of black tattoos. Br. J Plast Surg 36:455–459

Chemical Face Peeling

Paul S. Collins

Introduction

Chemical peeling even in the best of hands can be a trying experience, fraught with unexpected results. Expertise only reduces the incidence of unexpected results to a tolerable level and prepares the physician for the seemingly impossible task of reversing the untoward sequelae of chemical peeling. The ideal patient, one with fair skin, no pigmentary abnormalities, and moderate actinic damage, seldom creates a problem. Unfortunately, many patients who can benefit from chemical peeling do not have the ideal skin complexion. This group is susceptible to the untoward effects of peeling. One must therefore expect some of these individuals to experience complications from peeling. The object is to minimize or avoid those complications which are nonreversible and disfiguring while providing optimal effects of the chemical peel.

The extent of untoward results encountered is dependent upon the ability of the peeling chemical to produce both systemic effects through cutaneous absorption and its toxic effects on melanocytic function. The most widely used peeling agents are phenolic acid and trichloroacetic acid (TCA). Phenolic acid has the ability to produce toxic effects on melanocytic function and produce systemic symptoms when absorbed in sufficient quantities. In contrast, TCA has no systemic absorption and does not have a direct toxic effect on melanocytes. This chapter is divided into sections on the cutaneous effects common to all chemical peel agents, the cutaneous effects specific to phenol, the systemic effects of phenol, the cutaneous effects specific to TCA, and the specific effects of miscellaneous peeling agents. The general untoward effects of other acids such as the alpha hydroxy acids (lactic acid, pyruvic acid, and glycolic acid), retinoic acid, resorcinol, and salicylic acid can be correlated with those noted under the cutaneous effects of peeling agents, with notable exceptions as described under "Specific Effects of Miscellaneous Peeling Agents".

It is imperative the physician inform the patient of the more common and serious untoward sequelae. These include any systemic effects from absorption of the peeling chemical; cutaneous pigmentary abnormalities, and scarring. While there are other complications, these are the most common and disastrous and may require extended postoperative care and recovery. They are also the usual problems that result in litigation. It is better that the patient realize such problems can occur and decide not to undergo the procedure than to proceed with reckless abandon.

Cutaneous Effects Common to All Chemical Peel Agents

Recrudescence of Herpes Simplex Infection

Recrudescence of a herpes simplex infection is common after a chemical peel (Fig. 1). Fortunately, this usually does not cause scarring, but if it is extensive, it may produce pigmentary changes. It is important to differentiate the viral infection from impetigo caused by *Staphylococcus* or *Streptococcus* or a *Pseudomonas* folliculitis. Infection can cause scarring if left untreated or from the associated pruritus and scratching.

Typically a herpetic infection is manifested by the appearance of superficial, exquisitely tender ulcerations. Characteristic vesicles do not form due to the effects of the chemical peel upon the epidermis. The appearance of superficial ulcerations can mimic the results of a deep peel, but the presence of pain should clue the physician as to the etiology. Bacterial infections may also produce superficial ulceration but in contrast are not accompanied by pain initially. Involvement can be widespread, covering the entire upper lip and portions of the cheeks. The discomfort and pain responds rapidly to acyclovir.

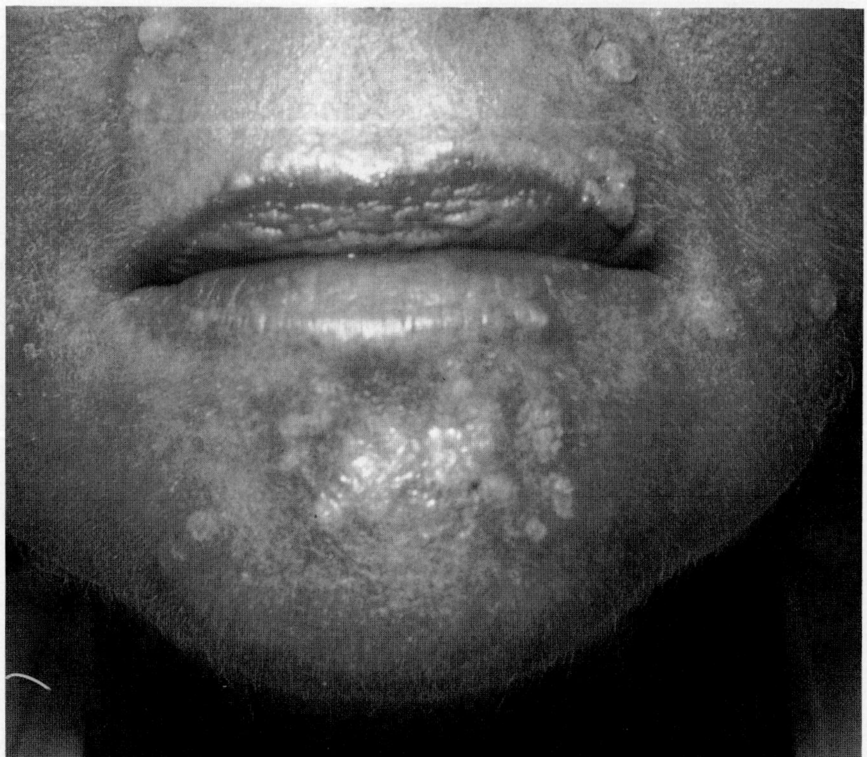

Fig. 1. Flare of herpes simplex with dissemination to the cheeks 5 days after a phenol peel.

Herpes can appear as late as a week after a peel and may delay healing for several weeks.

Acyclovir may prevent an outbreak of herpes simplex in a patient with a history of recurrent herpetic infections. A prophylactic dose of acyclovir 400 mg b.i.d. or 200 mg t.i.d. starting several days prior and continuing for 5–7 days after surgery may prevent outbreaks. A herpetic simplex infection should be treated immediately with acyclovir 400 mg q.i.d.

Facial Swelling

All peeling agents may cause facial swelling. Typically it is mild, unless phenol has been used (discussed below). Deeper peels of the face or a regional peel of the forehead may result in upper eyelid edema. The edema occurs 24–72 h after the peel and may actually swell the eyes shut. The edema is worse in the morning and improves with ambulation. It may be debilitating if the patient had planned on driving or working. It is certainly frightening if unexpected, and thus the patient should be warned of this possible complication. The eyelid edema may take several days to resolve.

Infection

Acids are germicidal, and therefore infection is less likely to follow application. Accumulation of tissue debris and occlusion with ointments such as vegetable fat, Vaseline, or similar nonantibacterial moisturizers can promote the development of folliculitis by *Staphylococcus, Streptococcus,* or *Pseudomonas.* The use of topical antibiotic ointments as moisturizing agents minimizes this complication but may produce a contact dermatitis. The patient should be instructed to cleanse the face to prevent accumulation of molting skin and debris which lends to bacterial overgrowth. Contact should be avoided with any individual with streptococcal pharyngitis or skin infections. The denuded facial skin is susceptible to infection by a streptococcal impetigo. Once infection is noted, appropriate penicillinase-resistant antibiotics should be promptly initiated.

Fortunately scarring does not always result from the skin infection. A neglected, unrecognized, or traumatized infection can produce scars and pigmentary changes. Pruritus may occur with any cutaneous infection and accidental excoriation can promote scarring. Pruritus should be treated by antihistamines such as diphenylhydramine or hydroxyzine.

Hypertrophic and Contracture Scars

Chemical peeling is not an all-or-none phenomena [1]. The physician can vary the depth of penetration and tissue destruction given the same concentration of acid and similarly prepared skin. Repetitive application of the acid enhances penetration. More acid is applied and tissue coagulation becomes universal and complete. Vigorous rubbing of the acid into the skin also increases penetration by removing the superficial debris which can block penetration. Such technique enhancements may be desirable when treating deep rhytides or skin with hyperkeratosis. Conversely, these techniques may increase the incidence of scarring. The physician must individualize the application of acid to the area treated to obtain optimal results and minimal complications. Facial areas with the highest incidence of scarring are the perioral, mandibular, and lower eyelid regions.

The mandible is prone to scarring due to the thinness of the overlying skin and the torsion produced as the edematous facial skin is stretched across the bone. Acid should be applied here carefully and not as vigorously. Since this is not an area that manifests significant rhytides and actinic changes as compared to the upper lips, cheeks, and forehead, it does not require as deep a peel.

The perioral region is an area of significant aging changes in women and is thus one of the more important, if not the most important, area requiring improvement from chemical peeling. The upper lip may be disproportionately aged with marked basophilic degeneration, cobblestoning, and rhytidosis when compared with the rest of the face. This scenario is usually seen in smokers. Unfortunately, the upper lip is also an area that is resistant to significant improvement by many modalities. Heroic attempts at improvement must be tempered to avoid scarring and other complications. Taping of the peeled area may induce scarring, and therefore many physicians avoid it or tape 0.5 cm above the vermilion lip. Zealous treatment complicated by a herpes simplex infection may also produce scarring. A combination of modalities such as dimethylsiloxane augmentation, repetitive milder peels (remember phenol and phenol formula peels can also be applied very superficially), and superficial dermabrasion can produce good and possibly excellent results with less hazard.

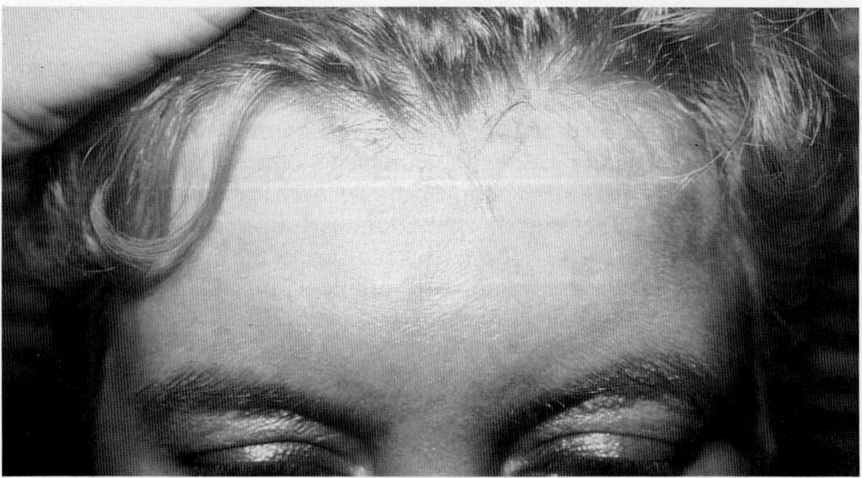

Fig. 2. Atrophic scarring at the hair line after a Baker's phenol peel. During healing the hair lay over this site. Just prior to the peel the patient had a hair permanent.

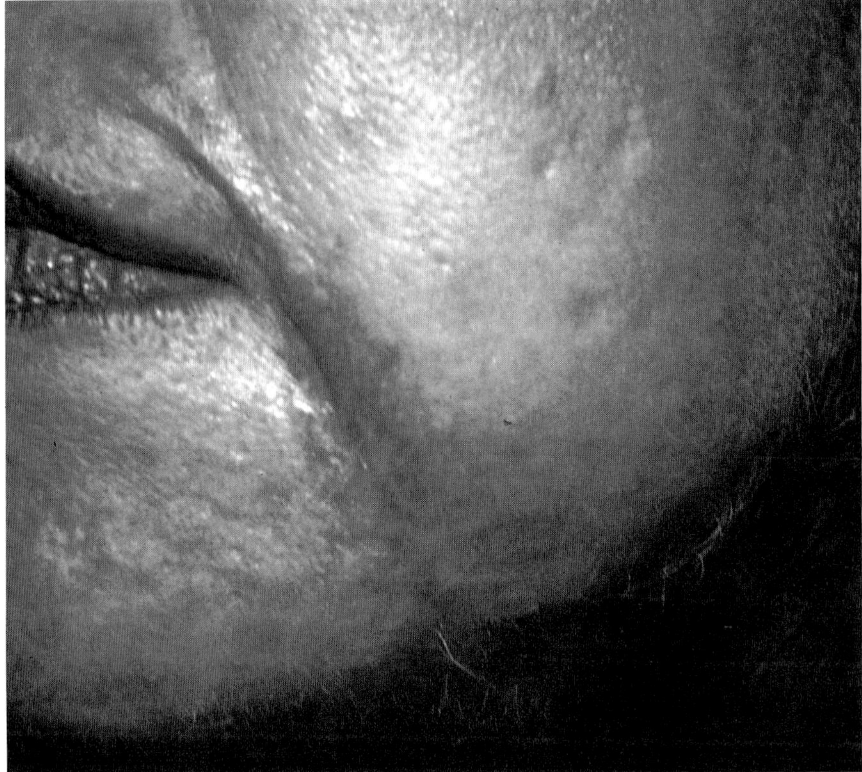

Fig. 3. Perioral hypertrophic scar occurring after a herpetic flare post phenol peel. Scarring after a herpes simplex flare is unusual.

The integrity of the lower eyelid must be carefully evaluated. Tissue tightening or scar contracture along the lower eyelid can eventuate in ectropion. Unusually, laxity of the lower eyelid as evidenced by abnormal horizontal lid excursion and lid lag, subclinical ectropion, or a history of previous blepharoplasty should alert the physician. Minimal application or even avoidance of the acid solution on the susceptible eyelids should be done and duly recorded in the operative note. Should a mild ectropion develop, message of the eyelid and taping up of the lateral lid at bedtime may resolve the problem. Topical steroids and careful diluted doses of intralesional steroids are also helpful.

Unlike the face, other areas of the skin such as the hands, neck, and upper chest do not have the appendage density often necessary for full recovery without scarring. Therefore these areas cannot tolerate deep peeling agents, and they slough and scar. Caution dictates the use of weaker peeling agents in lower concentrations and repetition of the peel treatments.

An area of persistent erythema or the appearance of an area of erythema especially along the mandible or cheek should alert the physician to the possible development of hypertrophic scarring. Scratching and excoriations can traumatize healing skin and also lead to scarring. Application of a topical steroid early is very effective in reducing or eliminating hypertrophic scars. The author's preference is to use both a topical steroid ointment (Aclovate) with a topical antibiotic ointment (Polysporin). Steroids, administered either orally or intramuscularly may relieve scar formation or tissue contracture. Intralesional steroids are also effective, but the physician must be aware of possible steroid atrophy at the injection site. Intercurrent infection may add to tissue injury and enhance scarring. When there is abnormal tissue sloughing, it is advisable to treat for possible secondary infection with topical and, if necessary, oral antibiotics.

Finally a word of caution: all peeling agents can induce scarring. The use of alpha hydroxy acids has recently been promulgated as relatively safe. The author is aware of litigation arising from the production of scarring and pigmentary abnormalities from the use of alpha hydroxy acids.

Erythema

Erythema is common after phenol application and usually persists for 6–8 weeks before fading. Persistent erythema can occasionally occur with facial redness lasting for months before slowly resolving. A special problem area is the perioral region. Phenol formula peels (Baker's or Litton's) are very effective in removing perioral rhytides. However, the expected erythema may be marked and persistent for many months. When the upper lip is the only area peeled, the intense redness is difficult to mask with cosmetics.

The erythema seen after TCA is less severe. A common area of involvement is the periorbital cheek on and above the medial zygoma. Any persistent erythema (lasting more than 1 week) must be carefully observed as it may be the first sign of hypertrophic scarring. This is especially true when it occurs on the cheeks. Early use of a topical steroid ointment is advisable.

Corticosteroids accelerate the resolution of the universal erythema. Upper lip erythema can, however, be stubbornly persistent. The author's preference for treatment of persistent universal erythema as seen with use of phenol is celestone soluspan 1.0–1.5 cm^3 intramuscularly. While topical steroids are also effective, prolonged use may be associated with the appearance of telangiectasia.

The erythema can also be accompanied with dermographism and pruritus. Dermographism associated with intense pruritus may cause the patient, especially during sleep, to excoriate the healing tissue, eventuating in scarring and pigmentary changes. Hydroxyzine 25 mg qhs quickly resolves these symptoms. It should be continued for 7 days to prevent a relapse of symptoms. Recommended is diphenylhydramine 25–50 mg qhs or as needed to minimize or prevent the hyperactivity and nervousness that occasionally occurs with the use of intramuscular celestone soluspan. It can be given in conjunction with hydroxyzine at qhs.

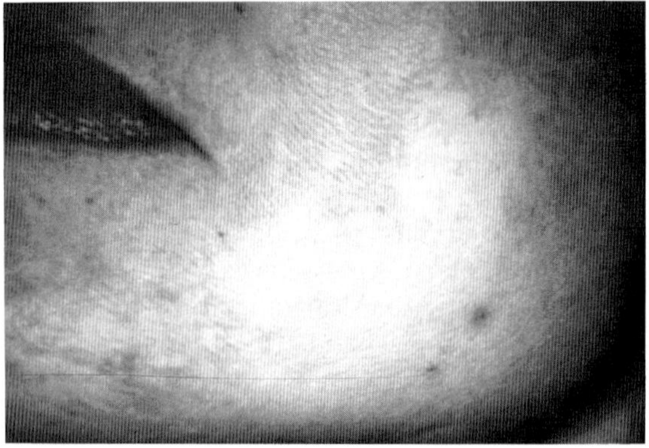

Fig. 4. Streaking hyperpigmentation in an individual of Oriental extraction. This is not unusual occurrence. In most cases the pigmentation will resolve but takes months. Often retreatment will only aggravate or prolong the time until recovery.

Mottled Skin Texture

The most common cause of mottled pigmentation is the patient's inherent tendency to respond nonuniformly to the peeling agent. However, blotchy or streaked skin texture and pigmentation may be due to faulty technique, improper cleansing of the skin, inadequate mixing of the solution suspension, nonuniform application of the chemical solution, tearing, or uneven application and nonuniform occlusion of the tape mask. The result is differences in the depth of peel with variations in the skin texture and color.

It is necessary to cleanse the skin thoroughly of all cosmetics, debris, and heavy oils which inhibit penetration. Examination of the cleansing gauze for lack of discoloration caused by oils and residual cosmetics of the skin is an adequate determination that the skin is now clear and ready for peeling. The skin, including the pores, must be thoroughly cleansed of all scales, sebum, moisturizers, dirt, cosmetics and other debris. Poor, inconsistent or uneven skin cleansing results in incomplete penetration of the acid. No cosmetics should be worn the day of the peel and preferably not for several days prior. Thick layers of cosmetics may be difficult to remove from skin creases and pores regardless of the cleanser. The physician in attempting to obtain complete skin frosting may erroneously apply too much acid to an area. The poorly prepared skin finally frosts, but it does so at the expense of a deeper acid penetrance in adequately cleansed adjacent skin. Pigmentary changes and scars may occur in these areas.

Phenol solution (Baker's or Litton's) does not stay in solution but must be mixed. Failure to apply a thoroughly mixed solution results in variation in the depth of the peel. Simply swirling mixture into solution prior to dipping the Q-tip prevents this problem. Meticulous cleansing of the skin and especially all rhytides with even application of the chemical solution produces a consistent uniform peel. Sensitivity to sunlight exacerbates this condition.

Birth control pills, extrogens, sunlight, photosensitizing medications, and pregnancy can also cause postpeel hyperpigmentation. Pigmentation can be in-

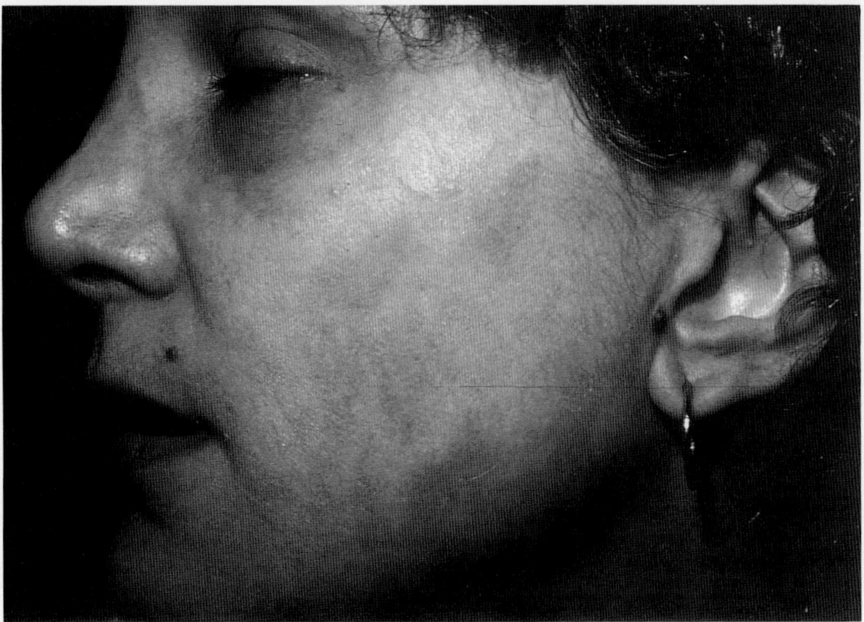

Fig. 5. Hyperpigmentation occurring after a Baker's phenol peel in a patient on estrogen replacement post hysterectomy. The pigmentation recurred after a spot peel. Only after the estrogen was stopped did the hyperpigmentation resolve. After several months the estrogen was restarted without incident.

duced months after the peel, during which time the melanocyte remains hypersensitive. It is advisable to avoid or eliminate any inducer of pigmentation both prior to and after a peel. Postinflammatory hyperpigmentation may respond to treatment only if the exacerbating factor is eliminated.

Treatment may require the entire area to be repeeled. Application of a hydroquinone may fade the hyperpigmentation but does not help any hypopigmentation. Strict avoidance of sunlight and fluorescent lighting and liberal daily use of wide-spectrum sunscreens are necessary. If the cause is poor skin selection, the pigmentation may correct itself in time without treatment.

Facial Swelling

The patient and any individual who administers postoperative care must be warned of the subsequent appearance. While any peeling agent may induce edema and facial swelling, phenol-induced facial swelling can be extreme, with the face ballooning to hideous proportions. The addition of the phenol chemical burn can produce a terrifying effect. While the appearance may look painful, it typically is not. The uninitiated may construe the appearance as a threatening

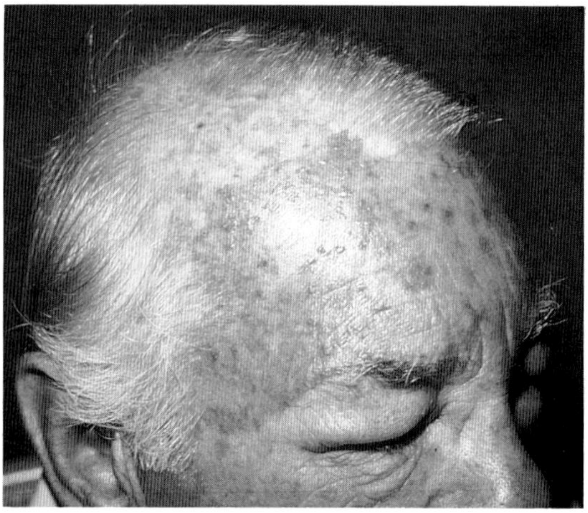

Fig. 6. Marked periorbital edema occurring four days after a 35% trichloroacetic acid peel. The edema lasted five days before subsiding.

complication and seek medical care elsewhere. The real danger lies when an uneducated physician negligently misinforms the patient and initiates grossly inappropriate treatment.

TCA can produce periorbital edema. The swelling may close the eyelids and inhibit normal vision for work or driving. The edema can persist for several days and is typically worse upon awakening. Consumption of salty foods probably exacerbates the condition. Firm pressure with cool compresses may hasten resolution.

Milia

Development of small facial inclusion cysts is common and is aggravated by the use of ointments after peels. The use of retinoic acid prior to and after peeling may reduce the number of milia. However, in susceptible individuals, retinoic acid can produce a cutaneous burn, induce hyperpigmentation, and interfere with cutaneous wound healing [2] if initiated too quickly. The author resumes use of retinoic acid 1 week after a peel.

Cutaneous Effects Specific to Phenolic Acid

Pain

Application of phenol is painful. The pain experienced is described as being similar to a hot grease burn. Phenol-induced skin pain may induce one of several different courses. In all cases there is an extreme burning sensation noted within seconds after application. At times the burning sensation reaches its peak immediately and remains for several hours before disappearing. Others may have an immediate burning sensation that dissipates after several minutes. However, within 30–60 min the discomfort returns and remains for approximately 8–12 h. An occasional patient may experience discomfort for several days.

The intensity of pain that patients experience varies greatly, from mild to the "worse pain I have ever had." The pain may not be controlled by either oral or intramuscular narcotic medications. Patients should be warned that discomfort is unavoidable during the first 24 h lest they consider it a harbinger to complications or an inappropriate or incorrect treatment. Midazolam's ability to produce amnesia is helpful; although the patient may experience pain, its discomfort will not be remembered as an unpleasant aspect of the surgery.

Removal of the Facial Tape

Taping after a phenol peel is loosing its popularity. Application of a moisturizing agent such as Vaseline, vegetable fat, or aquaphor is now more commonly practiced. Normally the tape is removed 24–48 h after the peel. If a marked serous exudate develops within this time, the tape literally floats off the face. Removal is easy because the tape does not adhere to the facial skin, and there is minimal pain. Unfortunately, not all patients produce a copious exudate. The tape remains adherent to the skin, producing pain as it pulls the peeling but incompletely separated skin off the face. Administration of narcotics may be necessary prior to attempting removal. Soaking the tape and face facilitates removal and minimizes trauma to the deeper layers of the newly exposed skin. The physician should apply the tape carefully and avoid taping hair.

Hypopigmentation

The bleaching effect of phenol is to be expected although it may not be noted until many months later. Indeed, as the erythema is fading, the skin appears refreshed with a healthy tint, giving a false impression of the final skin tone. This phase may take months before fading completely into the porcelainlike hypopigmentation. Proper patient selection can avoid most problems associated with loss of pigmentation. Sunbathers or individuals who are not accustomed to wearing cosmetic makeup do not appreciate the new color tone. The facial skin tone appears lifeless and ghostly. In contrast, a fair-complexioned individual who shuns sun exposure and skin tanning, and who is accustomed to utilizing makeup finds this pigmentary change perfectly acceptable, except for the expected line of demarcation.

The procelain white is due to hypopigmentation and depigmentation [3]. Melanocytes are not decreased, as was formerly believed, and may actually increase in number. The melanocytes can still synthesize melanin and distribute the melanin granules to epidermal cells. This is why some patients

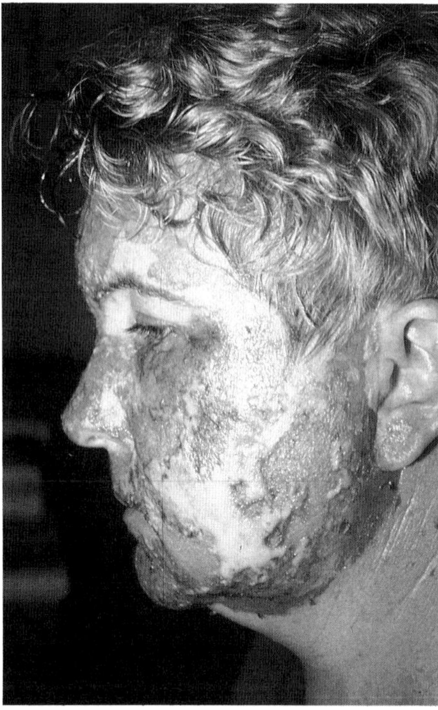

Fig. 7. Thick exudate in a Baker's phenol peel patient non taped who applied vaseline. The exudate took, two weeks to slough off. No scarring occurred but postinflammatory erythema remained for approximately four months. The erythema decreased but did not dissipate when treated with IM Celestone 1.5 cc given three times at 2 to 3 week intervals.

exhibit mild freckling and uneven pigmentation of the skin after excessive sun exposure. To avoid these changes the face should be protected with the daily use of sunscreens.

Hyperpigmentation

Hyperpigmentation after a phenol peel is unusual. Pigmentation is usually due to medications such as estrogen, progesterone and phenothiazine, which are known to produce hyperpigmentation in susceptible individuals [4]. These medications may need to be stopped before the hyperpigmentation resolves or responds to therapy such as a topical depigmentary agent or a second phenolic peel.

It is mandatory to emphasize the importance of avoiding exposure to the sun. It may also be necessary to limit exposure to fluorescent lighting. Although phenol produces hypopigmentation, it does not destroy the melanocyte. Pigmentation, usually mottled, can be induced from sun exposure. Wide-spectrum sun blockers for both UVA and UVB lighting should be worn. Photoplex provides adequate UVA protection and when used in conjunction with UVB blockers such as PreSun 39 or Shade 44 gives wide-spectrum protection. Hydroquinone with or without the addition of retinoic acid and topical steroid is effective and should be used promptly at the first appearance of hyperpigmentation.

Demarcation Lines

An obvious line of demarcation forms between peeled and nonpeeled areas. This is most commonly seen along the mandible, but it may also appear around the lips or hairline. Cosmetic makeups are necessary to camouflage the mandibular demarcation line, and patients who do not use makeup are not suitable candidates. Should the patient undergo a facelift, this line of demarcation, which formerly was hidden just below the mandible, is raised onto the cheeks. Obviously the greater the extent of solar dermatitis with its associated pigmentary changes, the greater is the contrast that is created.

Chemical peeling with phenol and phenol formulas is not an all-or-none phenomena. By lightly stroking a damp Q-tip in a zig-zag motion on the neck, a lessening of the demarcation line can be created. This is the same principle advocated for the use of a W-plasty versus a straight-line excision and scar formation camouflage. The neck tolerates phenol if applied very lightly and nonrepetitively. In men the line of demarcation is easily hidden in the bearded skin especially if the phenol is applied in a zig-zag pattern on the neck.

Another common mistake is the omission of phenol on the vermilion border of the lips. Unless the peel is carried onto the lips, an unsightly border of aged skin remains surrounding the lips. This same mistake can be made along the hairline unless phenol is correctly applied into the scalp hair.

Telangiectasia

Telangiectasias are relatively common and can be quite prominent. Superficial telangiectasia can be amendable to phenolic peeling and indeed can literally disappear after the peel. The majority of telangiectasias, however, are located deeper within the skin and may become more prominent. The peel strips the overlying aged skin thus bringing the telangiectasia closer to the surface and visual prominence. Patients should be warned prior to surgery that the presence of facial telangiectasia may become more noticeable and widespread. The appearance of so many prominent telangiectasia may make it difficult to camouflage with makeup. The pulse dye laser can effectively remove the telangiectasia if necessary.

Systemic Effects Specific to Phenolic Acid

Phenol is metabolized in the liver and excreted by the kidneys. It is a potential hepatorenal toxin. Avoid preoperative dehydration; the administration of intravenous hydration during and after the procedure accelerates the excretion of phenol. This decreases the incidence and severity of systemic toxicity.

Cardiotoxicity

Potentially the most serious complication of phenolic acid is its immediate cardiotoxic effect. Truppman and Ellenby [5] and later Gross [6] described arrhythmias including premature ventricular contractions, ventricular bigeminy, ventricular tachycardia, and premature atrial tachycardia that occurred in patients undergoing full face phenol peels. Significantly, the arrhythmias occurred even in the presence of a normal preoperative electrocardiogram. There was no apparent relationship to sex, age, phenol serum levels, administration of oxygen, or use of either saponified (Baker's formula) or nonsaponified (Litton's formula) phenol peel formulas.

Phenol is absorbed into the blood stream through both the skin and respiratory tract. Phenol is excreted by the kidneys and lungs. Absorption through the skin and thus toxicity is directly related to the quantity applied to the skin, the total surface area treated, the time of application duration, and the rate of excretion [7]. Restricting application to a single facial section, such as the forehead or the right cheek, and then waiting 15 min before treatment of the next section limits absorption. This probably prevents cardiotoxicity in an adequately hydrated patient without renal, hepatic, or significant cardiac disease.

It is recommended that any patient, while undergoing a full-face phenol formula peel, receive cardiac and blood pressure monitoring and be fully hydrated. Administration of intravenous Fluids (Ringer's lactate), 500 ml preoperatively and 500–1000 ml during and after the peel ensures adequate hydration and rapid diuresis of the absorbed phenol molecule. Upon appearance of an arrhythmia the physician should immediately suspend further application of phenol. Assuming that the arrhythmia resolves immediately, a timely delay befora additional application is advisable. Cessation of the procedure and administration of lidocaine may be required for persistent arrhythmias.

The respiratory tract may also be a source of phenol absorption. The physician should not idly hold the phenol-soaked applicator in front of the patient's nose. The room should be well ventilated for both the patient and physician's safety. A small fan in the room aids in the flow of room air.

Cutaneous Effects Specific to Trichloroacetic Acid

Complications of TCA are essentially limited to the skin. There is no systemic absorption. No preoperative blood evaluation is necessary because of this lack of absorption. It can be used in patients with myocardial, hepatic, or renal disease without cardiac monitoring [8] provided the patient can tolerate the discomfort of acid application. Remember: pain can induce cardiac arrhythmias.

Penetration of the epidermis by TCA can be easily influenced by many variables. Depending on the concentration of TCA used, manipulation of these variables may produce divergent and unexpected results. Among the major variables that may determine the depth of TCA peel produced include: the concentration of TCA utilized; the technique of acid application; prior and continued utilization of retinoic acid; the effectiveness of prepeel skin preparation and degreasing; sebaceous gland density and activity; the thinness of the epidermis and dermis from atrophic actinic changes; ingestion of any agent that causes epidermal sloughing and thinning such as vitamin A, beta-carotene or accutane; and the application of prepeel keratolytic agents and solutions [9].

Individual variation in any of the above factors can result in disparate peel results. Although the application of trichloroacetic acid is simplistic, the controlling factors that determine acid penetration are not. They must be standardized in order to obtain consistent effects. The common denominator behind any complication with acid peels is the assumption that all skin reacts equally. There is no single standard TCA concentration for peeling. Each individual patient must be evaluated before choosing the appropriate concentration. Thick sebaceous male facial skin may easily tolerate a TCA solution concentration of 50%, whereas scaring may result it the same solution is applied to the thin, fine facial skin of an elderly woman. Furthermore, any substance that reduces the thickness of the horny layer enhances the depth of destruction by TCA. Consequently, a seemingly weak concentration of TCA may produce a cutaneous burn deeper than expected with possible disastrous results [9].

Hyperpigmentation

Of all the possible complications that can occur from TCA peels, uneven hyperpigmentation is the most common and unpredictable. Its frequency is especially high in patients with brown skin. Not all individuals with Oriental, Latin, Indian, Mexican or Mediterranean heritage may exhibit brown skin; however, they still retain the ability to develop postinflammatory mottled hyperpigmentation. The pigmentary problems encountered in this group may be mottled, persistent, and inconsistently responsive to all treatments. Indeed treatment may actually exacerbate an already difficult pigmentary complication.

A test spot peel is reasonable in patients who are anxious or are apt to develop hyperpigmentation because of their skin color. While a negative test result is encouraging, it does not assure that hyperpigmentation will not develop. Development of hyperpigmentation in the presence of a negative test result may cause the patient to question the physician's peeling procedure while, conversely the physician may suspect that the patient has been exposed to an exacerbating factor such as excessive solar exposure. The author utilizes testing to discourage peeling in susceptible patients.

With weaker peeling agents such as TCA and the alpha hydroxy acids, it is imperative to eliminate or reduce exposure to any agent that can induce pigmentation. Birth control pills, estrogens, sunlight, photosensitizing medications, and pregnancy can also cause postpeel hyperpigmentation. As noted previously, postinflammatory hyperpigmentation may respond to treatment only if the exacerbating factor is eliminated.

Hypopigmentation

Very darkly pigmented individuals may not experience the phenomena of mottled hyperpigmentation. Uniform hyperpigmentation can occur, but this fades uniformly with time. However, hypopigmentation is of greater concern. If widespread, it may give the individual a pale, ghostly appearance. Patchy hypopigmentation may be the result of cutaneous scarring. It presents difficulty because it is not easily covered by makeup. Loss of pigmentation may thus be permanent and disabling in darker skin pigmented individuals.

Specific Effects of Miscellaneous Peeling Agents

Resorcinism

Resorcinol can cause a chronic poisoning resulting in paralysis, methemoglobinemia, and myxedema (10) along with damage to the capillaries, kidneys, heart, and nervous system. Resorcinol, like phenol, is a hydrocarbon with germicidal properties. Resorcinol is only one-third as potent as phenol and requires widespread application to approach the degree of toxicity of phenol. If applied extensively, resorcinol can produce systemic toxicity and symptoms similar to phenol poisoning.

Excess absorption can occur when several large areas are peeled such as the face and back or if the paste remains in contact with the skin for a long time. The author knows of no incidence of resorcinol toxicity, but the potential is present.

Salicylic Acid

Salicylism consists of a group of toxic effects due to excessive dosage with salicylic acid or its salts, usually marked by tinnitus, nausea, and vomiting. Salicylic acid is used in Jessner's or Comb's formula, is utilized as one of several ingredients in several types of peeling pastes and lotions [4]. The combination of oral ingestion of aspirin and widespread application of a paste containing salicylic acid may in theory produce symptoms.

Conclusions

Essentially two cutaneous complications cause the majority of disabling, untoward effects of chemical peeling. They are pigmentary alterations and scarring. Proper patients skin tone selection with the correct peeling concentration and procedure can avoid most of these difficulties. Many of the other additional peeling complications can usually be easily treated with minimal patient disability.

References

1. Stegman SJ (1980) A study of dermabrasion and chemical peels in an animal model. J Dermatol Surg Oncol 6:490–497
2. Hung VC, Lee JY, Zitelli JA, Hebda PA (1989) Topical tretinoin and epithelial wound healing. Arch Dermatol 125(1):65–69
3. Kligman AM, Baker TJ, Gordon HL (1987) Long-term histologic followup of phenol face peels. Plast Reconstr Surg 75:652–659
4. Collins PS (1987) The chemical peel. Clin Dermatol 5:57–74
5. Truppman ES, Ellenby JD (1978) Major electrocardiographic changes during chemical face peeling. Plast Reconstr Surg 63:44–48
6. Gross BG (1983) Cardiac arrhythmias during phenol face peeling. Plast Reconstr Surg 73:590–594
7. Wexler MR, Halon DA, Teitelbaum A et al. (1984) The prevention of cardiac arrhythmias produced in an animal model by the topical application of a phenol preparation in common use for face peeling. Plast Reconstr Surg 73:595–598
8. Stagnone, GJ Orgel MG, Stagnone JJ (1987) Cardiovascular effects of topical 50% trichloroacetic acid and Baker's phenol solution. J Dermatol Surg Oncol 13:999–1002
9. Collins PS (1989) Trichloroacetic acid peels revisited. J Dermatol Surg Oncol 15:933–940
10. Thomas AE, Gisburn MA (1961) Exogenous onchronosis and myxedema from resorinol. Br J Dermatol 73:378–381

Nail Surgery

Eckart Haneke and Robert L. Baran

Introduction

Nail operations are usually not difficult, but they are delicate. The nail organ may easily be damaged if the surgeon is not familiar with the anatomy, physiology, and pathology of the nail apparatus. Many dermatologists are reluctant to perform nail surgery except for nail avulsions, which are carried out far too often without an indication and as a substitute for correct diagnosis. On the other hand, nail surgery is often a sad example of surgeons performing an operation without having the faintest idea of the organ that they are operating on or the diagnosis for which this intervention is intended. Very often they do not even try to obtain minimal knowledge about the nail. Textbooks on "minor surgery" frequently provide schematic illustrations that demonstrate the author's lack of knowledge.

Like any other surgical operations, those on nails must be carefully planned in advance. It must first be clear why an operation is intended; there must be a working diagnosis or suspicion. Even operations for diagnostic purposes demand at least some idea of the altered structures to allow a biopsy of the correct portion of the nail. The aim of the operation must be reasonable; for example, it is absolutely impossible to make an unsightly, brittle, fragile or soft nail more beautiful by avulsion.

The most common complications of nail surgery are pain, bleeding, oedema, haematoma, necrosis, infection, recurrence, nail dystrophy, and unsightly scarring as well as failure to achieve the intended result and a variety of unpredictable complications.

Nail surgery is usually aimed at curing a disease that cannot be treated successfully by conservative means, at making or confirming a diagnosis, at alleviating pain, at eradicating tumours, at preventing irreversible damage, and at correcting traumatic abnormalities and nail deformities.

Prerequisites for nail surgery are in-depth knowledge of the nail's structure, its functional and surgical anatomy, its growth behaviour, and its response to acute (surgical operation) and chronic injury (delayed healing), as well as aseptic surgical conditions, surgical skills and a head magnifier lens.

Surgery on the Nail

Surgical Anatomy of the Nail

Four different structures are found in and around the nail:
a) The nail organ in the strict sense: matrix, nail bed, nail plate, hyponychium, lateral and proximal nail grooves and folds, the latter with the cuticle and eponychium;
b) ridged skin of the digital pulp with a rich innervation;
c) "common" skin on the dorsal aspect of the terminal phalanx; and
d) the bone of the terminal phalanx, which is mainly responsible for the gross shape of the nail.

A normal nail is formed only when all these structures cooperate normally; thus, damage to any of them may alter the nail.

The matrix is the sole structure to produce the nail plate. A longitudinal defect inevitably produces a defect in the nail plate because the epithelium covering the scar cannot form a normal nail. Incisions as well as biopsies must be performed transversely and without injuring the lunula-nail bed border. The nail bed has an unique pattern of rete ridges arranged in a parallel longitudinal fashion. Biopsies and incisions must be carried out longitudinally. Biopsies from the proximal nail fold must avoid either defects of its free margin or asymmetrical defects. Wounds through the proximal nail fold, nail plate and matrix usually result in a cicatricial pterygium as well as deep cuts in the pulp and hyponychium may result in a pterygium inversum.

Between nail plate and hyponychium there is a thin layer of dense connective tissue containing many nerves, vessels and glomus bodies. Vertically oriented collagen fibres connect the nail bed with the bone. Any volume augmentation such as oedema or haemtoma therefore causes considerable pain.

The nail organ is supplied mainly by the volar branches of the digital arteries, which are connected to the dorsal branches by collateral arteries and form arterial arches in the matrix and nail bed. This rich blood supply allows operations such as nail flaps [12] and the complete dissection of entire nail apparatus from the bone to correct congenital malalignment [1] without risk of necrosis.

Patient History and General Condition

Patients with nail alterations must be examined for general diseases as causes of their nail problems.

Alterations in the nail's shape and size usually reflect the shape of the underlying bone. A radiograph, preferably xeroradiography with magnification, should be taken; this allows evaluation of the both the bone and the soft tissue since this technique also shows the shade of the nail and of hypertrophic nail walls.

The condition of peripheral blood circulation is of utmost importance. Peripheral arterial insufficiency due to endangiitis obliterans, atherosclerosis, diabetic angiopathy, heavy smoking, Raynaud's disease and scleroderma may make any nail operation a disaster. Diabetes mellitus renders the patient more susceptible to infection, hence perioperative antibiotic prophylaxis may be considered. Elderly and incapacitated patients in poor general health have delayed wound healing. Peripheral neurological disease is commonly associated with poor vascular adaptation to surgical injury. Venous stasis and lymphoedema also cause problems in nail operations. Clotting disorders and drugs interfering with blood clotting increase the risk of postoperative bleeding and delayed healing; however, heparin may be given to prevent thrombosis. Care must be taken with drugs that may increase smooth muscle contraction.

Preoperative Measures

The nail operation begins with a thorough explanation of the surgical procedure and the intended outcome. On the evening and morning before operation, a careful cleansing of the fingers or toes is necessary: a 5-min surgical srub using povidone iodine or another disinfective soap is recommended. There is usually a heavy bacterial colonization of the nail bed in onychomycoses and onycholyses. Antibiotic prophylaxis is useful when one biopsies or operates on such a nail. It is strongly recommended to prohibit smoking starting from the day before surgery.

Surgical Instruments

Surgical skills, careful tissue handling, avoidance of crushing, kinking and tearing, limiting anaemia to a minimum of time are more important for preventing complications than are particular instruments specifically designed for nail surgery. A head magnifier loupe or microscope greatly aids in fine operations.

Anaesthesia

For most if not all nail operations a digital block is optimal. About 2-3 ml of plain 2% prilocaine, xylocaine, or mepivacaine are needed. A volume of 0.2–0.3 ml is injected around the dorsal digital nerve and 1 ml to the volar digital nerve by inserting the needle into the dorsolateral aspect of the digit's base just distal to the metacarpo-/metatarso-phalangeal joint. Any volume greater than 5 ml may interfere with the blood circulation, as may the addition of vasoconstrictors such as adrenaline (epinephrine), noradrenaline (norepinephrine), or ornipressin. A distal peripheral ring block has no advantage and is contraindicated in infections of the terminal phalanx. A metacarpal block may decrease the risk of compression from too great a volume, but it is more difficult to perform and takes longer until complete anaesthesia.

Surgical Operation

Lack of successful surgical results is commonly due to insufficient or wrong planning or to technical faults. Very often a wrong indication is due to wrong or absent diagnosis. Not infrequently there is no idea what the operation is intended for, and what can at best be achieved. Faults in the surgical procedure may have started with insufficient patient information. Full aseptic conditions are essential for all demanding nail operations. Anaesthesia must be complete and must not interfere with important structures or increase the risk of infection. Regional anaemia must be sufficient but should not last longer than 15 min; if 15 min is insufficient, anaemia must be released for some minutes every quarter of an hour. Hydropneumatic tourniquets are much less traumatizing than rubber strings or metal bands. For fingers, a sterile disposable rubber glove may be used. It is put on, a small hole is cut in the end of the corresponding finger, and it is then pulled back a little and finally rolled to the base of the finger. To release this particular tourniquet, it is simply rolled forward to the finger tip. The operation must be carried out atraumatically and with fine instruments. Periungual stitches may be put through the nail bed but usually not through the matrix. Crushing of nail structures must be avoided. At the end of the operation, blood remnants are removed with hydrogen peroxide, and disinfection should be repeated. A thickly padded dressing not constricting the digit is applied to absorb both blood from the wound and pain from any inadvertent shock. It is changed after 24 h in case of apparent bleeding or after 48 h. The outer layers of the dressing are removed first until clotted blood renders the procedure painful. The digit, hand or food is then immersed into a luke-warm bath with a disinfective soap solution until the rest of the dressing floats off. The wound is cleaned of clotted blood with hydrogen peroxide compresses. A non-adherent dressing with an antibiotic ointment is applied and may be left for 5–7 days depending on the wound condition.

Immediate postoperative pain may be intense and can be reduced by consistently raising the extremity above the head. Nonsteroidal antiinflammatory drugs may be started the day before operation; this reduces not only pain but also postoperative swelling, which is the major cause of pain after nail surgery. Again, the importance of stopping smoking cannot be overemphasized to reduce the risk of postoperative gangrene.

Particular Complications of Nail Surgery

Nail Avulsion

The surgical procedure that is performed most often is nail avulsion. It is not a treatment per se but may enable consecutive therapy to be effective. Distal nail avulsion is usually carried out; this leaves a more or less injured nail bed. In onychomycosis, the nail bed and matrix must be carefully curetted to remove keratoses rich in infectious fungi and bacteria. After a few days of treating the denuded nail bed and matrix as a vulnerable wound, oozing stops and reepithelialization begins. At this moment the specific treatment must be instituted, for example, antifungal or antibacterial therapy. Repeated nail avulsions often result in permanent nail dystrophy such as poor nail plate growth, onycholysis, scarring of the nail bed, cicatricial pterygium, nail deviation or overcurvature.

Nail avulsion of the great toe often results in the formation of a distal nail wall interfering with the nail plate's growth over the hyponychium. In the early stage, this may be reversed by consistent downward-plantarward massage of the distal nail fold. Recalcitrant cases must be corrected by a crescentic wedge excision, as proposed by Howard in 1899 [4, 6, 10].

Nail Biopsies

Other complications may result from nail biopsies. A medial longitudinal nail biopsy usually results in a split nail. A lateral longitudinal nail biopsy gives as good a specimen as medial biopsy; however, it leaves a nail that is only about 2 mm narrower but without split. Using back stitches to elevate the lateral aspect of the terminal phalanx restores the normal contour of the lateral nail fold [5, 6]. Biopsies of the proximal nail fold may be performed as crescentic excisions, median V-shaped excision or as a punch; the latter must leave the proximal nail fold's free margin and cuticle intact to avoid a consecutive defect [8, 9].

Matrix biopsies must not be performed with longitudinal incisions. A punch with a diameter of 3 mm leaves a barely visible reddish band in the nail, but any larger punch leads to a noticeable band-like nail dystrophy. Punch biopsies must respect the lunula border.

Nail bed biospies must be carried out with a small punch or as a longitudinal spindle-shaped excision. When the nail plate has not previously been avulsed, immersing the digit into water for 10–15 min softens the nail so that the punch or pointed scalpel may cut through it. Biopsies of the nail bed reaching the hyponychium may leave a small area of onycholysis or even a cicatricial pterygium inversum.

Any secondary infection of a biopsy may cause neurovascular dystrophy of the digit with consecutive decalcification on the bone. Early treatment with calcium blockers, calcitonin injections and blockades of the stellate ganglion may then be necessary.

Recurrence

Another problem in nail surgery is recurrence. This is most common in the treatment of ingrown toenails by the wedge excision technique. This method has some decisive disadvantages.
a) None of the schematic illustrations of this technique shows exactly how much of the nail organ's proximal portion must be removed to excise the matrix horn entirely. Recurrences are thus invited.

b) Furthermore, it includes excision of the lateral nail fold and groove from their beginning to the hyponychium. These are very important structures that cannot be substituted by scar tissue. The wedge excision for the treatment of ingrown nails must therefore be considered obsolete [4, 6].

Transverse Overcurvature

Transverse overcurvature leading to pincer nail (tubed nail, ungius contringens) is a common ailment. Two varieties can be distinguished. The symmetrical form probably genetically determined; it is usually associated with lateral deviation of the hallux nail's long axis and with symmetrical involvement of other toes, the axes of which are deviated medially. Radiography virtually always shows a very broad base of the bone of the terminal phalanx and lateral osteophytes at the base of the hallux which are larger tibially than fibularly. The non-symmetrical form is associated with acquired foot deformation; this is not genetically determined.

Repeated nail avulsions have been recommended for the treatment of pincer nails [13]. However, this does not alter the aetiology and usually worsens the condition, as sample experience with more then 50 patients has shown.

Split Nails

The surgical correction of split nails is often shown with sophisticated schematic illustrations demonstrating how to excise the scar in the matrix and nail bed which is the origin of the split in the nail. However, even the finest sutures, removal of 1 mm more of each side of the nail plate to allow additional nail plate sutures to further coapt matrix and nail bed, rarely succeed in avoiding a new split.

Dorsal Finger Cysts

Dorsal finger cysts are, in reality, myxoid pseudocysts secondarily connected with the distal interphalangeal joint [9]; they are not herniations of the synovia. Surgical treatment must therefore dissect all tissue with myxoid degeneration; otherwise recurrences will occur, as is commonly observed after simple excision, needling and expression, electrosurgery, etc. The intraarticular injection of 0.1 ml sterile methylene blue solution into the distal interphalangeal joint via the distal volar joint crease shows the true extent of this pseudocystic lesion. An operation microscope allows one to trace and dissect all extensions of this process to safely cure the disease [7].

Warts

The recurrence of warts, whether in subungual or periungual location, is as frequent as in other sites. Treatment if these benign infectious tumors should be careful to avoid both loss of nail structures and scarring.

Glomus Tumors

Recurrences may occur after extirpation of glomus tumors. This may be due to too careful an excision or to primary multiple glomus tumors.

Longitudinal Melanonychia

Longitudinal melanonychia in Caucasians tends to be rather malignant than benign [2, 3, 11]. The total removal of the lesion giving rise to the pigmented streak in the nail should therefore be aimed at. Since the histopathological evaluation of incipient subungual melanoma may be extremely difficult even when serial and step sections are performed, a reexcision is necessary in case of recurrence.

Other Complications

Specific risks may be associated with cryosurgery, electrosurgery and laser treatment.

Cryosurgery in the nail region is usually associated with considerable postoperative oedema and throbbing pain. Care must be taken not to damage the matrix when treating lesions of the proximal nail fold.

Electrosurgery may readily injure the matrix with consecutive scarring and nail dystrophy. Defects in the proximal nail fold have also been observed.

Laser surgery is most elegant, particularly the carbon dioxide laser for the treatment of periungual and subungual warts. Excessive carbonization must be avoided to prevent scarring. The neodymium-YAG laser produces deep necroses which develop during the first 3–5 postoperative days; the extent of the necroses can hardly be foreseen. This laser is therefore not generally recommended for dermatological use.

References

1. Baran R, Dawber RPR (1990) Guide médico-chirurgical des onychopathies. Arnette, Paris, pp 131–132
2. Baran R, Haneke E (1985) Diagnostik und Therapie der streifenförmigen Nagelpigmentierungen. Hautarzt 36:359–365
3. Baran R, Kechijian P (1989) Longitudinal melanonychia (melanonychia striata): diagnosis and management. J Am Acad Dermatol 21:1165–1175

4. Haneke E (1979) Chirurgische Behandlung des Unguis incarnatus. In: Salfeld K (ed) Operative Dermatologie. Springer, Berlin Heidelberg New York, pp 185–188
5. Haneke E (1985) Behandlung einiger Nagelfehlbildungen. In: Wolff HH, Schmeller W (eds): Fehlbildungen, Nävi, Melanome,. Springer, Berlin Heidelberg New York, pp 71–77 (Fortschritte der operativen Dermatologie 2)
6. Haneke E (1986) Surgical treatment of ingrowing toenails. Cutis 37:251–256
7. Haneke E (1988) Operative Therapie der myxoiden Pseudozyste. In: Haneke E (ed): Gegenwärtiger Stand der operativen Dermatologie. Springer, Berlin Heidelberg New York, pp 221–227 (Fortschritte der operativen Dermatologie 4)
8. Haneke E (1991) Operationen am Nagelorgan – Planung, Durchführung, Fehlermöglichkeiten und ihre Vermeidung. Z Hautkr 66 (Suppl 3):132–133
9. Haneke E, Baran R (1990) Nails: surgical aspects. In Parish LC, Lask GP (eds) Aesthetic dermatology. McGraw-Hill, New York, pp 236–247
10. Howard WR (1899) Ingrown toenail; surgical treatment. NY Med J 579
11. Kopf AW, Waldo E (1979) Melanonychia striata. Australas J Dermatol 21:59–70
12. Schernberg F, Amiel M (1987) Lokale Verschiebelappen des Nagels. Handchirurgie 19:259–262
13. Zaias N (1980) The nail in health and disease. MTP, Lancaster

Collagen Implantation

MELVIN L. ELSON

Soft tissue augmentation with injectable collagen materials has now been available for more than a decade. Their safety record is exemplary, and very little difficulty has been reported with these materials, now available in 30 countries around the world. Side effects, of course, do exist as do side effects with all materials for soft tissue augmentation and indeed all cosmetic procedures.

One of the most common side effects of collagen injection is the unrealistic expectation on the part of the patient [1]. It is imperative on the part of the physician to explain to the patient that this procedure, just as any other cosmetic procedure, has its specific uses and limitations. It is not meant to take the place of rhytidectomy nor other cosmetic procedures but to soften the features, augment such areas as the lips, and specifically to treat expression lines.

Once the patient understands the purpose of injectable collagen, other possible side effects must be explained to the patient. Some of these are mere nuisances and are short lived, although some may be significant.

Discomfort during the injection is minimized by the addition of 0.3% lidocaine (with the exception of the material in France, where mixtures of substances are not allowed). Icing the area to be injected prior to injection and keeping the material cold until immediately before injection also alleviates some of the discomfort. Some physicians have found Hurricaine jelly, eutectic mixtures of local anesthetics such as EMLA, and nerve blocks to benefit the patient, especially in painful areas of injection such as the lips [2].

Needle marks may occur, but these are short lived. To avoid these one must be as gentle with the skin as possible when injecting. In addition, a new form of collagen injectable material (Zyderm FL) allows the use of a 32-gauge needle, and marks are much less frequent with this size needle. Bruising may also occur, lasts 3–5 days, and disappears; this can be avoided by slow injection into the skin as well as not allowing the patient to take aspirin at least 48 h prior to a session.

Beading after the injection is a frequent complaint on the part of patients and can be virtually eliminated by obtaining a certain degree of skill in the use of the material, so that the injector allows the material to flow smoothly into the superficial skin rather than placing small beads into the area to be augmented [3].

Transient erythema after the injection session occurs in fewer than 10% of patients, disappears within hours, and is of no consequence. Some patients (fewer than 1%) do experience episodes of erythema and occasionally edema upon exposure to vasodilatory substances such as alcohol, exercise, sun exposure, flare-ups of hay fever and sinusitis, emotional upset, and menses [4]. The episodes are self-limited, and it should be noted that these patients do not have anti-Zyderm antibodies, are not experiencing adverse reactions, and may continue to undergo collagen replacement therapy without untoward sequelae. The mechanism of this phenomenon has not been delineated at this time.

A single episode of partial blindness in one eye has been reported [5], occurring during injection of the glabellar area, probably due to retrograde embolization. This is not a side effect of collagen injection itself but of the injection of this particular area, having been reported with the injection of other substances under pressure in this area on very rare occasions.

Infection is an extremely rare occurrence and is not an inherent side effect of the injection of this sterile material; however, infection may occur at the same rate as with any other transcutaneous injection. It should be noted that these materials are all sterile upon arrival from Collagen Biomedical, but once opened they are no longer so. The practice of recapping syringes by the physician for the patient for use at a later injection session should be avoided.

All patients considering soft tissue augmentation with injectable collagen materials must undergo skin testing prior to augmentation. Although the package insert enclosed with the material states that the patient must have a single test administered in the volar forearm and observed for 4 weeks prior to undergoing augmentation, almost all surgeons using this material perform double skin testing prior to injection. This significantly reduces both the rate and severity of the most common of the significant problems with injectable collagen, i. e., adverse reaction.

Adverse reactions are defined as sensitization reactions of an immunologic nature that occur at the treatment site after the patient has demonstrated clinically negative skin test results [6]. The incidence of these reactions is reported to be 1%–6%, probably occurring in less than 3% of patients undergoing augmentation [7]. The vast majority (89.6%) occur with the first treatment [8]. This also supports the concept of double skin testing, which essentially makes the first exposure after the first skin test, a second skin test in the arm, rather than a treatment in the face. Adverse reactions may begin to occur within hours but may be delayed by several weeks. They may last from a few weeks to many months (the average is probably around 6 months).

Adverse reactions are characterized by erythema, induration, pruritus or pain that may be intermittent or constant [9] (Fig. 1). Generally speaking, when the symptoms are intermittent, the precipitating events are the same as those causing intermittent erythema discussed above, i. e., vascular phenomena – such as alcohol, menses, and emotional upset. Sometimes the discomfort associated with these reactions is significant, and relief may be obtained by the application of ice and 10 grains acetylsalicylic acid by mouth every 6 h. Antihistamines are totally ineffective in relieving any of the symptoms. Topical steroids are of very little benefit, and although systemic steroids help significantly, the dose and length of time that treatment is required for the adverse event prevents the use of this modality. Some authors have advocated the use of intralesional steroids,

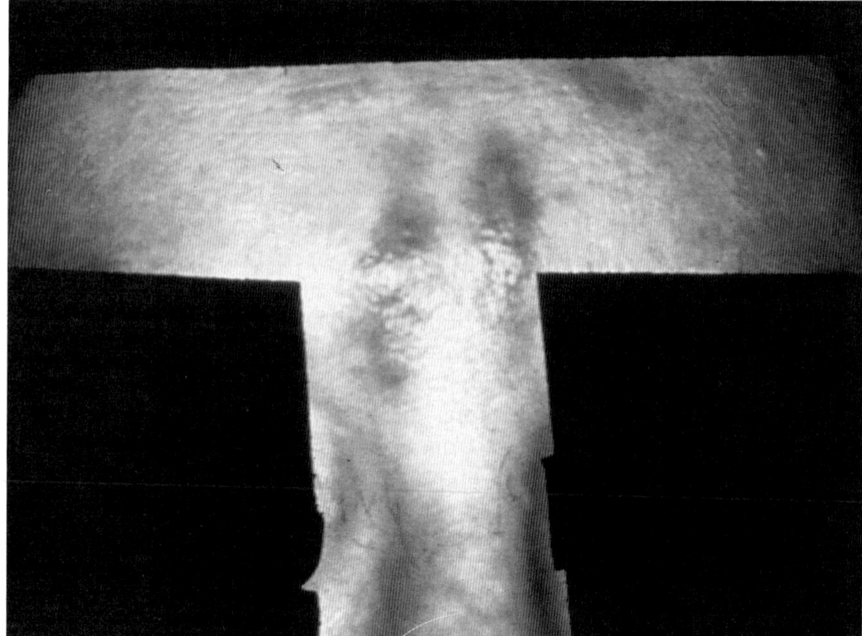

Fig. 1. Typical adverse reaction

but I have found this to be of little benefit; the results are short lived, and repeated injections may lead to atrophy.

In the past year or so some patients with adverse reactions have been undergoing treatment with propranolol 10–40 mg by mouth daily, taking into consideration that a great deal of the problem with the reaction is not simply immunologic but involves local vascular phenomena as well. The few patients who have been treated in this manner so far appear to have benefited; however, the series is not yet large enough to draw any conclusions.

These adverse events are usually associated with elevated titers against bovine collagen by ELISA [10] and anti-bovine antibodies can also be found by radioimmunoassay [11]. These antibodies are species specific and do not cross-react with human antibodies [12]. Titers do not necessarily correlate with the severity of the reaction or with their duration but may be used as a tool to contribute to the overall determination as to whether soft tissue augmentation with these materials should proceed [13]. The best method of performing double skin tests has yet to be determined. I perform a skin test in the right arm, read at 48–72 h, read and perform a skin test in the left arm after 2 weeks, and read both skin tests after another 2 weeks. If results of both are negative, soft tissue augmentation is carried out. Some physicians perform the skin test, wait 4 weeks, test again, and wait 48 h before proceeding to augmentation. The point is to give the immune system a second look at the material before proceeding with injection in the face in an attempt to reduce the incidence of this side effect.

Obviously, as there is no particularly effective treatment for adverse reactions, the physician should do his utmost to try to prevent such an event. Double skin testing does not eliminate every adverse reaction, but it eliminates most of the serious ones and certainly decreases the incidence somewhat. No one should undergo soft tissue augmentation with injectable collagen materials before undergoing two skin tests.

In the original study regarding the use of double skin testing, 200 patients underwent single testing while 200 were double tested. The groups were comparable as to sex, age range, and diagnoses. Group 1 underwent skin testing according to the protocol in the package insert: receiving 0.1 cm^3 Zyderm injected into the volar forearm and observed at 48–72 h and over a 4-week period. Five (2.5%) showed positive skin test results and did not undergo augmentation. Of the 195 who did, 6 developed allergic reactions. Of the 200 patients undergoing double testing in the manner outlined above, the first test in the right volar forearm was positive in 5 (2.5%). Of the 195 who received a second test in the other arm, 7 (3%) developed a positive reaction while the first remained negative. The 171 patients who had two negative skin test results and decided to undergo augmentation were then treated with injectable collagen material. None had an adverse reaction [10].

In addition, systemic complaints have been reported to the manufacturer by fewer than 0.1% of patients. These have consisted of nausea, rash, arthralgia, myalgia, and headache. Although these complaints are reported to the manufacturer following collagen injection, there is no documentation of the relationship of these systemic complaints and the injection of collagen material. A single anaphylactoid response has been reported that did include an episode of hypotension and difficulty in breathing [9].

As more and more patients are injected, side effects that are not very common and depend upon sheer numbers for their emergence will come to the fore. Two of these are abscess formation and local necrosis. The rate of local necrosis based upon adverse reports to Collagen Biomedical from physicians and using the amount of material sold as the basis of possible reactions, is currently placed at 9/10 000, or 0.09% [14]. Although this incidence is quite low, there appeared to be an increase in the rate of this side effect with the introduction of glutaraldehyde cross-linked collagen implant material (Zyplast) in late 1985. Local necrosis following the injection of Zyderm/Zyplast results from an interruption of the vascular supply of the area injected and is not dependent upon the material itself. The material may compress or injure the blood vessels in the area of injection to compromise oxygen flow, leading to the slough. The first manifestation is a blanching of the area, followed by a duskiness, which gives way to bruising with necrosis developing over the next day or so. This may take up to 2 weeks to heal and may eventuate in scarring.

According to Collagen Corporation 56% of all reported instances of this side effect have occurred in the glabella (Fig. 2). It is theorized that this occurs due to the lack of collateral vessels in this area, which is midline and tends to be supplied by fewer and smaller vessels. Hanke et al. [14] reported that when the skin of the forehead is reflected in the cadaver, the bilateral supratrochlear and

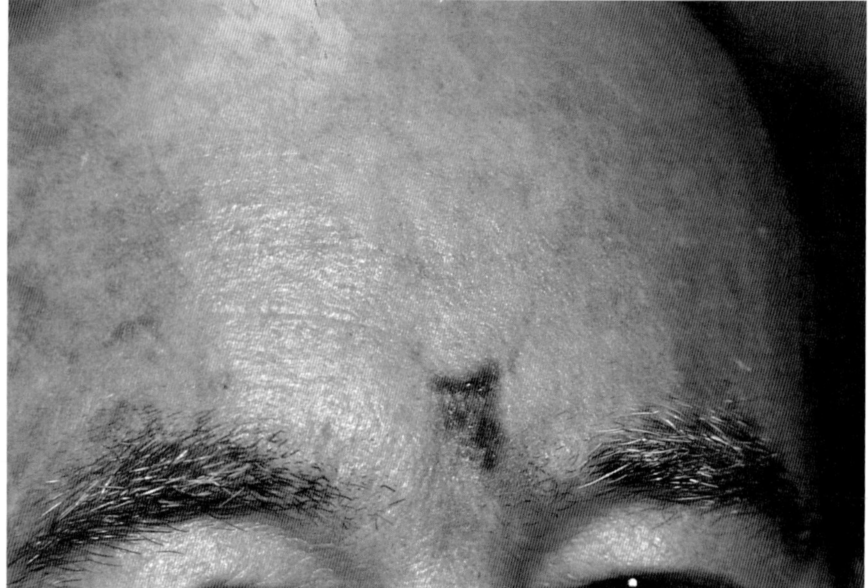

Fig. 2. Slough in the glabellar area with Zyplast

supraorbital arteries, which are branches of the ophthalmic, lie in the superficial fascia and ascend the forehead in company of the supratrochlear and supraorbital branches of the ophthalmic nerve. In addition, they stated that the bilateral symmetry of the superficial neurovascular bundles is carried over into the deeper hypodermis of the glabella. Sections taken from the glabella reveal large-caliber vessels on either side of a median fat pad. The absence of large vessels in the midline dermis and hypodermis suggests that the perfusion of midline tissues is dependent on small branches of these larger lateral vessels.

The vessels are in close proximity to the glabellar crease, and for this reason interruption of the large or small vessels of the region is certainly a possibility during soft tissue augmentation. Zyplast is injected deeper into the dermis and undergoes less syneresis than Zyderm [15]; therefore vascular compromise and the resultant slough are more likely to occur with the cross-linked material.

It is important to remember that vascular compromise with the resultant slough may still occur with Zyderm I or II and may occur in areas other than the glabella (Fig. 3). It is the higher incidence of problems associated with Zyplast in this area that has led to the recommendation that Zyplast not be used in the glabellar area (Collagen Biomedical, communication to physicians).

Once it is apparent that there is pressure on a vessel in the area of injection, be it glabella or otherwise, it is prudent immediately to discontinue the injection and to massage the area. Some physicians also advocate the use of ice, some heat, and some nitroglycerin paste. All the data regarding the use of these modalities are anecdotal, and further study is necessary for a conclusion to be reached. Suffice it to say at the moment, that if blanching and bluish discolora-

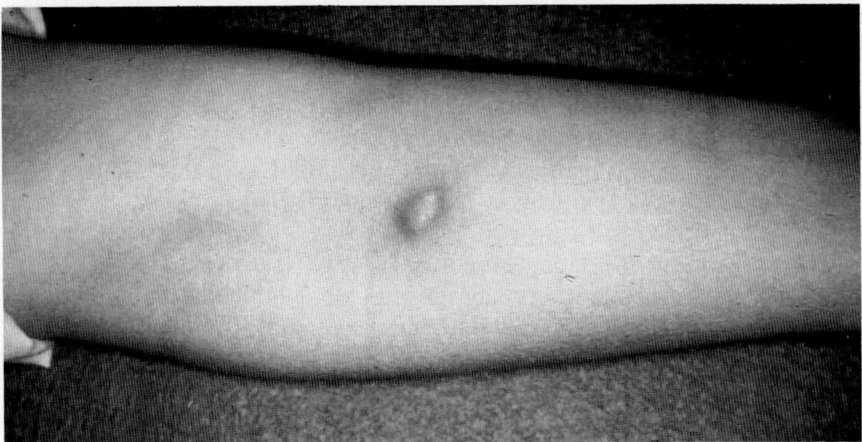

Fig. 3. Slough in a skin test with Zyderm I (skin test material)

tion occur in an area that is being injected, the session should be discontinued. If the patient continues on to frank necrosis, good wound management is in order until the wound is healed. Any scarring that may result can be treated with light dermabrasion, scar revision, or filling materials including collagen implants.

Abscess formation is the most serious complication of injectable collagen. The incidence of this severe reaction to collagen injectable materials is currently reported at 4/10 000, or 0.04%, and apparently has remained at a steady level of reporting since 1981 with the introduction of the first of the injectable collagens (Zyderm I) [14]. This reaction can occur upon the first exposure to collagen, but it may also occur upon any subsequent exposure. Onset is delayed, but the delay may be as short as 7 days or as long as 22 months after injection. There is also a great deal of variability reported in the clinical description of the reported event – from a small draining lesion at the site to severe fluctuant lesions surrounded by a great deal of induration and erythema. These reactions differ from routine hypersensitivity reactions to collagen implants in that, although the adverse reaction may be indurated and erythematous, they are not fluctuant.

Hanke et al. reported that in many patients not all injection sites react; however, this is also characteristic of allergic reactions to collagen materials in general. There may be long periods of remission followed by exacerbation without a precipitating event that is detectable. The severity of the reactions tends to decrease over a period of time. Sometimes the abscesses drain spontaneously; culture results are either negative or yield *Staphylococcus epidermidis*. Significant pain may be associated with these lesions. All the available evidence at this point indicates that this reaction is dependent upon hypersensitivity, as 86% in the original study had elevated titers against bovine collagen as determined by ELISA. Others have also reported that these titers tend to be very high.

Treatment consists of drainage of the lesion, which usually affords considerable relief. Intralesional steroids may be used, and if response is evident they may be given at weekly intervals until resulution. One should wait 6 months following resolution before attempting to revise the resultant scar. Scar revision may be performed utilizing any of the modalities available to the dermatologic cosmetic surgeon, with the exception of injectable collagen.

Although there has been a great deal of publicity in the United States regarding injectable collagen materials and the alleged link with the production of autoimmune diseases (particularly dermatomyositis/polymyositis), there is no scientific basis for this in any way.

There have been 107 patients reported by physicians through the Collagen Corporation adverse reporting system as of 15 May 1991 who have had collagen injections and have some type of rheumatoid disease of an autoimmune nature such as rheumatoid arthritis, scleroderma, or dermatomyositis/polymyositis. Although, this is well within the expected numbers of these diseases to be reported in a population of 650 000, there has been much furor due to litigation and publicity by a few individuals. In addition, it has recently been reported that the United States Food and Drug Administration has approved a labeling change "which warns that some cases of connective tissue disorders have been reported in patients who have had collagen injections" (AAD/ASDS, communication to physicians). Despite this, there remains to date no evidence to link collagen injections with this type of disease process or any other.

In fact, bovine collagen has been used in the manufacture of biomedical devices for decades, first in the form of resorbable sutures and agents for hemostasis [16]. The use of injectable collagen was approved by the Food and Drug Administration in 1981, but clinical trials were begun in a multicenter study involving more than 5000 patients in 1976 [17]. The subsequent data regarding adverse sequelae in the more than 650 000 patients who have received these injections are discussed above; although some problems are of cosmetic significance, and some systemic symptoms have been reported, no significant disease process has been described.

The actual term of collagen vascular disease is a misnomer that was originally used in the medical literature to denote the organ systems of major involvement in these disease processes; it incorrectly implies that collagen and the vasculature are involved in the development of rheumatologic diseases. In actuality, these diseases are disorders involving an altered state in the immune system with the production of autoantibodies, the specific antibody varying from state to state, and the incipient factors to this point remain basically unknown. The role of collagen in causing of these disorders has not been delineated. There are at least ten different genetically distinct types of collagen; however, the primary source of biomaterials has been dermal collagen because of its abundance and ready availability.

There is a vast literature relating to the safety of these products as biomaterials. A review by DeLustro et al. in 1990 summarized this well, reminding us that the low incidence of immune response to the materials must not be construed as more than they are [12]. The earliest clinical studies with Zyderm/Zyplast indicated a 3% reactivity rate to the initial skin test, indicating presensitization to bovine collagen most likely through dietary exposure. Following skin testing another 1%–3% developed localized hypersensitivity responses [10, 11, 13]. Antibodies to bovine collagen correlated well with these reactions, and the picture histologically was the typical immune reaction in the skin with a lymphohistiocytic infiltrate. The clinical picture has been described previously. Antibodies in the sera of these patients are specific for bovine collagen and do not cross-react with human collagen. In addition, immunohistology demonstrates host antibody in the infiltrating plasma cells and bound to bovine dermal collagen implant material but not to surrounding host dermis.

An additional study utilizing another form of injectable bovine collagen (Atelocollagen, Koken, Tokyo) [11] concluded that in the extensive study and follow-up of 705 patients there was some cross-reactivity to bovine collagen type II as well as types I and III, but that the reactivity remained species specific. Indeed, it was suggested that those patients who exhibit elevated levels of antibodies to bovine collagen implant might benefit in the future from human collagen implants.

The review by DeLustro et al. [12] concludes that an immune response to xenogeneic collagen has been demonstrated in both the animal and human, and that the data clearly demonstrate immunity per se not to be associated with any significant adverse sequelae in vivo.

Lyon et al. in 1989 reported the largest series of patients with dermatomyositis/polymyositis (DM/PM), attempting to determine causation and incidence of the disease [18]. The overall incidence is between 5.0–9.6/million per year. In regards to etiology, no correlation was found with infection or any allergic phenomena. Emotional stress was considered to be a significant factor preceding the onset of the disease, as was antecedent heavy muscular exertion. This study indicates that the incidence of DM/PM in patients who have received augmentation with injectable collagen materials is well within the expected range, and that the lack of antecedent events that could possibly be related to these injections is also obvious.

A statement issued by The American College of Rheumatology on 1 April 1991 stated that as of 30 August 1990, 100 cases of autoimmune disease had been alleged in the United States and Canada in the 500 000 patients receiving these injections. Of these, 11 cases were alleged to be of PM/DM. The latest epidemiologic studies have indicated that between 12 and 23 cases of PM/DM would be expected by chance alone among these 500 000 patients. According to The American College of Rheumatology "the alleged cases of PM/DM are less than would be expected for the population."

This news release also points out that studies using both antibodies and histology have failed to show a cross-reactivity between bovine collagen and human collagen. It concludes that all the evidence at the moment indicates collagen injections to be safe.

A panel of experts made up of dermatologists, rheumatologists, immunologists and observers from the Food and Drug Administration regarding the issue of collagen injection and the alleged link to autoimmune diseases (7 October 1989) concluded that "there are no current data to suggest that immunity to xenogeneic dermal collagen can precipitate autoimmune disease" and that "there are considerable data that are inconsistent with the hypothesis of a relationship between injectable collagen and autoimmune disease" [19].

In summary, there is no evidence from clinical data, ongoing research, epidemiology or any other source to suggest any relationship between the injection of bovine collagen and the development of autoimmune diseases, specifically DM/PM.

References

1. Elson ML (1991) Communication is imperative regarding side effects of soft-tissue augmentation. Cosmet Dermatol 4(3):8–12
2. Elson ML (1990) Techniques for lip augmentation discussed. Cosmet Dermatol 3(11):16–19
3. Klein AW, Rish DC (1984) Injectable collagen update. J Dermatol Surg Oncol 10:519–522
4. Stegman SJ, Chu S, Armstrong R (1988) Adverse reactions to bovine collagen implant: clinical and histologic features. J Dermatol Surg Oncol 14 Suppl:39–49
5. Cucin RL, Barek D (1983) Complications of injectable collagen implants. Plast Reconstr Surg 71:731
6. Swanson NA, Stoner JR, Siegle RJ et al. (1983) Treatment site reactions to Zyderm collagen implantation. J Dermatol Surg Oncol 9:377–380
7. Elson ML (1988) Clinical assessment of Zyplast implant: a year of experience for soft tissue contour correction. J Am Acad Dermatol 18:707–713
8. Cooperman L, Michaeli D (1984) The immunogenicity of injectable collagen. II. A retrospective review of seventy-two tested and treated patients. J Am Acad Dermatol 10:647
9. Zyderm/Zyplast package insert (1991) Collagen Biomedical, Palo Alto, California
10. Elson ML (1989) The role of skin testing in the use of collagen injectable materials. J Dermatol Surg Oncol 15 3:301–303
11. Charriere G, Bejot M et al. (1989) Reactions to a bovine collagen implant. J Am Acad Dermatol 21:1203–1208
12. De Lustro F, Dasch J, Keefe J, Ellingsworth L (1990) Immune responses to allogeneic and xenogeneic implants of collagen and collagen derivatives. Clin Orthop 260:263–279
13. De Lustro F, Smith ST et al. (1987) Reaction to injectable collagen: results in animal models and clinical use. Plast Reconstr Surg 79:581
14. Hanke CW, Higley HR et al. (1991) Abscess formation and local necrosis after treatment with Zyderm or Zyplast collagen implant. J Am Acad Dermatol 25:319–326
15. McPherson JM, Ledger PW, Sawamura S et al. (1986) The preparation and physicochemical characterization of an injectable form of reconstituted, glutaraldehyde cross-linked, bovine corium collagen. J Biomed Mater Res 20:79–92
16. Pachence JM, Berg RA, Silver FH (1987) Collagen: its place in the medical device industry. Med Device Diagn Ind 9:49
17. Knapp TR, Kaplan EN, Daniels JR (1977) Injectable collagen for soft tissue augmentation. Plast Reconstr Surg 60:398–405
18. Lyon MG, Bloch DA, Hollak B et al. (1989) Predisposing factors in polymyositis-dermatomyosities: results of a nationwide survey. J Rheumatol 16:1218–1224
19. Stegman S, Bauere, Fries J et al. (1989) Summary of panel review of systemic complaints in patients receiving injectable collagen. Collagen Corporation internal memo Collagen Corporation, Palo Alto, CA, USA

Treatment of Telangiectasias

Eugene L. Bodian

Sclerotherapy has proven to be an excellent tool for the treatment of spider veins and telangiectasias of the lower extremities. At present the use of sclerosing solutions is more advantageous than any other method when treating the lower extremity. Tunable dye lasers have advantages when treating telangiectatic lesions on the face. The key to avoiding most complications is the development of a fine technique. Serious problems are few when sclerotherapy is performed correctly.

Storage

One must store hypertonic saline separately from local anesthetics so that there is no chance of mistaken substitutes. Labels should be conspicuous, and sclerosant should be away from all other injectables. If an accident occurs, and hypertonic saline is injected into the intracutaneous tissue, it causes a slough and ulcer. Therefore, it must be diluted to physiologic skin concentrations by injecting ten times the presumed amount present in the tissues using 1% procaine solution or water for injection. The use of 0.9% saline solution adds more salt to the site. After injection of dilutent, massage is helpful to dissipate the bolus of saline.

Infiltration

It is almost unavoidable to leave a small bleb of saline inside the vein when the needle is withdrawn from the skin. Gentle kneading and massage – not rubbing – usually avoids any serious sequela. A small brown spot may result which gradually disappears within a few weeks. Some cramping pain can occur immediately after injection. Patients are told that this can occur, and that it disappears in a few minutes. Kneading and massage of the calf and thigh is very helpful. The cramping pain is probably due to irritation of the muscle by the sclerosant. This cramping is present in almost all patients who receive injections around the ankles, and they should be so warned. Edema of the dorsum of the foot can occur when a large amount of saline or polidocanol is injected around the ankle or dorsum of the foot. This occurs within 24 h and may last for a week or more.

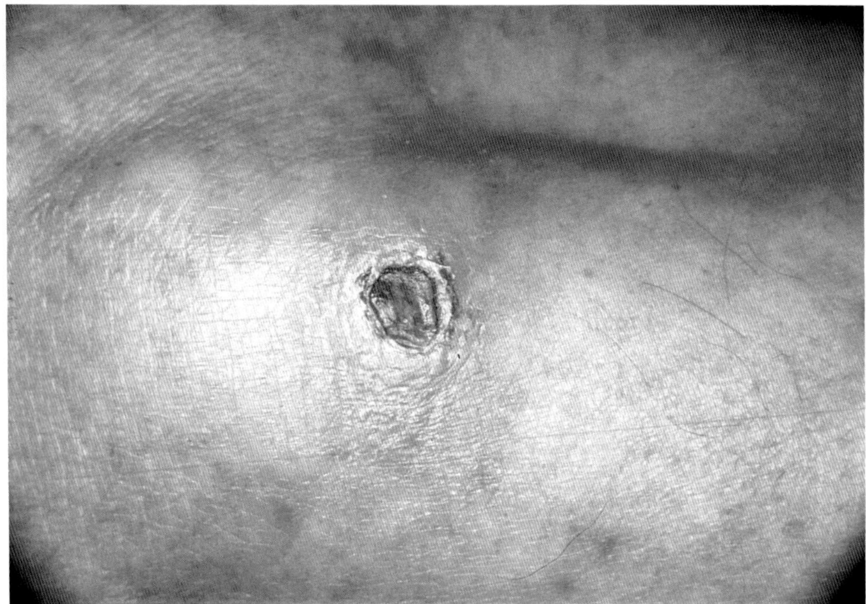

Fig. 1. Ulcer 3 weeks after 0.25% polidocanol

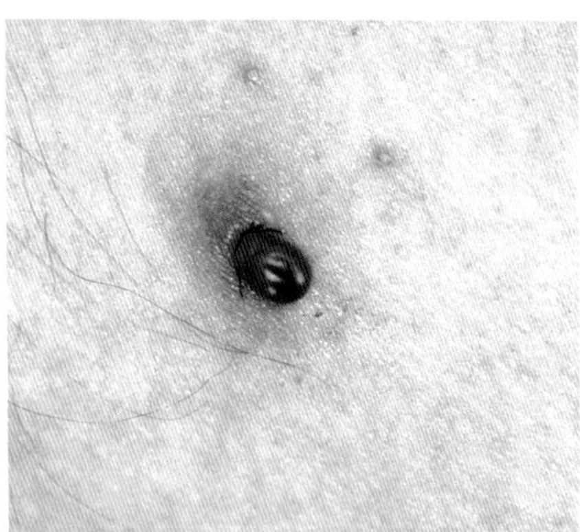

Fig. 2. Ulcer 4 weeks after injection
of hypertonic saline

More serious is the extravasation of a large amount of saline outside the
lumen of the venule. Although most problems of this sort are due to poor technique, some extravasations are due to rupture of a weak venule wall. The first indication of this is a complaint from the patient of acute pain and burning. This
may last 24–48 h. Aspirin and ice packs are helpful in alleviating the discomfort.
The skin may look porcelain white. When this occurs, tissue concentration must
be promptly diluted to normal levels. Ten times the amount of saline must be in-

jected with 1% procaine or water. Prolonged kneading can help to dilute the concentrated bolus if both are done immediately. Some surgeons may attempt to use small amounts of diluted triamcinolone (1 mg/cm^3) to reduce inflammation, but the dilution and kneading seem to work better. The area may appear porcelain white, but if kneading is started early enough along with dilution, an ulcer may be avoided. The kneading and massage may have to be done for 5–10 min before any color is restored. With all of this, ulceration may still not be avoidable. Small amounts of extravasate can cause small ulcers, while large amounts can cause large ulcers with significant scarring.

An undetected extravasation can result in a hemorrhagic bulla. By the time that this occurs, there is probably no way to avoid a slough. Polidocanol can also cause sloughs and ulcerations, but they are not caused by simple extravasation. Ulceration may be due to vessel spasm or ischemia and is not predictable. It may be extensive. Ulceration on the face and ankles is about twice that of the upper legs when using polidocanol. Small amounts and great care should be exercised when using polidocanol on the face. Ulcers can be treated with moist dressings such as Vigilon or Duoderm and topical antibiotics. The use of 20% benzoyl peroxide powder into the wound has helped to speed healing by stimulating granulation tissue formation.

Patients must be informed before treatment that ulcers can occur with sclerotherapy. An actively sympathetic and encouraging attitude can make a painful and disappointing experience somewhat more bearable. Most ulcers heal surprisingly well, leaving a scar similar to a vaccination.

Allergic Reactions

If saline solution is used, there is no risk of allergic reaction. Acute urticaria, generalized urticaria and even anaphylactoid reactions can occur with all other sclerosants except saline. Appropriate treatment must be instituted. Polidocanol should not be used in patients with bronchial asthma for fear of causing allergic broncho spasm. Scleremo is a chrome derivative and may cause reactions in patients (and physicians) with chrome sensitivity. Allergic reactions and anaphylaxis have been reported with the use of sodium morrhuate and sodium tetradecyl sulfate.

Hyperpigmentation

The most common and annoying sequela to sclerotherapy is hyperpigmentation. It may occur in greater than 20% of patients. This pigment is not melanin but hemosiderin. Many biopsies have been carried out and have yielded positive results for iron and not melanin. The pigment is unsightly and may disappear after a few months, but it may last longer than 5 years. Preparations containing hydroquinone are useless since the pigment is not melanin. Attempts to remove the pigment with trichloracetic acid have been only modera-

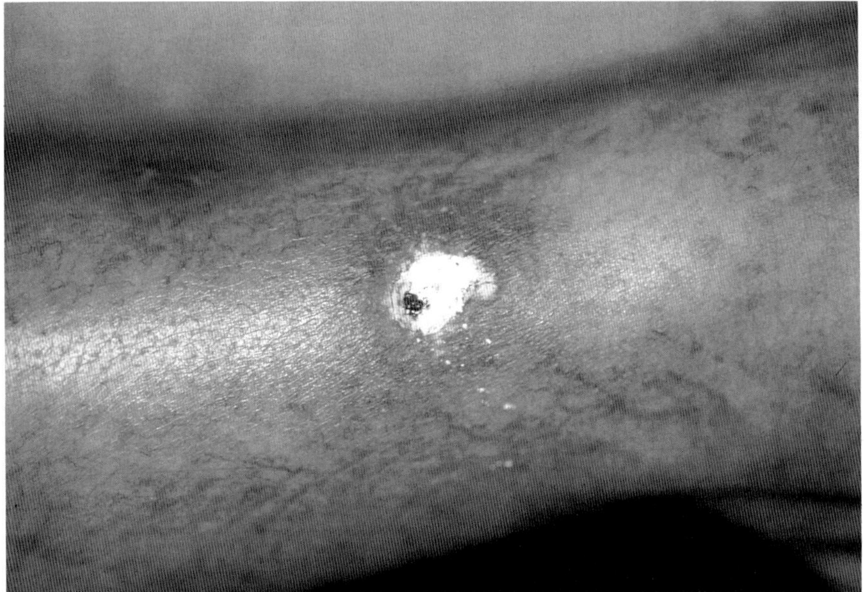

Fig. 3. Ulcer treated with 20% benzoyl peroxide

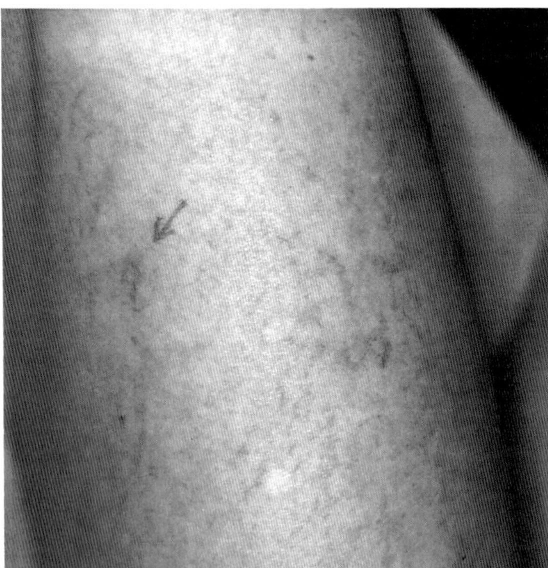

Fig. 4. Vaccinationlike scar of healed ulcer

tely helpfu. Liquid nitrogen has not helped. Baker's phenol solution and plain liquid phenol, when used cautiously and lightly over several months has given some encouraging results. Polidocanol seems to cause more pigment problems than saline.

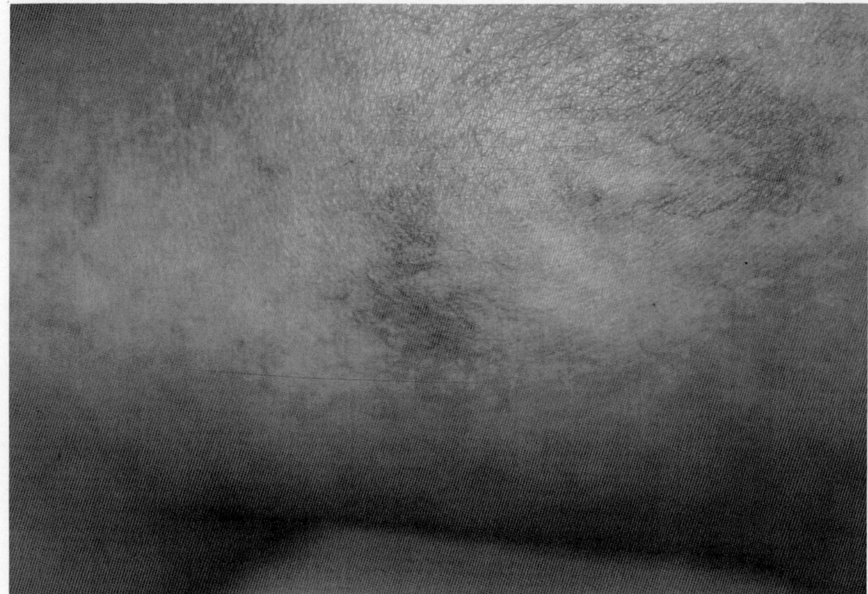

Fig. 5. Telangiectatic mattes 3 weeks after surgery

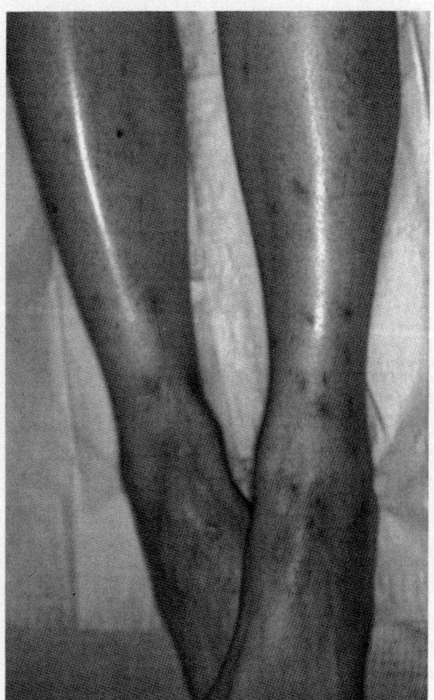

Fig. 6. Pigment 1 year after surgery

Telangiectatic Matting

The occurrence of fine tiny venules peripheral to, adjacent to, and composed of vessels much smaller than the venules treated is called matting. They usually occur 2–3 weeks after successful injection of the venules. The patient returns in 2–3 weeks complaining of redness of "recurrence" of the venous blemishes. Examination reveals a dusky pink area, usually above the knee on the medial aspect of the thigh. Closer inspection shows that this is made up of many tiny blood vessels. Although the true etiology is unknown, various unconvincing theories such as high volume of injection, high pressure of injection, lack of compression hose, and other rather weak hypotheses have been made. In my opinion, compression hose has little influence on spider vein sclerotherapy. Perhaps, when we better understand neoangiogenesis, we will better understand this phenomenon. It occurs in about 25% of patients, but approximately 10% must be treated. The others disappear spontaneously. The remaining mattes can be treated with care, patience, and a number 33 needle.

Other Complications

Other side effects that accompany normal office procedures can occur. These include rare and transient cardiac arrhythmias, syncope, vasovagal reflex, and hypoglycemia. Patients should be advised to have a substantial breakfast or other meal before treatment. This prevents most of the above.

Scintillating scotoma has been but rarely reported, with the patient complaining of momentary "flashing lights." Some of these patients have a history of migraine headaches. Shortness of breath, which disappears promptly when the patient sits up, has been seen in elderly patients injected with saline.

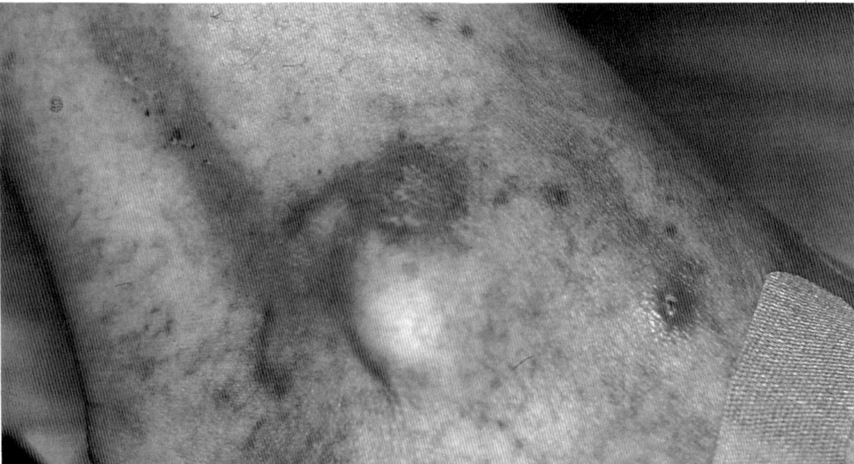

Fig. 7. Pigment 5 years after surgery

References

1. Alderman DB (1977) Therapy for essential cutaneous telangiectasia. Postgrad Med 61:91–95
2. Alderman DB (1975) Surgery and sclerotherapy in the treatment of varicose veins. Conn Med 39:467
3. Allen EV, Barker NW, Hines EV Jr (1972) Peripheral vascular disease. Saunders, Philadelphia
4. Bodian EL (1983) Sclerotherapy of sunburst varicosities. Dialogues Dermatol 13:3
5. Bodian EL (1985) Techniques of sclerotherapy for sunburst venous blemishes. J Dermatol Surg Oncol 11:7
6. Brauer EW (1970) Cosmetic management of selected skin changes of the legs. South Med J 63:1190
7. DeFaria JL., Moraes JN (1963) Histopathology of telangiectasia associated with varicose veins. Dermatologia 127:321–329
8. Duffy DM (1988) Small vessel sclerotherapy – an overview. Adv Dermatol 3:221–242
9. Foley WT (1965) Office treatment of varicose veins and ulcers. Gen Pract 31:3, 90–99
10. Foley WT (1975) The eradication of venous blemishes. Cutis 15:665–668
11. Goldman et al. (1987) The treatment of telangectasia. J Am Acad Dermatol 17:167–182
12. McPeeters HO, Anderson JK (1938) Treatment of varicose veins and hemorrhoids. Davis, Philadelphia
13. Orbach EJ (1979) Hazards of sclerotherapy of varicose veins, their prevention and treatment of complications. Vasa 8:170–173
14. Shields JL, Jansen TG (1982) Therapy for superficial telangiectasia of the lower extremities. J Dermatol Surg Oncol 8:10

Shave Excision

Daniel W. Collison and Roger I. Ceilley

Introduction

Shave excision is one of the simplest techniques used in dermatologic surgery. Despite its simplicity, shave excision can be performed crudely or with elegance. Expertise in this method is amply rewarded since it is used in the diagnosis and therapy of a variety of conditions. Mastery of shave excision requires both fine manual skill and good clinical judgment. Skillfully performed, a shave excision usually leaves barely a scar, leaving patients pleased with the results, especially since sutures are not required.

Shave excision is an excellent technique for the extirpation or biopsy of many lesions of epidermal or superficial dermal origin

> such as acrochordon, actinic keratosis, benign adnexal tumor, basal cell carcinoma, Bowen' disease, melanocytic nevus, pyogenic granuloma, rhinophyma, elevated scar, seborrheic keratosis, skin biopsy, split-thickness skin graft harvesting, and verruca.

Faced with a clinical lesion, the physician should know the thickness of epidermis and dermis at that site and whether the histopathologie features of the lesion make shave excision an appropriate modality. Intelligent integration of manual technique with knowledge of local skin characteristics and the histopathology of the clinical lesion keeps complications to a minimum.

Because the term "shave" may have pejorative connotations or may be misunderstood as being an incomplete form of treatment, we often use the phrase tangential excision; alternative terms such as laminar excision, subcision, or subsection have also been suggested [1]. In shave excision, tissue is excised with a blade directed nearly tangential to the skin. The excision produces a defect that is either flush or slightly concave in comparison with the adjacent skin. The wound heals by second intention. Our discussion of shave excision is limited to the use of the scalpel, the single-edged razor blade, and the double-edged razor blade (both plain and flexible varieties). Other modalities used to excise or destroy the epidermis and superficial dermis include:

> blistering agent (e. g., cantharidin), chemical peel, cryosurgery, dermal currette, dermatome, dermabrasion, electrosurgery, laser (e. g., defocused CO_2 laser), scissors (especially pedunculated lesions), topical 5-fluorouracil, and ultrasound devices (experimental).

Three variables determine the extent, depth, and shape of the shave excision: (a) the angle of the blade with respect to the skin; (b) the lateral margin of the blade with respect to the lesion; and (c) forces of compression or distension applied to the tissue being cut. Increasing the angle of the blade to the skin surface increases the concavity of the defect. Shallow shave excisions may be described as tangential excisions (Fig. 1 a, level A), whereas deeper angles of excision result in so-called "undercut" or "deep" shave excisions (Fig. 1 a, level B) or "saucerization" excisions (Fig. 1 a, level C). Modifying the clearance margin around a lesion results in partial excision at one extreme (Fig. 1 b, level A) or complete excision with a clearance margin at the other (Fig. 1 b, level B). Applying forces to the tissue, such as compressing it between the fingers (Fig. 1 c) or distending it with subjacent infiltration of local anesthetic agents (Fig. 1 d) results in deeper defects once these forces are released. Massaging an area of edema caused by anesthetic agents disperses the fluid and reduces the distending forces.

Prevention and Management of Complications

The complications of shave excision are similar to those occurring with other surgical modalities:

> infection, contact dermatitis, excessive granulation, scarring, postinflammatory pigmentary changes, bleeding, pain, paresthesia, inadequate biopsy, incomplete excision, persistent pigmentation, and persistent hair.

Infection is rarely a complication of shave excision. Standard surgical sterile technique with lengthy scrubs, draping, and strict asepsis, as practiced in major surgery, is not necessary and not cost-effective for most shave excisions. However, clean surgical technique is obviously important and decreases the incidence of infection. A 10-s scrub with 70% isopropyl alcohol [2] followed by a no-touch shave excision has little risk of wound contamination. Scalpel blades and razor blades, even those used for shaving, are sterile when removed from their package [1]. Appropriate wound care, as discussed below, with written and verbal wound care instructions to the patient, also decreases the chance for infection. Areas with greater colonization by gram-negative organisms, such around the ears and in body creases, may benefit from the addition of 1/4% acetic acid compresses to the wound care regimen. Any suspected infection should be handled according to standard protocol for infectious diseases, including cul-

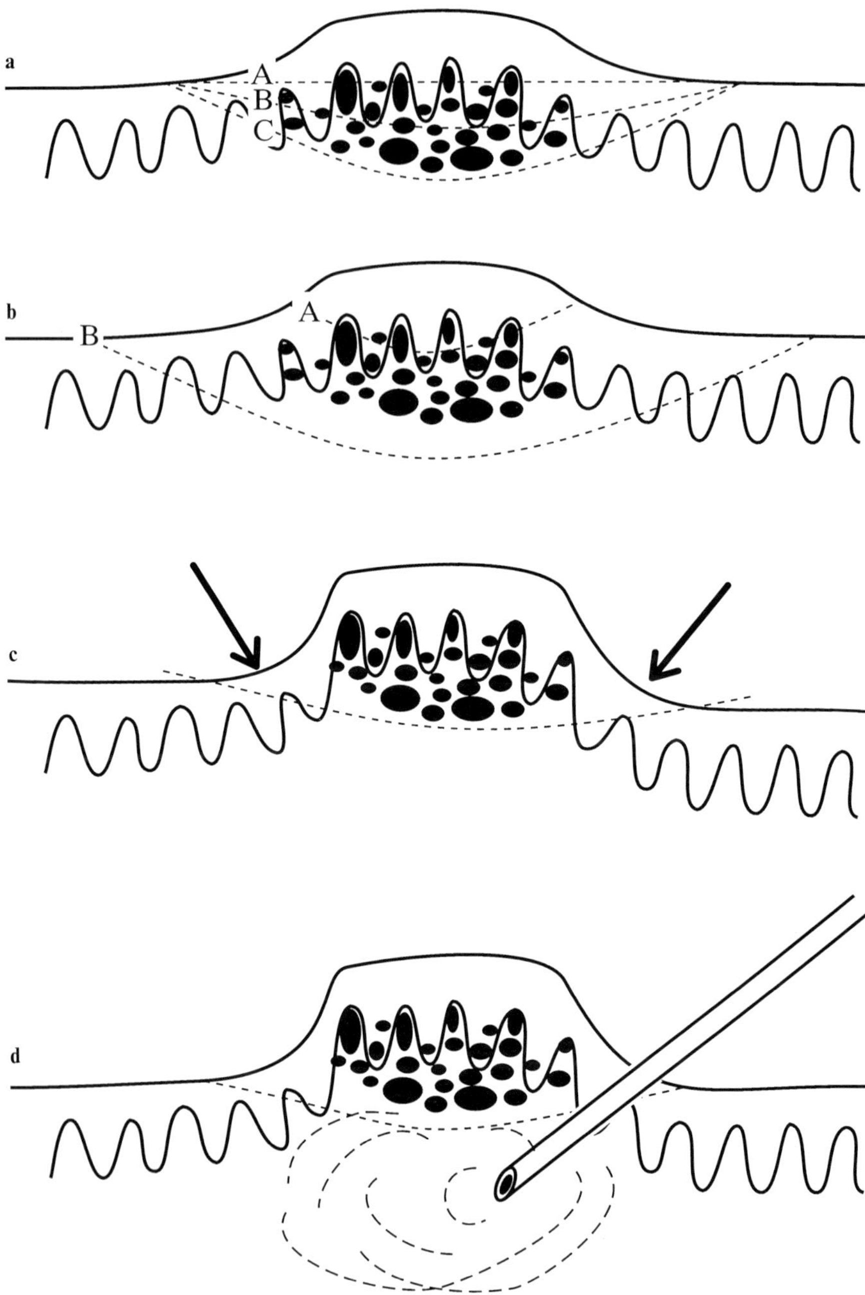

Fig. 1 a.–d. Cross-sectional diagram of nevus. **a** Various angles of shave excision *(A–C).* **b** Various degrees of clearance margin *(A, B).* **c** pinching forces of fingers *(arrows)* resulting in upward distension of reticular dermis; deep excision results, comparable to *level C.* **d** Infiltration of anesthesia distends the reticular dermis; deep excision results, comparable to *level C*

ture of wound exudate, empiric administration of oral or topical antibiotics, and definitive antimicrobial therapy based on sensitivities of culture isolates.

Contact dermatitis, of both the irritant and allergic types, may mimic infection. The shave excision site may appear erythematous, swollen, and moist. The offending agents are usually wound care agents such as antibiotic ointments or dressing adhesives. In our experience, bacitracin zinc ointment has the least potential for complications, although it too can sensitize [3]. Contact dermatitis is treated by discontinuing the offending agent; topical steroids or compresses may be indicated to reduce inflammation.

Excessive granulation tissue may develop at a shave excision site, especially in areas that receive, are exposed to, or are subject to trauma. These sites can be treated by silver nitrate chemocautery, curretage or electosurgery, followed by application of 1% aqueous gentian violet.

Preventing or minimizing significant *scarring* is the goal of any surgeon. In most cases scarring is barely perceptible following shave excision, but the patient should be forewarned of possible results. The visibility of scarring increases with deeper angles of incision since the scar rim is sharper and the defect deeper. The depth of a shave excision and resultant scarring may be adjusted according to the surgeon's goal. For example, most compound or intradermal nevi may be excised with better cosmesis if partial, relatively shallow excisions are performed [4]. The cosmetic result from the partial excision is usually more desirable than the scar resulting from complete extirpation, even if a full-thickness fusiform excision of the nevus is done. If a shave-excised nevus recurs to an unacceptable degree, it may always be reexcised, while a linear scar or deep saucerization scar is often more unsightly than the original nevus.

Poor blade control may result in an irregular excision and unwanted scarring. Maintaining adequate tension on adjacent skin while excising is essential. The contralateral hand or an assistant can stretch the skin to provide firm tissue for cutting (Fig. 2). The eyelids and similar sites with thin or lax skin often cannot be made taut enough for shave excision, and other instruments, such as scissors, must therefore be used. Finer control of a blade can be achieved by keeping the arm fixed and using the wrist and fingers to make sweeping motions with the blade. Advancing the blade steadily in the same plane while keeping even contact with the tissue being cut helps to prevent a ragged, sawtoothed excision. An even excision is more easily achieved with a sharp blade; when excising multiple lesions from the same patient, a blade may be dulled even after a single excision [1].

Proper blade selection is essential for optimal blade control. Single-edged razor blades are the least expensive and are ideal for exophytic lesions on a fairly flat or convex surface, and some feel that they are easier to control than the flexible variety. Some dermatologists find, however, that the unmatched sharpness of a flexible razor blade makes it the blade of choice. Also, they feel that the U-shaped contour of a flexible razor blade bent between the guiding fingers or attached to a blade holder provides a more easily controlled excision; this is especially true when excising lesions from concave surfaces such as the nasofacial angle. A number 15 blade on a scalpel handle is also convenient for concave surfaces or if a more carefully sculpted saucerization is desired. For large lesions, a

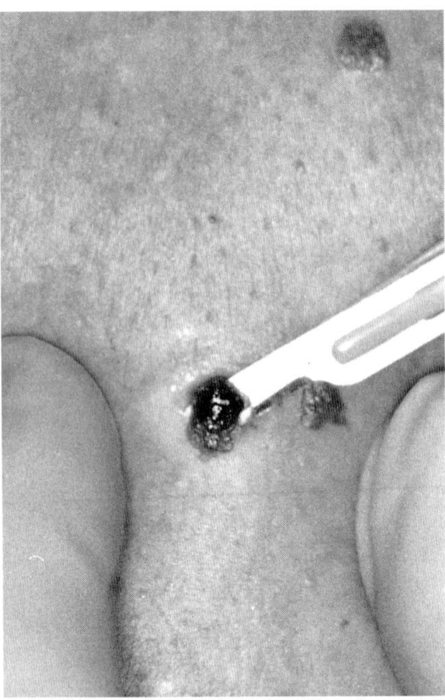

Fig. 2. Shave excision of a seborrheic keratosis using a 15 scalpel. Contralateral hand stretches the skin, providing optimal tissue consistency for cutting

number 10 blade may be easier to control than a number 15 blade, for example, when excising a large seborrheic keratosis or a large palque of superficial basal cell carcinoma. Beginners may find practicing on a grapefruit or pigsfoot helpful in determining the cutting characteristics of each blade type and size.

Scarring may be less obvious if the rim of the excision is blended in with surrounding skin. Blending or "feathering" may be done with very light electrosurgery (Fig. 3) or with a dermal curette, which is especially useful with seborrheic keratoses in which fragments of tissue may persist at the edge of the excision. However, since curettage or electrosurgery also causes further tissue destruction, they should be used judiciously.

Hemostasis of shave excisions can usually be accomplished by applying 35% aqueous aluminum chloride. Monsel's solution may rarely leave permanent iron tattooing but provides excellent hemostasis. Electrosurgery may be required for persistent bleeding; low-power electrodessication of pinpoint sites of bleeding is usually sufficient. Battery-powered hand-held electrocautery devices provide convenient pin-point hemostasis; since the electrocautery tip becomes red-hot, it is also self-sterilizing. Some practitioners avoid all forms of hemostasis except direct pressure, believing that electrosurgery and styptic agents produce significantly more tissue destruction and poorer cosmesis.

Wound care also influences scar outcome. Effective wound care decreases the incidence of infection, which may lead to greater inflammation and scarring and also decreases eschar formation, which may impede epithelialization. A variety of methods for wound care may be successfully employed. The simplest wound

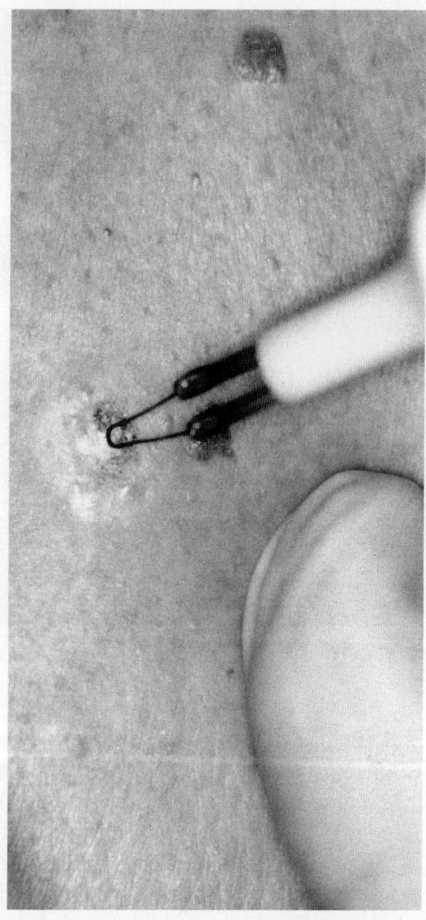

Fig. 3. Blending in the rim of a shave excision using light electrocautery with a battery-powered cautery unit

care is to let an eschar form and fall off without further intervention; this may give as good a result as the most sophisticated semiocclusive dressing. Certainly, excellent healing also results from twice-daily cleansing with soap and water or hydrogen peroxide. Some supplement cleansing with the application of antibiotic ointment. Application of antibiotic ointment and an adhesive bandage is inexpensive and provides moist occlusion, which may speed healing. However, if the patient is not scrupulous about regular dressing changes, adhesives and antibiotic ointments may cause a contact dermatitis or macerate the skin and complicate healing. With semiocclusive membrane dressings, the added cost and inconvenience must be weighed against the potential benefits of improved healing.

In addition to these preventive measures, there are a variety of ways to improve a scar that has already formed. *Hypertrophic or keloidal scarring,* although less likely to occur with shave excisions, are complications of any type of cutaneous surgery, especially on the chest, deltoid area, and foot (Fig. 4). Hypertrophic

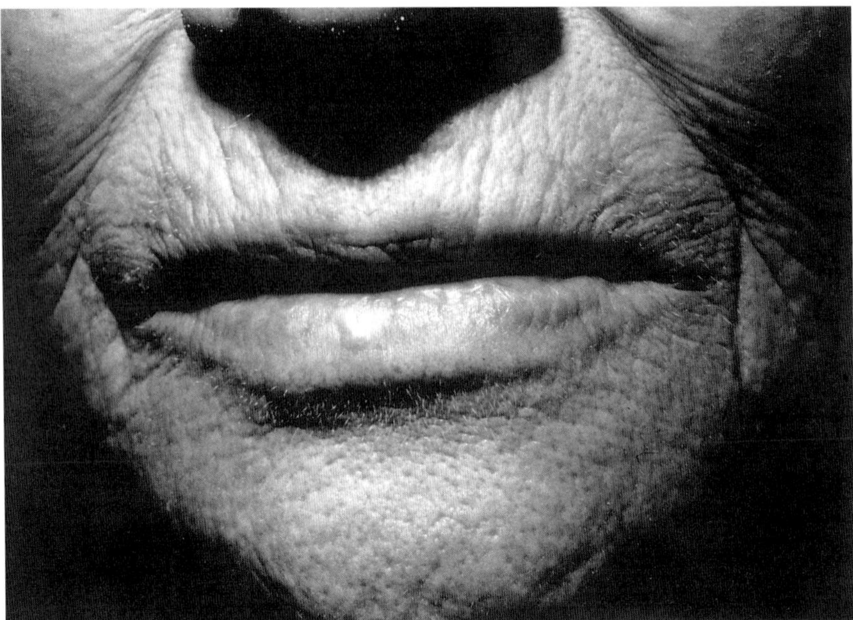

Fig. 4. Hypertrophic scar at shave excision site

scarring often improves with time but may be treated by a variety of methods, such as intralesional corticosteroids, topical corticosteroids (including those impregnated in tape, e. g., Cordran tape), cryotherapy, pressure therapy, or massage [5]. These techniques are most effective if instituted as soon as the untoward healing is recognized, while collagen formation is still in progress. Injections of low concentrations (2.5 mg/ml) of triamconolone acetonide are almost always sufficient in reducing scar hypertrophy while collagen formation is active; however, like most modalities, this is less effective in reducing mature scar. Increasing the concentrations of intralesional corticosteroids increases the risk for atrophy or telangiectasia. Massage therapy is effective when performed for a few minutes several times a day over several weeks. Keloidal scars respond less effectively to these techniques; excision of the keloid with institution of postoperative intralesional corticosteroid injections to prevent repeat keloid formation is sometimes performed.

Filler substances, for example, injectable collagen, Zyderm, Zyderm II, Zyplast, Fibrel or silicone, may be used to elevate *depressed scars.* In some instances, surgical scar revision may be indicated. Techniques include dermabrasion, punch lifting, punch graft replacement or full thickness excision with sutured closure.

Patients should be warned that *postinflammatory pigmentary changes* may affect shave excision sites. Soon after excision, the site may be more erythematous than normal; later, the healed skin may become hypopigmented or hyperpigmented. Darker skinned patients are more likely to have postinflammatory hypo- or hyperpigmentation, and they should be forewarned. Sun screen, especially in the 1st year following surgery, may prevent or minimize pigmentary changes. Many pigmentary changes improve with time. If not, makeup is the simplest method of camouflage. Flesh-colored pigments may be used for hyper- or hypopigmentation, while light application of green-based makeups masks redness. Yellow-light pulsed tunable dye laser also can be used to reduce scar erythema.

Bleeding, pain, and *paresthesia* are unusual complications of shave excision, but patients should be forewarned of their potential. In their written wound care instructions, patients should be told what to do if their wound bleeds. Chemocautery, electrosurgery and vascular ligature stop bleeding. Pain from shave excision is usually minor but may be greater if the wound is infected. Paresthesia of the surgical site should resolve over months; if it persists, it is usually minor.

Inadequate biopsy material is not a complication per se, but if shave excision is being performed for purposes of diagnosis, the physician must anticipate whether adequate tissue is being removed for histopathologic study. An inadequate specimen may result especially when a lesion unexpectedly turns out to be malignant. For example, if the shave excision is superficial, the depth of an unexpected squamous cell carcinomas or melanoma cannot be assessed. Deep saucerization, punch or fusiform excisions are often better choices for biopsy if malignancy is suspected. Obviously, shave excisions are not indicated for biopsy of diseases suspected to have involvement of middle to deep dermis or subcutis.

Inadequate excision may be an untoward result, although it also is not a true surgical complication. It commonly arises if lesions have a dermal component. Deeper and wider excisions obviously increase the likelihood of complete excision. Incompletely excised lesions that are malignant, or that may have malignant potential should be retreated with a definitive modality. The patient with a persistent nevus should be warned that further biopsy of the lesion may reveal pseudomalignant changes, and that any physician performing surgery on the lesion should be informed of the previous surgery [6]. Inadequate excision should not be confused with incomplete excision. Sometimes, as in treatment of certain nevi for cosmetic reasons (discussed above), incomplete excision is the expected result.

Persistent pigmentation or *persistent terminal hairs* may be seen in incompletely excised melanocytic nevi (Fig. 5), the former especially in areas surrounding hair follicles. Depending on the extent of the residual melanocytes, treatment consists of further shave excision, spot electrosurgery, or spot cryotherapy. Persistent hairs may be effectively treated with shaving, plucking, epilation, or electrolysis.

In summary, the complications of shave excision can be minimized when skillful manual technique is used for lesions of epidermal or superficial dermal origin. Complications that do occur can be effectively managed by a variety of methods well known to the practicing dermatologist.

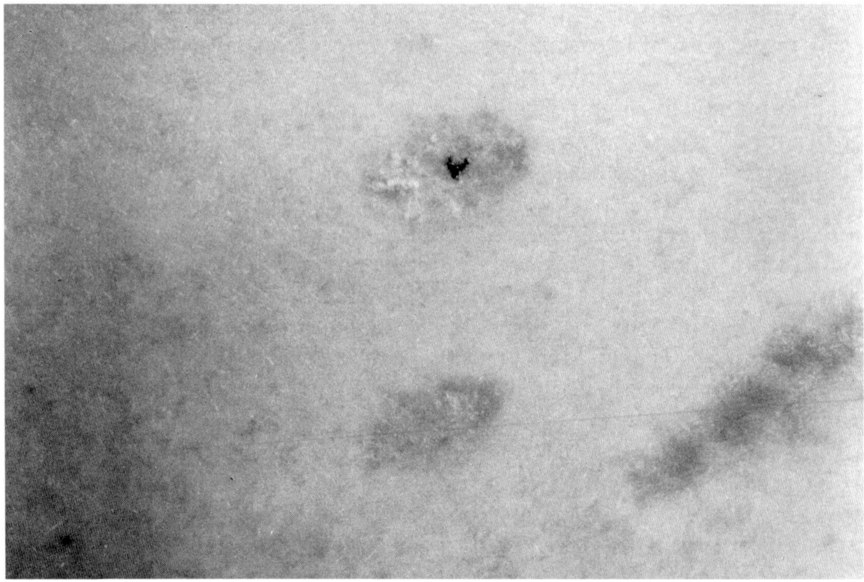

Fig. 5. Persistent pigmentation at site of melanocytic nevus following shave excision

References

1. Shelley WB (1982) Razor blade surgery. In: Epstein E, Epstein E Jr (eds) Skin surgery, 5th edn. Thomas, Springfield, pp 320–330
2. Dzubow LM, Halpern AC, Leyden JJ, Grossman D, McGinley KJ (1988) Comparison of preoperative skin preparations for the face. J Am Acad Dermatol 19(4):737–741
3. Held JL, Kalb RE, Ruszkowski AM, DeLeo V (1987) Allergic contact dermatitis from bacitracin. J Am Acad Dermatol 17(4):592–594
4. Ceilley RI (1987) Surgical treatment of nevi. In: Epstein E, Epstein E Jr (eds) Skin surgery, 6th edn. Thomas, Springfield, pp 564–571
5. Ceilley RI (1987) The treatment of hypertrophic scars and keloids. In: Epstein E, Epstein E Jr (eds) Skin surgery, 6th edn. Thomas, Springfield, pp 580–586
6. Park HK, Leonard DD, Arrington J III, Lund HZ (1987) Recurrent melanocytic nevi: clinical and histologic review of 175 cases. J Am Acad Dermatol 17(2):285–292

Mohs' Micrographic Surgery

Pearon G. Lang, Jr.

Despite the fact that the cutaneous malignancies managed by Mohs' micrographic surgery (MMS) often prove quite invasive and extensive, and that many of the patients are elderly, the procedure is amazingly free of complications. This is true even when a multidisciplinary approach under general anesthesia is required either to rid the patient of his tumor and/or to reconstruct the surgical defect [1]. Many of the potential complications of MMS are not unique but are common to all surgical procedures involving the skin. These have been reviewed by others [2] and are also discussed elsewhere in this volume. Because other authors discuss the complications associated with the repair of surgical defects, and because these are no more likely or different in the MMS patient, I omit these from my discussion.

Fixed-Tissue Technique

The fixed-tissue technique [3–5] has been largely supplanted by the fresh-tissue technique. For historical reasons, however, as well as the fact that the fixed-tissue technique is still occasionally employed it should be discussed.

The application of the zinc-chloride fixative may be associated with significant edema, particularly in areas such as the periorbital area (Fig. 1). Once surgery is completed, this resolves; however, sleeping with the head elevated and using ice packs hastens its resolution.

As the tissue is fixed, the patient may experience significant pain which may require oral or parenteral narcotics for relief. This is true especially if the cancer is extensive or in a sensitive area.

Incorrect use of the fixative can lead to an unnecessary full-thickness defect in the nose or ear; thus the surgeon using MMS should be well versed in its use. Even when used correctly, with a deeply penetrating tumor the patient may develop a full-thickness defect when the residual fixed tissue separates. Also if the tumor extends to the perichondrium or periosteum – unlike in the fresh-tissue technique, where granulation tissue forms without further intervention – with the fixed-tissue technique it might be necessary to remove cartilage on bone to encourage granulation tissue to form. Because it is more tissue sparing, the fresh-tissue technique has become preferred over the use of the zinc-chloride fixative. Moreover, with the fixed-tissue technique one

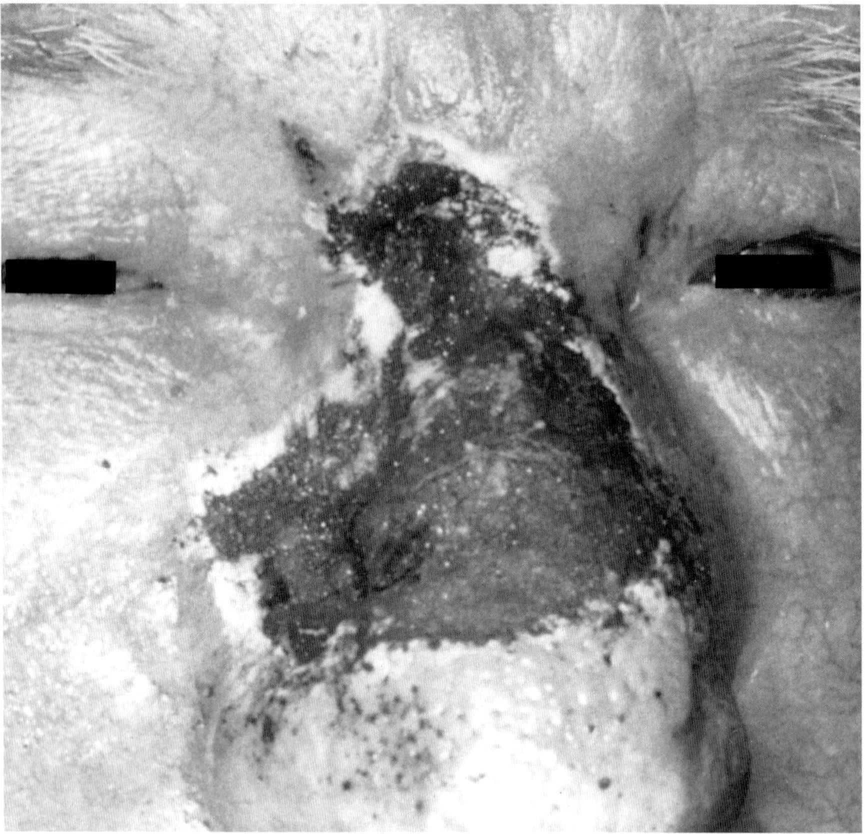

Fig. 1. The zinc chloride fixative has been applied to the wound bed following removal of the gross tumor. Note the resultant edema

must wait until the final layer of fixed tissue separates before the wound can be repaired.

Although several stages of MMS can sometimes be performed in a single day employing the fixed-tissue technique, it was more common to leave the fixative in place overnight and perform only one stage of surgery per day. This, coupled sometimes with significant pain and a delayed repair, could cause the procedure to be exceedingly prolonged and arduous for the patient. These negative aspects of the procedure may have been responsible for delaying the wider acceptance of MMS and are certainly further reasons why the fresh-tissue technique has replaced the fixed-tissue technique.

If a large vessel is present in the wound bed as the residual fixed tissue separates, severe hemorrhaging may occur. To prevent this the vessel should be ligated at the completion of MMS.

A transient low-grade fever which may accompany the use of the fixative can be treated with acetaminophen.

Fresh Tissue Technique

General Medical Considerations

At the time that the patient is scheduled for surgery his general medical status is reviewed, along with the list of his current medications. Allergies and intolerance to medications are noted. The patient is also asked whether he has a history of problems with bleeding, healing, or unusual scarring. If the answer is yes, this is further discussed in the context of the impending surgery, and appropriate preoperative evaluation and management of any potential problems are carried out. If the patient has a medical problem such as hypertension, diabetes mellitus, or congestive heart failure, and if the problem appears poorly controlled, he is referred to his primary care physician for reassessment. Surgery is postponed until the problem is brought under control [6, 7].

Preoperative chest X-rays, electrocardiograms, and blood studies are usually not obtained unless:
a) they are performed by the primary care physician to assess a medical problem, for example, diabetes;
b) general anesthesia and an interdisciplinary approach is planned;
c) the patient is at risk for metastatic disease; or
d) the patient is on sodium warfarin.

Although aspirin, nonsteroidal anti-inflammatory drugs (NSAID), sodium warfarin, and dipyrimadole increase intraoperative bleeding and the risk of postoperative bleeding, I leave it to the patient and his primary care physician to decide whether these agents are discontinued prior to surgery. In patients on sodium warfarin, I do require that determination of a protime (PT) be obtained just prior to surgery, and that it be in the proper therapeutic range.

The need for prophylactic antibiotics in patients with valvular heart disease, those with prosthetic heart valves, and those with orthopedic implants has been questioned. In patients undergoing surgery for noninfected tumors, the incidence of bacteremia is low, and it is currently recommended that only patients with prosthetic heart valves receive prophylactic antibiotics [7, 9]. However, one finds that many patients with valvular heart disease (including mitral valve prolapse) and those with orthopedic implants have been told that they need prophylactic antibiotics to prevent bacterial seeding of their implant or damaged heart valve. In such circumstances I leave the decision to the patient and his family physician (or cardiologist or orthopedic surgeon). It has been suggested that for patients with prosthetic heart valves at least 60 days old that a first-generation cephalosporin be given in a dose of 1–2 g orally 1 hour before the procedure and in a dose of 500 mg every 6 h for one or two doses following completion of the procedure [8, 9]. If the valve is less than 60 days old, because of the increased risk of infection with diptheroids, parenteral vancomycin should be given [9]. Because MMS may be an all-day procedure, and the patient may be left with an open wound, I routinely start patients on 500 mg cephalexin every 6 h, 24 h before surgery and continue it for 24 h following the completion of surgery.

Although most patients are anxious about having surgery, some are more so than others. If extreme anxiety is anticipated, I usually administer 10 mg diazepam the night before surgery and 1 h before surgery. This can be continued throughout the day if necessary. If the patient's anxiety does not manifest itself until he presents for surgery, I will give 10 mg diazepam sublingually. If the patient's blood pressure is markedly elevated because of anxiety, I give 10 mg nifedipine sublingually. This usually brings the blood pressure to a normal range within 10–15 min. If the patient begins to hyperventilate, he is told to take slow, deep breaths.

Occasionally a patient experiences a vasovagal episode. This can be quite alarming, with the patient exhibiting tonic, convulsive movements in addition to being pale and sweaty. If a patient begins to feel faint, warm, or nauseous, or if a full vasovagal episode occurs, he should be placed in a reverse Trendelenburg position, with cool cloths placed on the face, neck and wrists. He should be left in this position until he fully recovers. When surgery is completed, the head of the surgical table should be raised slowly and the patient allowed to sit for a while before returning to the waiting room. He should be escorted to the waiting room so that he does not hurt himself if he faints.

Orthostatic hypotension leading to a syncopal episode may occur in the elderly with significant arteriosclerosis or in patients on antihypertensive medication. With such individuals, the head of the surgical table should be raised slowly and the patient allowed to sit before trying to ambulate. Such patients should be escorted to the waiting area.

Patients with coronary artery disease may experience angina during surgery, probably as a result of anxiety. Such patients usually have nitroglycerin tablets with them and should be allowed to take these. Supplemental oxygen via a nasal cannula may be used if the angina is severe or slow to resolve. If the angina is severe and persistent, a cardiology consultation should be sought. In patients with a history of severe coronary artery disease, I may omit the epinephrine from the local anesthesia or dilute it to 1:200,000. In the anxious patient, preoperative diazepam may also be helpful. Patients with a history of cardiac arrhythmias are placed on a cardiac monitor during surgery.

As already noted, despite the fact that many of our patients are elderly and often infirm, MMS is relatively free of complications. However, no one knows when a patient may experience a cardiac arrest, myocardial infarction, cardiac arrhythmia, or untoward reaction to a medication. The surgeon and staff performing MMS should be prepared to deal with such emergencies. Appropriate drugs and equipment should be available, and the surgeon and assistants should know how to use these.

Local Anesthetics

One of the greatest causes of anxiety in patients undergoing MMS is fear of the injection of the local anesthetic. The patient's anxiety is best allayed and his discomfort minimized by:

a) using a 30 gauge needle,
b) injecting the anesthetic slowly,
c) adding sodium bicarbonate to the anesthetic if it contains epinephrine, and
d) performing nerve blocks when possible prior to local infiltration of the surgical site [6, 10].

If after all these maneuvers the patient still finds the injection of the anesthetic intolerable, I block the area at the completion of the surgical session with a long-acting anesthetic such as bupivacaine to minimize the discomfort of reanesthetizing the area should additional surgical sessions be necessary.

Some patients are extremely sensitive to epinephrine and become tremulous, develop a marked tachycardia, and become very anxious. In such patients I may use an anesthetic not containing epinephrine or may lower its concentration to 1 : 200,000. A similar course of action may be pursued in patients with poorly controlled hypertension or severe coronary artery disease whose disease or symptoms may be aggravated by the epinephrine [6].

Digital blocks should not be performed with anesthetics containing epinephrine for fear of causing severe ischemia and resulting gangrenous changes. Even local infiltration with anesthetics containing epinephrine may cause tissue necrosis in acral areas (especially the digits and ears) in patients with severe vascular insufficiency (e. g., diabetics). In these patients an anesthetic not containing epinephrine should be used.

Documented IgE-mediated allergic reactions to injected local anesthetic preparations, especially the amides, are rare, but when they occur, they may represent a reaction to the anesthetic or "inert" ingredients (parabens, bisulfites). Most reported reactions to local anesthetics are probably vasovagal in nature or related to the epinephrine mixed with them. However, if it is not clear whether the patient had a true allergic reaction, further evaluation is required. It is said that cross-reactions do not occur between the amide group and ester group of anesthetics; however, if the patient is sensitive to a preservative common to the two preparations, he will experience a reaction. Thus empirically switching to a different class of local anesthetics does not guarantee safety. A patient strongly suspected of having had an IgE-mediated reaction to a local anesthetic should therefore undergo skin testing (scratch and intradermal) to the anesthetic and any preservatives contained within it. If results of the skin tests are negative, subcutaneous challenge(s) should be performed. False-negative skin tests are rare, but false-positive tests are seen in approximately 15% of patients undergoing testing. Cross-reactivity between various members of the amide group of local anesthetics may or may not exist. Thus the patient should be skin tested and challenged to the anesthetic that one intends to use. If the patient has a history of contact sensitivity to a local anesthetic, it should not be used for infiltration. If the patient experiences an anaphylactic reaction to a local anesthetic, it should be managed appropriately (e. g., adrenaline, and antihistamines) [11]. If a patient is unable to tolerate any of the usual local anesthetics, an antihistamine may be used. Promethazine and pyribenzamine appear the most effective for this purpose [12].

Idiosyncratic responses may also occur to local anesthetics, for example, cardiovascular collapse as the result of the inadvertent intravenous administration of bupivacaine or methemoglobenemia secondary to the use of benzocaine or prilocaine [11].

Systemic toxic responses may occur in association with the use of local anesthetics, and thus careful attention must be given to patient selection, the total amount of anesthetic used, and the avoidance of direct intravascular injection. Local anesthetics may induce drowsiness or cause restlessness and twitching. As toxicity increases, seizures and cardiovascular collapse may occur, and coma may ensue. The amide anesthetics are metabolized in the liver, and their half-life, and thus the risk of toxicity, is increased in patients with liver disease or cardiac failure and in those on propranolol and cimetidine [11].

Epinephrine as noted may cause tachycardia and aggravate hypertension and angina. It also may induce arrhythmias and should be used with caution in patients with cardiac disease [11].

Bleeding

With the advent of the NSAIDs and the common use of aspirin (ASA) to prevent cardiovascular accidents, intraoperative and postoperative bleeding [6, 7] is a greater problem in patients undergoing MMS. It is also not unusual to encounter patients on sodium warfarin. Although ideally it would be best to stop these drugs prior to MMS, it is not always feasible to do so, and I leave this decision to the patient and his primary care physician. As noted in patients on sodium warfarin, I do require that a PT be determined just prior to the time of surgery, and that this not exceed the limits of proper anticoagulation. With careful attention paid to the proper ligation and electrocoagulation of blood vessels intraoperatively, I find no increased incidence of postoperative bleeding in these patients. ASA, because of its irreversible effect on platelets, needs to be discontinued 10–14 days prior to surgery to be beneficial. NSAIDs with a long half-life also must be stopped well in advance of MMS even though their effects on platelets are reversible. In my experience, intraoperative nuisance-type bleeding with persistent oozing is a significant problem with the NSAIDs and ASA but much less so with sodium warfarin.

When performing surgery on a digit or the penis, many physicians use a rubber band or rubber drain to control bleeding. This is a very acceptable practice as long as the tourniquet is periodically released. However, if the tourniquet is left in place too long, ischemic necrosis may occur. I have found that if my assistant squeezes tightly that the same benefit can be achieved but with greater safety since invariably the assistant must release their hold because of fatigue or cramping. In managing intraoperative bleeding and preventing postoperative bleeding, small vessels may be electrocoagulated, but larger vessels (e. g., branches of the superficial temporal artery) should be ligated with an absorbable suture (e. g., 5–0 coated polyglactin). We routinely pack the wound with oxidized cellulose (Oxcel) following completion of MMS since we feel that this also decreases the risk of postoperative bleeding. A generous coat of antibiotic ointment needs to be applied over this because bleeding ensues the next day when the dressing is changed if the bandage is adherent to the oxidized cellulose. A pressure dressing is also used for several days to discourage bleeding. Postoperatively we ask patients for 1 week to avoid strenuous activities as well as bending and to avoid alcoholic beverages, ASA, and NSAIDs for 24–48 h. If bleeding does develop we instruct our patients to hold firm and constant pressure for 15 min. If bleeding resumes after doing this, we ask that they contact us.

A large vessel that was unknowingly nicked, or whose supporting tissues were removed occasionally ruptures postoperatively, leading to significant hemorrhage. To prevent this I often ligate and divide such vessels at the completion of the surgery. If a prominent vessel is exposed, it should be kept well covered and moist; otherwise, it desiccates and may rupture.

Often, when a patient presents for postoperative bleeding, the bleeding has stopped. If there has been significant bleeding and clot formation, I will remove the clot and probe vigorously with a Q-Tip to discover the source of bleeding. If this is not done, bleeding may resume once the patient has returned home.

In sutured wounds, hematoma formation may lead to wound dehiscence and/or infection. For small hematomas, I use moist heat to promote their absorption and/or make a small incision along the suture line and attempt to evacuate the hematoma. When bleeding is brisk, a large painful hematoma may develop. In these instances, the wound must be opened, the source of bleeding identified and controlled, and the wound resutured. To decrease the likelihood of wound infection, I give these patients 500 mg cephalexin (or its equivalent) every 6 h for at least 24–48 h.

Although pacemakers, as regards external sources of interference, have been greatly improved, one must still be careful when using electrocoagulation to stop bleeding in these patients. These patients should be carefully monitored during electrocoagulation. If the patient's pacemaker is susceptible to electrical interference, following certain guidelines may be helpful in avoiding problems:
a) if the pacemaker is a demand type convert it to a fixed type;
b) a bipolar unit is safer than a monopolar unit;
c) keep the indifferent electrode as far from the heart as possible but as close to the active electrode as possible;
d) do not perform electrocoagulation over the heart or power source; and
e) electrocoagulate for less than 5 s at a time [13].

If the electrocoagulation does adversely affect the pacemaker, an electrocautery unit may be used safely since electrical current does not pass through the patient. Although there are electrocautery machines, I generally use the large, battery-operated, penlight type of disposable electrocautery unit.

Pain

Despite the fact that large defects are often left by MMS, severe postoperative pain is unusual [6, 7]. Most patients' pain is easily controlled with 650–975 mg acetaminophen taken every 3–6 h. However, occasionally, a patient may require acetaminophen with codeine or oxycodone for relief of pain. When MMS is performed on an extremity, elevating the limb for several days postoperatively decreases the severity of the patient's pain. This also decreases postoperative swelling.

Swelling and Bruising

Postoperative edema and bruising are not unusual especially in areas where the skin is loose, for example, the periorbital area and neck [6, 7]. A pressure dressing for several days and ice packs minimize this complication, and reassurance and ice packs are used to manage it. When surgery is performed on the forehead, periorbital swelling may require several days to manifest itself. Patients are often amazed at how far bruising may migrate, for example, from the neck onto the chest. Extensive bruising is much more likely when extensive undermining has been carried out.

Infection

Infection is very uncommon following MMS [6, 7] even if the wound is left to heal by second intention or is reconstructed. *Staphylococcus aureus* and *Streptococcus pyogenes* are the usual offenders, and antibiotic therapy should be prescribed accordingly. I usually prefer 250–500 mg cephalexin (or its equivalent) every 6 h for 10–14 days, but the semisynthetic penicillinase-resistant penicillins can also be used, as can erythromycin in patients unable to take the penicillins or cephalosporins. Moist heat and incision and drainage may be helpful or necessary in infected reconstructed wounds. The lower extremities and ears appear to be more susceptible to the development of postoperative infections.

A chondritis/perichondritis of the ear may be a particularly serious sequela of MMS, and for this reason some authors suggest that exposed auricular cartilage be covered (e. g., grafted; Fig. 2) [7]. In my experience these infections of the ear respond readily to a 2-week course of 500 mg cephalexin every 6 h; however, in a diabetic or immunocompromised patient, *Pseudomonas aeruginosa* may be the culprit, and often a culture should be taken. I start these patients on 750 mg ciprofloxacin twice a day [14]. Although a swab-acquired culture may be adequate, in patients not responding to treatment a biopsy of cartilage may need to be performed to elucidate the causative organism. Malignant external otitis, a dreaded complication seen in diabetics and the elderly and caused by *Pseudomonas aeruginosa,* may result in liquefaction of cartilage, with a resultant deformity of the ear, and in involvement of bone, cranial nerves and vessels, and even death. It

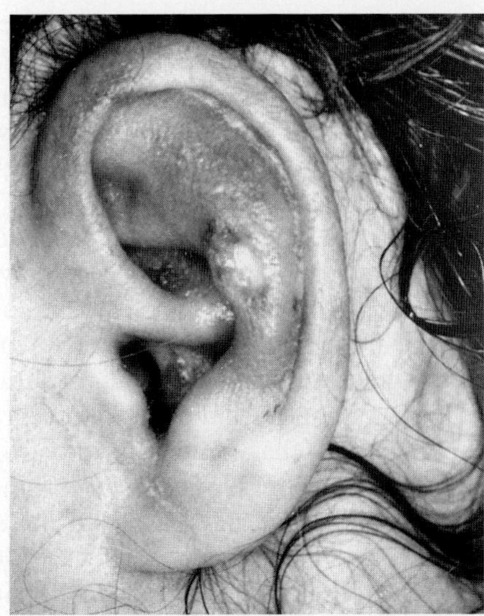

Fig. 2. Perichondritis surrounding a surgical wound. Note the exposed cartilage (Courtesy of J. D. Osguthorpe)

requires hospitalization, surgical débridement, and parenteral aminoglycoside antibiotics [7, 14]. To prevent this complication I do not operate on poorly controlled diabetics until their diabetes is under control, and I modify postoperative wound care for open wounds and use Burrow's solution compresses followed by gentamicin ointment (which is effective against gram-negative organisms as well as *Staphylococcus aureus)*.

Prophylactic antibiotics play a minor role in my management of patients. I use them primarily in patients undergoing a delayed repair of their defect or developing a hematoma postoperatively and whose reconstructed wound must be taken apart and resutured. If the delayed repair is anticipated, I will start the patient on 500 mg cephalexin every 6 h by mouth 24 h before their repair and continue it for 24 h thereafter. In patients allergic to the penicillins and cephalosporins, I substitute enteric-coated erythromycin in 250-mg tablets. If the repair is not preplanned, I give 1 g cefazolin intramuscularly 30–60 min prior to the repair. This is supplemented with 500 mg cephalexin every 6 h for 24 h. In patients unable to receive cephalosporins, 500-mg enteric-coated erythromycin is given 1 h prior to the repair and 250 mg is given subsequently every 6 h for 24 h. In patients requiring evacuation of a hematoma in the immediately postoperative period, either cephalexin or erythromycin are administered orally in a dose of 500 mg at the time of evacuation. These are continued in a dose of 500 or 250 mg, respectively, every 6 h for 48 h.

Some authors feel that surgical defects of the fingers and toes are more susceptible to infection, suggesting that they be closed whenever possible, and that prophylactic antibiotics be given [7]. As noted above, this author does not use prophylactic antibiotics in this setting. Whether or not the defect should be closed depends on the health of the patient, his healing ability, his reliability, and the size and depth of the defect. Large wounds with exposed tendons should usually be repaired, as should wounds in patients incapable of carrying out good wound care. In patients with significant defects of the extremities or digits I often substitute Burrow's solution or warm water and povidone iodine for hydrogen peroxide and have the patient change the dressing several times daily. If tendons are exposed, they need to be kept well covered and moist; otherwise they desiccate and become nonfunctional.

Good wound care is important to avoid infection. Our standard regimen for wound care in wounds which are left to heal by second intention include changing the dressing daily, cleansing the wound with hydrogen peroxide, and applying a topical antibiotic, usually bacitracin (see modifications noted earlier for ears, digits, and extremities). Although topical antibiotics are used to prevent infection, other than mupiricin, most topical antibiotic ointments may merely provide a moist environment to promote wound healing.

A problem that may arise with the use of topical antibiotics is the development of a contact sensitivity (Fig. 3). Gette et al [15] recently reported a 4.2% incidence of allergic contact dermatitis in their surgical patients. Although neomycin is still the most common cause of this problem, there are an increasing number of patients allergic to bacitracin. Katz and Fisher [16] reported their experience with bacitracin as a topical sensitizer. The zinc salt (Polysporin) appears to be less sensitizing than plain bacitracin, and therefore the latter should be used for patch testing. Coexisting sensitivity to neomycin and bacitracin does not represent cross-reactivity; however, because polymyxin B, like bacitracin, is derived from *Bacillus subtilis,* it may cross-react with bacitracin. In a patient with

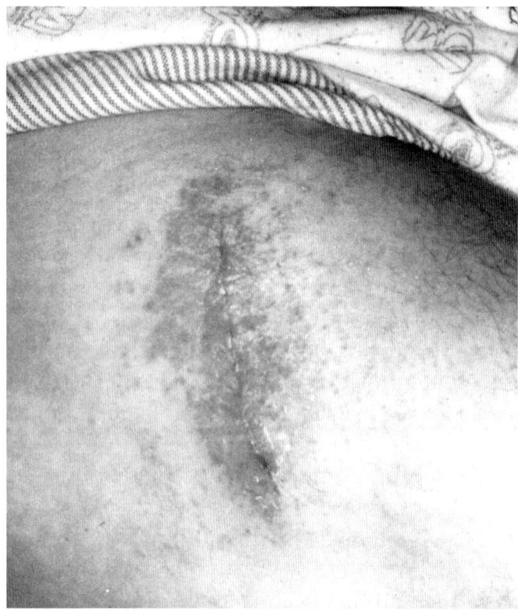

Fig. 3. Contact sensitivity to bacitracin which was used for postoperative wound care

bacitracin sensitivity the patch test to bacitracin may not show positive results before 96 h.

Rarely, anaphylaxis may develop following the topical application of bacitracin.

Nerve Damage

During MMS numerous small nerves are transected [6, 7]. As a result, the surgical site may remain numb for up to a year. As feeling returns, the patient may complain of itching, crawling sensations, shooting pains, and tenderness. This may be quite alarming to the patient, who fears the tumor is returning, or that the surgical site is not healing properly. Reassurance is sufficient to manage this problem. Although numbness may persist for a considerable time, generally there is enough overlap of cutaneous innervation that sensation eventually returns. Numbness may be remote to the surgical site. This is not uncommon when performing MMS for forehead lesions. These patients often complain of numbness in their scalp because of the interruption of nerve fibers which course through the forehead on their way to innervate the scalp.

Neuromas following MMS are extremely rare.

To avoid damage to critical superficial nerves an in-depth knowledge of surgical anatomy is crucial. In addition, ballooning out the overlying tissue with either local anesthetic or saline helps to prevent damage to the nerve.

In the head and neck area the facial nerve and spinal accessory nerve are the nerves most susceptible to injury. The temporal branch of the facial nerve as it crosses the zygomatic arch is very susceptible to damage (Fig. 4). Damage to this nerve results in the inability of the patient to wrinkle the forehead on this side.

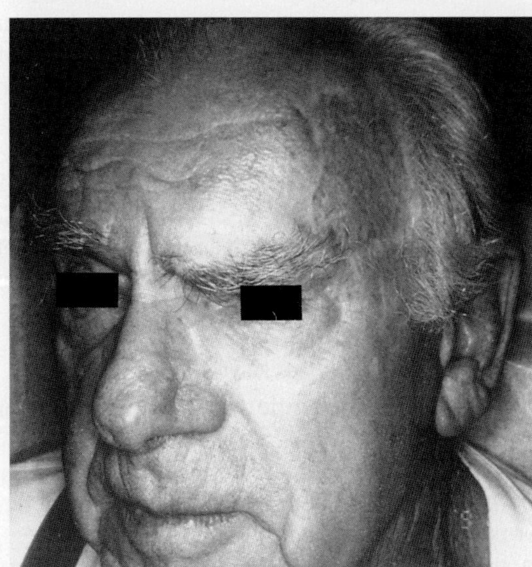

Fig. 4. Multiply recurrent deeply invasive basal cell carcinoma of the left temple which had been managed by MMS. The temporal branch of the facial nerve had to be sacrificed to rid the patient of his tumor. Note the sagging of the left forehead and eyebrow

The eyebrow droops, and this may require surgical correction for cosmetic as well as functional reasons (i. e., interference with vision). The mandibular branch of the facial nerve as it runs along the jawline is also susceptible to injury. The spinal accessory nerve courses superficially in the posterior triangle of the neck, and when injured the patient develops shoulder drop and pain, paresthesias, wasting of the trapezius muscle, and decreased ability to abduct the arm.

When it is anticipated that a major nerve may need to be transected or may be inadvertently injured during MMS (e. g., perineural squamous cell carcinoma; tumor invading the parotid gland), it is wise to consult with a head and neck surgeon. The head and neck surgeon may be able to dissect out the nerve and save it (e. g., the facial nerve) or perform a nerve graft once the patient is tumor free. This requires an interdisciplinary approach under general anesthesia. If an important nerve is inadvertently damaged, a head and neck surgeon should be consulted immediately. An undue delay (over 48 h) prevents the localization of the nerve by electrical stimulation and the successful grafting of the nerve (if feasible). If uninjured, but exposed, important nerves should be kept well covered and moist; otherwise, they will desiccate and degenerate.

Additional Postoperative Tissue Loss

If the tissue remaining on an ear or the nose is very thin following resection of a deeply infiltrating tumor, the area may undergo necrosis resulting in a full-thickness defect or loss of the ala rim. Other than good wound care, there is nothing that can be done to prevent this. If chondritis develops in the nose or ear, cartilaginous structure may be lost, resulting in further deformity. If extensive resection is required on a digit, and if the wound is circumferential, the remaining blood supply may be inadequate, thus leading to gangrenous changes. If feasible, doing the resection as a staged procedure may preserve the digit (i. e., operating on the tumor in segments and letting one area heal before removing another portion). If an extensive resection is anticipated, consultation with a hand surgeon may also be beneficial.

If periosteum or perichondrium is exposed, it must be kept covered and moist. If it desiccates, granulation tissue does not form.

Gaspari et al. [17] have reported a patient whose tendon ruptured several days after completion of MMS for a recurrent squamous cell carcinoma overlying the first metacarpophalangeal joint of the hand. Several factors may have contributed to this complication:
a) systemic corticosteroids,
b) wound infection, or
c) "nicking" of the tendon at the time of surgery.

The authors felt this complication may have been avoided if:
a) the patient had been placed on prophylactic antibiotics,
b) the wound had been repaired, and
c) the finger had been splinted.

Wound healing

Since its inception, MMS has continued to evolve. One of the greatest changes to occur in association with the technique has been the management of the surgical defect [6, 7, 18, 19]. Many more wounds are now repaired than previously. This has not only facilitated wound care and improved the overall cosmetic outcome in many patients but has probably also resulted in wider acceptance of the procedure by both patients and other physicians. However, accompanying the benefits of repairs are additional complications, such as loss of grafts, wound dehiscence, flap necrosis, hematomas, and seromas. Since these topics are covered elsewhere in this volume, our discussion is confined to healing by second intention.

Numerous studies have shown that a wound which is kept moist and occluded heals much more quickly. We have our patients change their dressings once or twice a day. Other than the exceptions noted above in the section on "Infection" we usually have our patients cleanse their wound with hydrogen peroxide. Subsequently, a dressing of gauze and bacitracin ointment is applied. If perichondrium or periosteum is exposed, white petrolatum is also applied. This procedure is continued until the wound is healed, at which point we have the patient lubricate and massage the area daily for 5 min until the scar matures. For periocular wounds, warm water and erythromycin ophthalmic ointment are used in place of hydrogen peroxide and bacitracin ointment. Some clinicians believe that transparent film dressings (e. g., Opsite, Bioclusive) may expedite the healing of MMS wounds and improve the cosmetic outcome [20].

Cartilage devoid of perichondrium and bone devoid of periosteum do not heal. To stimulate granulations to cover cartilage either the cartilage must be removed, or small holes (3 mm) must be made in the cartilage. On concave surfaces, cartilage may be removed but on convex surfaces only holes should be made since removal of cartilage predisposes to a depressed scar.

Although rare, exposed bone may develop osteomyelitis if left to desiccate, and granulation tissue is not stimulated [21]. To stimulate granulations to cover bone several methods may be employed:

a) the chiseling of bone at 3-to 4-week intervals [22, 23],

b) the application of zinc chloride fixative to the bone following completion of MMS and having the patient return in 3–4 weeks at which time with the aid of a chisel the fixed bone usually separates allowing the development of granulation tissue [4],

c) the use of power drills or a dermabrader to fenestrate the bone and encourage the development of granulation tissue [24], or

d) the use of the carbon dioxide laser to perforate the outer table of bone and allow the generation of granulation tissue [25].

Large wounds of the scalp, especially in the elderly may take months to heal or fail to completely heal or continue to break down once they do heal. Grafting may be required to complete healing or to yield a stable healed wound.

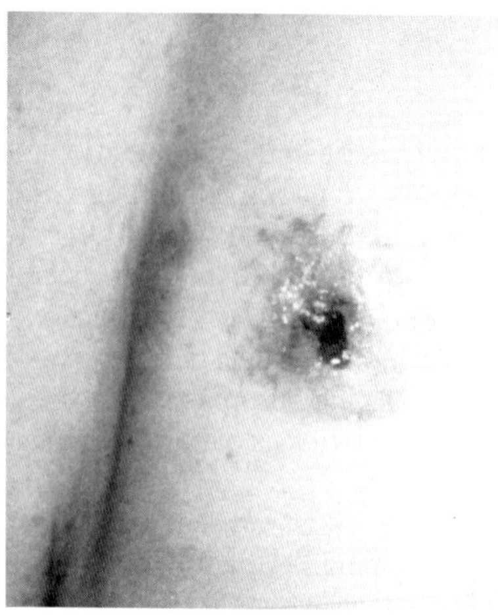

Fig. 5. MMS defect which was allowed to heal by second intention. Note the excess granulation tissue

Wounds with exposed perichondrium and periosteum and those located on the lower extremities also heal slowly.

Drugs which interfere with wound healing (e. g., corticosteroids), poorly controlled diabetes, nutritional deficiencies, arterial and venous insufficiency, impairment of the microcirculation, and prior irradiation may all adversely effect wound healing and should be corrected or improved if possible. Such factors which may influence wound healing are screened preoperatively and properly addressed – rather than dealing with their effects after the surgery is performed. Patients should also be asked whether they have a tendency for hypertrophic or keloidal scars. Wounds greater than 6–10 cm in diameter may not only take months to heal but may be unstable once they do heal. Such wounds require grafting.

The formation of excess granulation tissue is not uncommon, especially in large wounds (Fig. 5). Excess moisture and allowing hair to get into the wound contribute to this complication. Shaving the hair around the wound, letting air get to the wound for short periods of time, and minimizing the amount of antibiotic ointment applied help to prevent this problem. If the excess granulation tissue is not removed, wound healing is impeded. The simplest method of managing this complication is to curette away the excess granulation tissue. Once this is done, the patient may notice that wound healing resumes at a rapid rate.

As might be anticipated, small shallow wounds usually heal with better cosmetic outcome than large deep wounds. Since scars are often hypopigmented, they are less noticeable in fair-skinned individuals. Telangiectasias may form within the scar. These may be eliminated by electrodesiccation or pulsed dye laser treatment. In general, scars from second intention healing are less noticeable and cosmetically more acceptable in the elderly because of their lax skin, wrinkles, and irregular pigmentation. In young patients, the resultant scars tend to be more hypertrophic and sensitive and to remain red longer. Thick, porous,

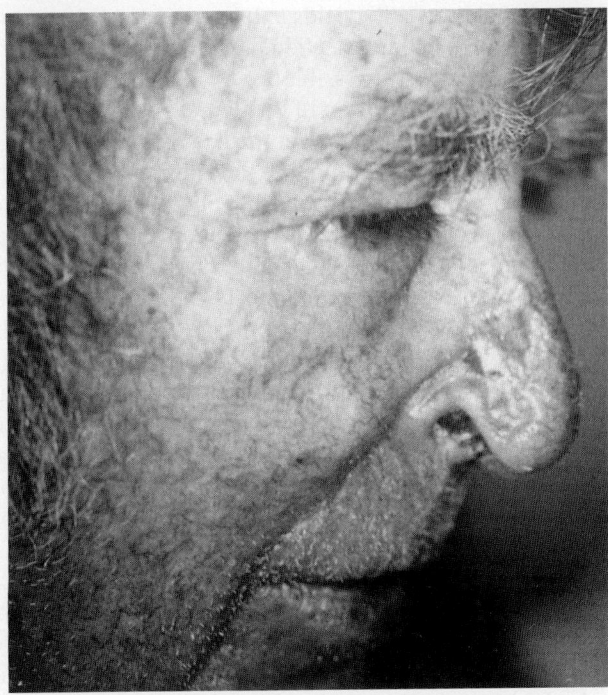

Fig. 6. Alar rim retraction following healing of a MMS defect by second intention

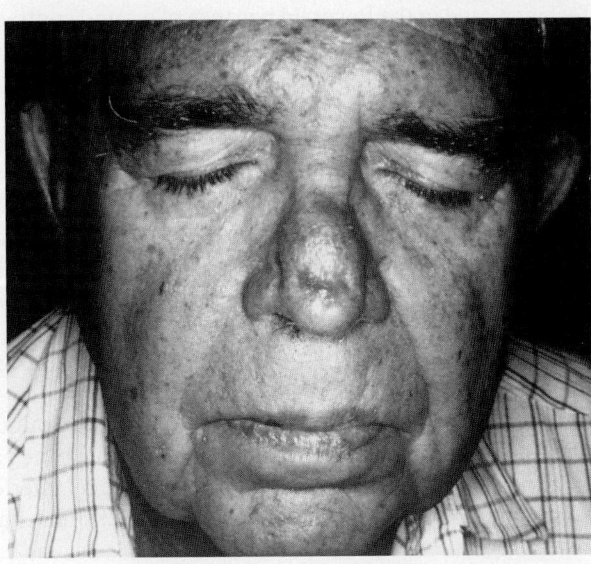

Fig. 7. Depressed and hypertrophic scar of the dorsal nasal tip following healing of a MMS defect by second intention

sebaceous skin usually yields a depressed scar whereas thin pale skin with fine pores often yields an excellent result. Wounds involving hair-bearing areas should be repaired if possible to avoid a "bald patch."

The anatomical location of the defect also influences the outcome of healing by second intention. Scars over the chest, shoulders, and back are more likely to be hypertrophic. Wounds on the lower extremities result in scars which stay red or violaceous for many months. In general, wounds on concave surfaces yield a better cosmetic result than those on convex surfaces, especially as regards the nose, periocular area, and ear. Even large wounds of the temple usually heal with excellent cosmetic outcome. The antihelix heals well if cartilage is not removed but heals with a depression if cartilage is removed. This is also true of the rim of the helix. Preauricular and postauricular wounds usually do well. Wounds of the ala crease and nasolabial fold usually heal with a good cosmetic outcome; however, if the wound impinges on the alar rim or involves a major portion of the ala, retraction and notching of the rim may occur (Fig. 6). If the wound involves both the nasolabial fold and cheek, webbing and blunting of the nasolabial fold may occur. Deep wounds on the convex surface of the distal nose/tip often heal with a depressed scar but may heal as a hypertrophic or flat scar (Fig. 7). Wounds of the forehead usually heal with a cosmetically acceptable scar; however, the convex surfaces of the cheeks and chin may heal as hypertrophic stellate scars or depressed scars. Large wounds of the forehead which impinge on the eyebrow may result in elevation of the eyebrow when healed.

In the inner canthus, if the wound lies equidistant above and below the medial canthal ligament, the wound heals with excellent cosmesis and no distortion of the lids. However, if the wound is asymmetric in relation to the medial canthal ligament, lid distortion may occur. If the medial canthal ligament is transected during MMS, a suture should be placed in the lids and anchored to the nasal bone to maintain the proper position during healing. If a full-thickness defect is created in the lower lid because of wound contracture and a hammocklike effect, the lid usually heals without ectropion. However, if only a partial-thickness wound is present, ectropion may result if the wound is allowed to heal by second intention (Fig. 8). Partial- and full-thickness defects of the upper lid usually require repair. Wounds of the nasal root, if left to heal on their own, often result in webbing. Wounds of the cheek located beneath the inferior orbital rim usually do not result in ectropion. Wounds of the mucous membranes usually heal well by second intention. Since wounds in the periocular area and those impinging on the vermilion may result in ectropion and eclabium, they should either be repaired or, if allowed to heal by second intention, guiding sutures should be placed to redirect the forces of wound contracture and prevent this complication [26]. Not only is an ectropion unsightly, it may lead to epiphora and exposure keratitis.

Wound contracture and loss of support in deep wounds of the ala results in prolapse of the nasal mucosa. Not only does this cause the patient anguish in terms of believing the tumor is returning, but it also may interfere with breathing.

Through-and-through defects of the cheeks and lip require repair to avoid fistula formation.

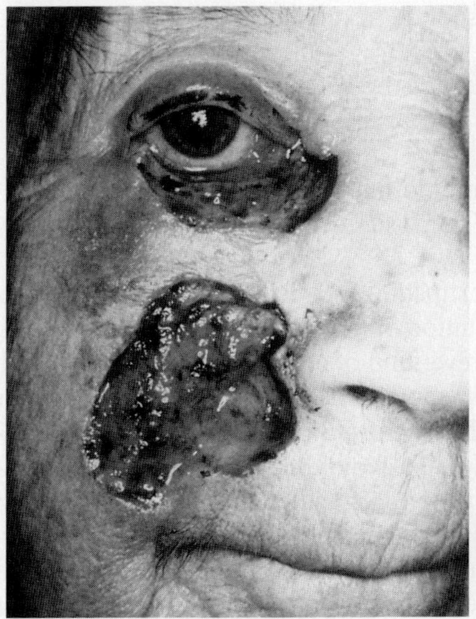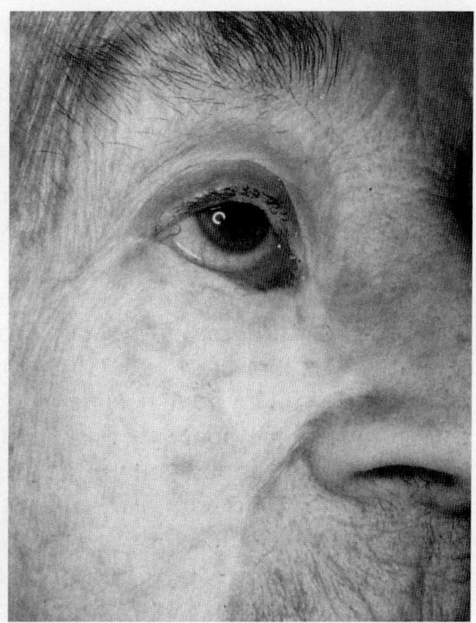

Fig. 8 a, b. MMS defect of the lower lid Ectropin which resulted when the wound was allowed to heal by second intention

Large wounds of the ear involving the external auditory canal or circumferential wounds of the canal usually require grafting to prevent stenosis [27]. However, Larson [28] has reported the prolonged use (6 months) of a hydroxylated, polyvinyl acetal wick to prevent stenosis when the wound is allowed to heal by second intention.

Depressed scars resulting from healing by second intention may be improved by the injection of bovine collagen [29], Fibrel [30], or autologous fat [31]. Dermabrasion also may be helpful.

Healing by second intention is an excellent means of wound management especially in the infirm, in situations in which outlying disconnected foci of tumor may be present, or in patients who are not certain that they want to undergo additional surgery to reconstruct a defect. If careful attention is paid to patient and wound selection, good to excellent cosmetic results are often achieved. However, even under the best of circumstances, the cosmetic outcome occasionally proves unsatisfactory. In these instances if after 1 year there has not been significant improvement, scar revision may be performed.

Special Anatomical Considerations

Penis. Unique complications and sequelae resulting from MMS include
a) paraphimosis which may require surgical intervention to prevent strangulation and necrosis of the penis;
b) urinary obstruction which requires catheterization;

c) urethral structure which usually responds to dilatation;
d) perforation of the urethra;
e) angulation of the penis and deviation of the urinary stream; and
f) painful intercourse.

Vulva. If the urethra is involved by tumor, urinary incontinence or urethral stenosis may be a consequence of MMS. Vaginal stenosis and dyspareunia also may occur following MMS.

Anus. Anal stricture with resultant constipation and rectal pain may be a sequela of MMS. Strictures may respond to dilatation or may require surgical correction.

Eye. The occurrence, sequelae and prevention of ectropion are covered above in the section on "Wound healing" and are not discussed further. However, other complications may arise as a result of MMS in the periocular area. One such complication is inadvertent damage to the eye. To avoid this, eye shields may be utilized [6, 32, 33]. This requires the use of a topical anesthetic which interferes with the corneal reflex; thus, the eye needs to be patched postoperatively until the corneal reflex returns [33]. At times the lacrimal system must be violated to rid a patient of their tumor. However, inadvertent damage should be avoided, and if there is minimal damage, an attempt should be made to preserve the system. Robinson [34] has described the use of a Johnson wire to avoid damage to the lacrimal ducts. If the lacrimal canaliculi are lacerated, a silicone tube can be inserted to preserve the duct [34, 35], and if not badly damaged, the lacrimal system may be repaired. In those cases in which it cannot be repaired a Jones tube can later be placed to drain the tears. The usual consequence of the loss of the lacrimal system is epiphora, which may be annoying and interfere with vision. However, in older patients, who often have minimal tear production, tearing may not be a problem.

In extirpating a tumor in the periocular area it may be necessary to remove a portion of the lid (or lids). Since the eyelids provide protection and lubrication for the eye, it is necessary to make sure that the eye is kept moist; otherwise, exposure keratitis may develop [36, 37]. If the lid defect is small, keeping the eye lubricated with artificial tears and an ointment such as Lacrilube is adequate. For larger defects, plastic film in conjunction with a topical antibiotic and eye pad may be used. This may be left in place for 12 h at a time. If a significant portion of the eyelid(s) has been removed, a temporary tarsorrhaphy may be required to protect the eye. If not enough eyelid remains to cover the eye, a bubble (moisture chamber) may be placed over the eye after an antibiotic ointment has been applied. This may be left in place for at least 12 h. Consultation with an ophthalmologist/oculoplastic surgeon should be sought if there is a significant defect to make sure the eye is adequately protected.

Tumor Implantation

Although the actual risk of tumor implantation is not known, it is best when dealing with tumors such as squamous cell carcinoma and melanoma to presume that it can occur [7]. Therefore, regional or field blocks rather than local infiltration should be utilized to avoid inoculating tumor cells deeper with a needle. Instruments should be cleansed and scalpel blades changed frequently during surgery. In removing the obvious tumor, an attempt should be made not to cut through tumor. At the completion of surgery, the wound may be cauterized with dichloracetic acid or irrigated with saline to destroy or remove any free-floating tumor cells.

The use of the fixed-tissue technique is another method of avoiding this potential complication.

Summary

Despite the advanced years of some of our patients and the size of the defects created by MMS, the procedure is relatively free of complications. Complications can best be avoided by appropriate planning, consultation, anticipation, and attention to details. Despite our best efforts, however, complications may still arise. When they do, the surgeon performing MMS should be available, attentive, supportive, and prepared to deal quickly and effectively with the problem. Consultation should be sought when appropriate. This approach minimizes the patient's anxiety and prevents further and possibly more serious harm and discomfort to him.

References

1. Lang PG Jr, Osguthorpe JD (1989) Indications and limitations of Mohs micrographic surgery. Dermatol Clin 7:627–644
2. Salasche SJ (1986) Acute surgical complications: cause, prevention and treatment. J Am Acad Dermatol 15:1163–1185
3. Lang PG Jr (1989) Mohs micrographic surgery. Fresh-tissue technique. Dermatol Clin 7:613–626
4. Braun M III (1981) The case for Mohs surgery by the fixed-tissue technique. J Dermatol Surg Oncol 7:634–640
5. Mohs FE (1978) Chemosurgical techniques. In: Chemosurgery. Microscopically controlled surgery for skin cancer. Thomas, Springfield, pp 7–29
6. Bailin PL, Ratz J, Wheeland RG (1988) Mohs micrographic surgery technique. In: Roenigk RK, Roenigk HH Jr (eds) Dermatologic surgery. Principles and practice. Dekker, New York, pp 833–852
7. Larson PO (1991) Surgical complications. In: Mikhail GR (ed) Mohs micrographic surgery. Saunders, Philadelphia, pp 193–206
8. Halpern AC, Leyden JJ, Dzubow LM et al. (1988) The incidence of bacteremia in skin surgery of the head and neck. J Am Acad Dermatol 19:112–116
9. Sabetta JB, Zitelli JA (1987) The incidence of bacteremia during skin surgery. Arch Dermatol 123:213–215
10. Stewart JH, Cole GW, Klein JA (1989) Neutralized lidocaine with epinephrine for local anesthesia. J Dermatol Surg Oncol 15:1081–1083
11. Glinert RJ, Zachary CB (1991) Local anesthetic allergy. Its recognition and avoidance. J Dermatol Surg Oncol 17:491–496
12. Bennett RG (1988) Anesthesia. In: Fundamentals of cutaneous surgery. Mosby, St. Louis, pp 194–239

13. Bennett RG (1988) Electrosurgery. In: Fundamentals of cutaneous surgery. Mosby, St. Louis, pp 553–590
14. Noel SB, Scallan P, Meadors MC et al. (1989) Treatment of Pseudomonas aeruginosa auricular perichondritis with oral ciprofloxacin. J Dermatol Surg Oncol 15:633–637
15. Gette MT, Marks JG Jr, Maloney ME (1991) Incidence of postoperative allergic contract dermatitis to topical antibiotics. Annual Meeting of the American College of Mohs Micrographic Surgery and Cutaneous Oncology, March 11–13, Orlando
16. Katz BE, Fischer AA (1987) J Am Acad Dermatol 17:1016–1024
17. Gaspari AA, d'Aubermont PC, Bennett RG (1984) Delayed extensor tendon rupture. A complication of Mohs surgery. J Dermatol Surg Oncol 10:721–723
18. Bernstein G (1989) Healing by secondary intention. Dermatol Clin 7:645–660
19. Zitelli JA (1983) Wound healing by secondary intention. A cosmetic appraisal. J Am Acad Dermatol 9:407–415
20. Hein NT, Prawer SE, Katz HI (1988) Facilitated wound healing using transparent film dressing following Mohs micrographic surgery. Arch Dermatol 124:903–906
21. Synder PA, Alper JC, Albom JM (1984) Osteomyelitis complicating Mohs chemosurgery. J Am Acad Dermatol 11:513–516
22. Vanderveen EE, Stoner JG, Swanson NA (1983) Chiseling of the exposed bone to stimulate granulation tissue after Mohs surgery. J Dermatol Surg Oncol 9:925–928
23. Mohs FE (1985) Avoidance of osteomyelitis after Mohs surgery. J Am Acad Dermatol 12:726–727
24. Latenser J, Snow SN, Mohs FE et al. (1991) Power tools to fenestrate exposed bone to stimulate wound healing. J Dermatol Surg Oncol 17:265–270
25. Bailin PL, Wheeland RG (1985) Carbon dioxide (CO_2) laser perforation of exposed cranial bone to stimulate granulation tissue. Plast Reconstr Surg 75:898–902
26. Albright SD (1981) Placement of guiding sutures to counteract undesirable retraction of tissues in and around functionally and cosmetically important structures. J Dermatol Surg Oncol 7:446–449
27. Buecker JW, Phelan JT (1986) Carcinoma of the external auditory canal. Removal and prevention of stenosis. J Dermatol Surg Oncol 12:598–600
28. Larson PO (1987) Stenosis of the external ear canal: prevention using hydroxylated polyvinyl acetal wicks. J Dermatol Surg Oncol 13:1121–1123
29. Bailin PL, Bailin MD (1988) Collagen implantation: clinical applications and lesion selection. J Dermatol Surg Oncol 14 Suppl 1:21–26
30. Millikan L, Multicenter Study Group (1989) Long-term safety and efficacy with Fibrel in the treatment of cutaneous scars – results of a multicenter study. J Dermatol Surg Oncol 15:837–842
31. Hambley RM, Carruthers A (1991) Microlipoinjection for elevation of depressed full-thickness skin grafts on the nose. Annual Meeting of the American College of Mohs Micrographic Surgery and Cutaneous Oncology, March 11–13, Orlando
32. Rabinovitz HS, Epstein G (1985) The corneal shield. J Dermatol Surg Oncol 11:207–208
33. Wheeland RG, Bailin PL, Ratz JL et al. (1987) Use of scleral eye shields for periorbital laser surgery. J Dermatol Surg Oncol 13:156–158
34. Robinson JK (1983) Prevention of intraoperative trauma of the lacrimal system. J Dermatol Surg Oncol 9:802–804
35. Dortzbach RK, Angrist RA (1985) Silicone intubation for lacerated lacrimal canaliculi. Ophthalmic Surg 16:639–642
36. Baylis HI, Cies WA (1975) Complications of Mohs chemosurgical excision of eyelid and canthal tumors. Am J Ophthalmol 80:116–122
37. Whitaker DC, Goldstein GD, Birkby CS et al. (1988) Post-operative techniques for corneal protection in Mohs micrographic surgery. J Dermatol Surg Oncol 14:951–955

Fusiform Excision with Primary Closure

MARWALI HARAHAP

Fusiform excision with primary closure is usually best suited for removal of relatively small lesions which are in an area where the resulting edges are easily approximated.

Dermal nevi, verrucous nevi, and basal cell carcinoma of the face are among the most frequently scheduled. Most of these lesions are excised in a fusiform pattern following the relaxed skin tension lines. In excising the fusiform, significant anatomical landmarks must be considered and not distorted by the closure. The length-to-width ratio of the excision is approximately 4:1 to allow for a smooth closure at the ends. The local tissue also determines to some extent the amount of standing cone or "dog ear" that occurs.

Complications in fusiform excision with primary closure are regrettably common but are in large part preventable. These include infection, bleeding and hematoma formation, dehiscence, and unsightly scar.

Wound Infection

It is important to differentiate wound infection from wound inflammation. Wound inflammation is characterized by mild, nonprogressive erythema in a narrow margin about a wound. It is often a benign process characteristic of the healing wound and resolves spontaneously, or it may be the result of suture tension as the skin edges swell postoperatively and subsiding as the swelling regresses. Other wound inflammation occurring because of collection of pus at the point of entry or exit of a suture (i. e., stitch abscess) is not a generalized wound infection.

Wound infection is characterized by discharge of pus with pain or redness in the scar, swelling, and throbbing in the wound. It is often surrounded by cellulitis, induration, lymphangitis or lymphadenopathy, and possibly even tissue necrosis. It may or may not be accompanied by fever and general malaise.

Causes of Wound Infection

General Risk Factors

The general risk factors which predispose to infective complications include diabetes mellitus and corticosteroid therapy. Diabetes mellitus is the most common condition that may be attented by retarded or poor healing of wounds due to impaired carbohydrate and fat metabolism [1]. The anti-inflammatory, anti-proliferative, immunosuppressive, and vasoconstrictive properties of corticosteroids would cause impairment of the healing process and increased susceptibility to infection [2]. Cytotoxic drugs may cause poor healing and are associated with infection, probably because of immunosuppression [3]. Experience in surgery has demonstrated that conditions which render wound hematoma more likely such as extreme obesity, bleeding disorders, and old age also increase the risk of surgical infection [4]. Malnutrition, particularly protein deficiency and calorie undernutrition, seriously hampers the patient's ability to mount a substantial antibacterial effect [5]. As a result, patients with protein deficiency may be at higher risk for wound infection. Vitamin deficiencies can have a similar effect, and vitamins A and C in particular are associated with natural immunity [6, 7].

Certain anatomic regions are more prone to infection. Perianal procedures are contaminated, and the moist environment of groins or axillae makes surgical wound more likely to become infected. Wound infection is found less frequently in the head and neck regions and on the hand because of the rich blood supplies of these areas.

Patient and Hospital Staff

Adjacent skin infection in proximity to the cutaneous lesion to be excised is readily detected.

Patients and hospital staff with active infections such as furuncles, carbuncles, dermatitis, psoriasis, draining sinuses, osteomyelitis, hydradenitis, ulcers of the skin, and unhealed wounds may be identified. Less obvious is that the patient himself and the hospital staff may be symptomless carriers of such bacteria as *Staphylococcus aureus* or may indeed be incubating a streptococcal throat infection. They present special risks in the airborne contamination of surgical wounds.

Approximately one-third of patients on admission and about one-half of hospital staff are carriers of *Staphylococcus aureus* [8]. The surgeon and his scrubbed assistants contribute to the bacterial contamination of the operating room, and they present the added risk to the patient of direct bacterial inoculation of surgical incision. Fortunately, this mode of wound contamination appears to be an unusual cause of wound infection, although it has been shown that wet operating gowns permit the transfer of bacteria from the surgeon's skin, and that 25% of surgeon's gloves are perforated by the end of the surgical operation [9].

Organisms

Most bacteria recovered from surgical wounds are opportunist pathogens. They are commensal organisms normally found in the hollow viscera or the skin surface, and they give rise to wound infections when inoculated in the wound in sufficient number. A minority of surgical wound infections are caused by pathogenic bacteria, and most of these are staphylococcal [10]. Wound infection by hemolytic streptococci *(Streptococcus pyogenes)* is less common than staphylococcal infection, and it is encountered chiefly in plastic surgery [11].

Wound infections in clean surgery generally appear from the 4th or 5th postoperative days, except in the head and neck where more rapid healing is ensured by the rich blood supply.

The development of wound infection depends on the extent of contamination, virulence of the organism, and existence of the correct conditions for multiplication or spread. However, the pathogenesis of wound infection is not determined simply by the degree of wound contamination. Evidence indicates that the physiological state of tissues within the wound is more important than the mere presence of bacteria.

Surgical Technique

Any local factor which interferes with the blood supply affects the local inflammatory response and favors bacterial growth. This may occur in several ways: extensive tissue destruction in traumatic wounds or tissue necrosis either by rough handling of the tissues, strangulation of tissues during the knotting of ligatures, or excessive use of surgical diathermy. Other local factors which affect the host resistance are hematomas, seromas, and foreign bodies. Poor surgical technique which results in an inaccurate hemostasis, retained blood clots, and a collection of serum in the wound play an important role in the development of bacterial infection. The most common foreign bodies are sutures. Generally, bulky braided suture materials are more likely to cause trouble than monofilament sutures. The use of mass ligatures or exposure of the wound to drying or pressure from retractors invites infection.

Wound Drainage

Wound drains also behave as foreign bodies in surgical wounds, and they may adversely effect host defenses. The use of drains is indicated to facilitate the drainage of blood, serum, or potentially infective material that are anticipated postoperatively.

Drains may be open or closed. In open drainage the wound is protected only by wound dressings, and secondary infection of the wound may occur through the drain site. In closed drainage the drain is connected to a collecting receptacle, and drainage may be aided by the use of vacuum suction; the risk of secondary infection is reduced.

Duration of Operation

As the duration of operation increases, a progressive increase in the infection rate generally can be expected. This is because the dose of bacterial contamination increases with time, wound cells are damaged by drying and retraction, and increased amounts of suture material and electrocoagulation reduce the resistance to infection. Moreover, longer procedures are more likely to be associated with blood loss and shock, thereby reducing the general resistance of the patient.

Prevention of Wound Infection

General Risk factors

A number of measures should be considered in the preoperative period for the prevention of postoperative infections in patients scheduled for elective surgical procedures. To achieve this goal the following methods are possible: controlling the patient's weight, identifying and treating established infection, correcting malnutrition, treating associated noninfectious conditions, and maintaining general cleanliness.

In obese patients preparing for elective surgery, it may be advisable to return the patient to acceptable weight prior to operation. Severe obesity was found to be associated with an increased postoperative infection rate of 18.1% [12].

The presence of any skin infection close to the lesion to be excised should be identified and treated. Any other active infection should be searched for and recognized prior to operation. These infections may be entirely unrelated to the disease of concern, but they may contribute to the risk of operave wound infection if unrecognized and untreated. The presence of an acute upper respiratory tract infection, chronic ear infections, furuncles, carbuncles and impetigo, chronic dermatologic disease, draining sinuses are strong reasons to consider deferring elective operations until control of such infections is accomplished. If the lesion to be excised is already infected, and surgery is essential, pus should be submitted for bacteriological examination by smear, culture and sensitivity.

For the malnourished patient, improvement in his state of nutrition is mandatory prior to elective surgery, as host resistance to infection may be impaired by protein and calorie undernutrition and vitamin deficiencies. Restoration of nutrition can rapidly bolster the patient's metabolic needs and increase resistance to bacteria.

Associated noninfectious conditions such as diabetes mellitus, uremia and cirrhosis require correction and treatment.

It is important to remove any dirt or soilage from the body surface through bathing, with special attention being given to the hair, fingernails, and toenails. A significant measure of benefit may also be gained by showering with antiseptic soap or hexachlorophene soap before the operation.

Hair at the Operation Site

There is considerable debate about the most appropriate method of dealing with hair in the area of the proposed operative incision. Seropian and Reynold in 1971 reported that the postoperative wound infection rate was 5.6% in those shaved with a razor, 0.6% in those not saved, and 0.6% in those in whom hair was removed by a depilatory cream [13]. Alexander et al. [14] in 1983 compared the influence of razor shaving and of clipping on the incidence of postoperative wound infection; they concluded that clipping the morning of operation is the preferred method [14].

If the hairs is to be removed, it should be done with care, avoiding iatrogenic skin trauma or irritation. Shaving or clipping may produce multiple superficial lesions containing exuded tissue fluids that favor or contain bacterial growth. The alternatives are shaving or clipping immediately prior to the time of the operation and the use of a depilatory cream.

Prophylactic Antibiotics

The routine use of prophylactic antibiotics is not indicated in all patients undergoing clean surgery but is recommended for patients who are known to be carriers of pathogenic microorganisms (e. g., nasal carriers), or who have existing infection distant from the operative site. This is also the case for patients with cardiac valve disease, with a foreign body in place (e. g., a pacemaker or artificial joint), or with impaired resistance to infection (e. g., those having diabetes mellitus or glucocorticoid therapy).

Broadly stated, the prophylactic use of an antibiotic is recommended in those preoperative surgical patients in whom the risk of postoperative wound infection is great, or in whom the consequences of each infection would be grave.

Prophylactic antibiotics are effective when the tissues that are be exposed to lodgment of microorganisms during the surgical procedure have protection against microbial colonization. Starting sometime after the operation has no value. Antibiotics should be initiated 1–2 h prior to operation to achieve adequate tissue levels in the incision. It need not be continued for more than 4 days after the operation, by which time the contaminating organisms should have been destroyed. Short-term antibiotic therapy is preferable as it is less likely to result in the emergence of antibiotic-resistant strains of hospital bacteria [15].

The indiscriminate use of prophylactic antibiotics must be avoided; it may do harm by creating the uncontrolled growth of resistant organisms, creating a false sense of security with resultant relaxation of aseptic precautions, the probability of side effects of the drug, and the additional cost to the patient.

The use of prophylactic antibiotics are not substitutes for careful surgical technique, which includes gentleness, preservation of vascularity, hemostasis, removal of devascularized tissue and foreign particles, anatomic closure without tension or dead space, and careful selection of suture material.

Hospital Staff

Hospial staff harboring pathogenic bacteria present a special hazard, and several outbreaks of staphylococcal wound infection have been attributed to this source [16, 17].

Staff with infected wounds or bacterial illness such as tonsillitis should be excluded from the operating room and from any contact with the hospital patient until a check by appropriate bacteriological swab has confirmed cure by either local or systemic treatment.

Movement, conversation, and sneezing in the operating room should be minimal. The more talking, the more frequent are coughing and sneezing, and the more movement, the greater the dissemination of bacteria. Any breach of personal hygiene should be recognized and corrected as soon as possible by changing gloves, recleansing, or redraping as required. If an unusual number of "cluster" of infections occur in patients, especially by the same organism, the appropriate staff should be temporarily restricted from contact with patients, clinical examination and bacteriological investigations by swabs of nares and fauces should be performed, and effective treatment must be given.

Facilities

The optimum environment for surgery is an operating room with plenum air ventilation, designed to minimize contamination, and minimum personnel traffic and thorough cleansing of the walls, floors and other surfaces between operations. The ideal environment is difficult to achieve and maintain in the major surgical suite, and it is vastly more difficult to achieve high standards of asepsis in the outpatient clinic. A rapid turnover of patients, and a relatively high incidence of contaminated wound and abscesses are factors which reduce the opportunity to maintain rigid control of environmental contamination in outpatient operations. In practice many minor surgical procedures are performed in a section of the outpatient department with the surgeon often operating in normal outdoor clothes. It is perhaps remarkable that with such facilities the incidence of infection is not increased. Presumably this is due to the use of non touch technique and to the very short duration of the operation. Although compromises become necessary, the surgeon should always endeavor to maintain as wide a field of sterility about his patient as possible.

Whenever the skin lesion requires more than a short procedure, every effort should be made to maintain an optimum environment for elective procedures in clean cases. It may be best to establish one operating room further from the entrance for elective outpatient surgery.

Duration of Operation

Prolonged duration of the procedure, in the range of 3 h, increases risk of infection and decreases the value of prophylactic antibiotics [18, 19].

Surgical Technique

Wherever the operation is performed, normal precautions of skin cleansing and draping are essential. For surgical procedure on the face, a scalp shampoo, oral hygiene, and removal of all cosmetics are routine. A male patient is preferably clean shaven on the morning of surgery. When the procedure is to be performed on the trunk or extremities, a shower bath before leaving home is advisable. Current practice requires the surgeon to scrub his hands, fingernails, and arms meticulously, using an appropriate degerming method immediately prior to the operation. The purpose is to reduce the bacterial population to the vanishing point, with reasonable assurance that it will remain miniscule during the operation. If a tear or puncture develops in the gloves, bacterial contamination of the wound should be minimal.

The surgical gloves are useful in preventing the transfer of organisms to or from the wearer. Surgical gloves are often perforated [20, 21]. There was no evidence that perforations increased the number of wound infection, but exposes surgeons to infections from patients [22]. Dermatological surgeons should consider the incidence of glove perforation when planning surgeries on patients with infectious diseases. Recent concern about transmission of deadly infective viruses has emphasized the use of intact surgical gloves for the protection of operating personnel. Specialized infectious disease precautions plus the use of double gloves and gown, one on top of the other, may be appropriate for operations on HIV-infected patients [23].

On the operating table, the operative area should be cleansed initially with soap or a nonirritating detergent solution. A degerming agent should then be applied. Degerming agents commonly used include iodine solutions, chlorhexidine, alcohol, quarternary ammonium compounds, and hexachlorophene. Appropriate draping should be used as a means of demarcating, maintaining, and protecting a limited area prepared for the operation by cleansing and degerming techniques.

Meticulous surgical technique is crucial to the prevention of postoperative wound sepsis. Although ample evidence shows that the number of bacteria involved play an important role in the development of bacterial infection, equally impressive evidence reveals that injury and hypoxia are also of crucial importance in the creation of bacterial infection. The exact number of bacteria needed to create a suppurative lesion varies according to the physiological state of the tissue. Therefore, incomplete hemostasis, retained blood clots, and necrotic or traumatized tissue can allow small numbers of contaminating organisms to create a suppurative wound.

Meticulous surgical technique is aimed at avoidance of tissue damage caused by mechanical injury or ischemia. Rough handling of tissues, ligatures or large "bites" of tissues, excessive pressure and tension from retractors impair circulation and predispose to bacterial colonization. Necrotic tissue or foreign substances must be avoided. Complete hemostasis reduces hematoma formation and minimizes tissue damage and is therefore indispensable. Tissues should be handled gently. The use of toothed forceps and clamps is kept to a minimum. Rough and prolonged retraction should be avoided. Fine skin hooks, used carefully, provide adequate exposure. If the electrocoagulator is used, the production of numerous areas of necrotic tissue [24] should be prevented, since these areas are more susceptible to bacterial growth and infection.

Thoughtful selection of suture material is required to reduce tissue damage and the quantity of foreign material left in a wound. Sutures should be used to approximate tissue accurately without causing strangulation. The types of sutures, their spacing, the depth of "bites" taken, and the degree of tension necessary to bring tissues into apposition are especially important. For skin closure, monofilament such as nylon is preferred to braided material such as silk. The finest gauge compatible with the wound should be used, ranging from 6/0 or 5/0 on the face to 5/0 or 4/0 elsewhere.

If meticulously adhered to, these principles of surgical technique provide a surgical incision with maximum resistance against bacterial invasion.

Accurate anatomic reconstruction of the wound is essential to the success of primary closure. If repair of the incision restores proper anatomic relationships and does not create spaces for the collection of blood or serum, healing proceeds at an optimal rate, and the risk of infection is minimal. Any factor that delays wound healing increases the risk of bacterial infection.

In postoperative management, local dressings, immobilization, prevention of venous or lymphatic congestion by elevation of the extremity and proper shielding of the wound from environmental bacteria continues to be important in preventing wound infection [25].

Management of Wound Infection

Where changes are limited to stitch abscess, a watching policy can be adopted. If erythema alone is present, simple observation is sufficient unless symptoms are severe. The peak incidence of the onset of symptoms and signs of wound infection occurs 5–10 days after surgery. The patient may complain of increasing discomfort or pain in the surgical incision. Fever may be present. On examination of the wound the skin is swollen and red, the wound is tender on palpation, and a purulent discharge may be present. It is sometimes necessary to remove the skin sutures, gently separate the edges of the skin incision with a sinus forceps, and probe the wound to encourage discharge of pus from the subcutaneous tissue (Fig. 1).

The wound should be irrigated to remove all debris. Warmed normal saline is often used, but where there is debris and slough, the bubbling action of hydrogen peroxide is particularly effective. Any resultant slough should be removed with forceps, for which process adequate analgesia is required. Most wounds clean very nicely with simpler dressings of saline. In general terms, the management of the infected wound adheres to the principles of free drainage, mechanical cleansing, and wet dressings to promote the separation of slough and the ingrowth of healthy granulation tissue.

Any pus obtained should be submitted immediately for bacteriological investigation. The contaminating organism must be isolated and identified by Gram-stained smear and culture. Microscopic examination of the Gram-stained direct smear is easy, inexpensive, and rapid, and it gives immediate information that is valuable as a guide to therapy until the results of cultures indicate the adjustments that should be made for maximum antibacterial effect. Its antibiotic sensitivity pattern must be determined and an appropriate antibiotic therapy selected.

To be effective in the treatment of wound infection [26] the antibiotic must be active against the infecting organism in a concentration that is bactericidal or bacteriostatic. Moreover, in achieving effective antimicrobial therapy contact

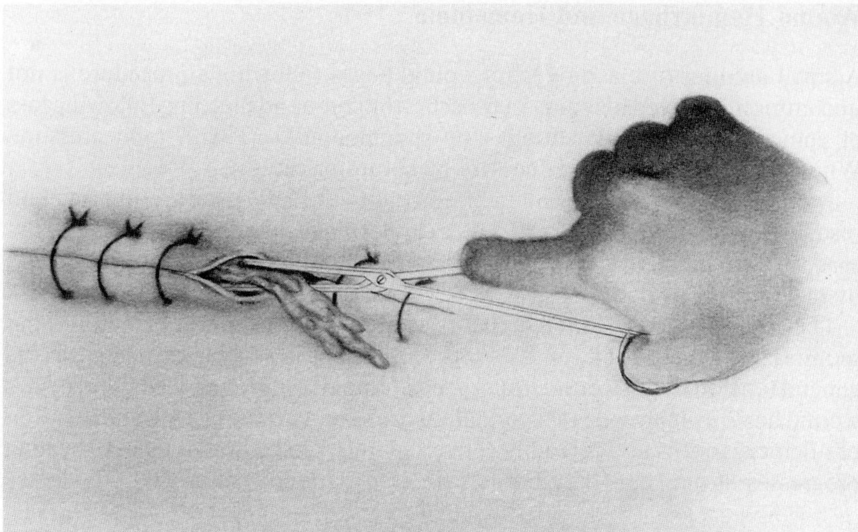

Fig. 1. After removing the skin sutures, the edges of the skin incision are gently separated with sinus forceps of hemostat and the wound probed to encourage discharge of pus

between microorganisms and an adequate amount of drug is one of the cardinal tenets. The method of administration and the route which the drug travels to make this contact are of importance. There should be no substance present that can inhibit action of the drug where its effect is desired; for example, the penicillins are inhibited by penicillinase and the cephalosporins and the sulfonamides by para-aminobenzoic acid. The drug should be relatively free from untoward consequences of therapy and the surgeon must be prepared to recognize and treat the unfavorable side effects promptly. Unsatisfactory response during treatment must be evaluated so that drug therapy can be tailored to the changing needs of the individual patient. Antibiotics are simply adjuncts to host resistance and surgical drainage; they do not replace them.

While localized reddening of the skin around the edges of an infected wound is not uncommon, a spreading cellulitis is unusual. Only certain bacterial species (B-hemolytic streptococcus and some staphylococci) usually spread through tissue as extending cellulitis. The constitutional symptom is usually mild, but the local manifestations are pain and local tenderness, swelling, and redness, without suppuration. Infections involving the extremities may have evidence of an associated lymphangitis.

Rest is an important element in the treatment of cellulitis. Penicillin should be given intravenously or by intramuscular injection on the assumption that the bacterial organism most likely to produce the classic picture of cellulitis is the hemolytic streptococcus. If this is the case, complete resolution of the symptoms and signs may be anticipated. For other bacterial species the choice of antibiotic is not as clearcut, and identification of the organism and its antibiotic sensitivity is required for effective therapy.

Wound Hemorrhage and Hematoma

A small amount of bleeding from wound edges following a procedure is not uncommon. Delayed bleeding may occur from rebound bleeding following loss of epinephrine effect. It should stop spontaneously or with mild pressure. Where it persists, it requires control by suture or cautery.

A smaller degree of self-limited bleeding into the soft tissue around a wound results in areas of ecchymosis, as does a similar small degree of bleeding into the space of a wound. Ordinarily they are not troublesome and do not require treatment.

The accumulation of blood in the space of a wound results in hematoma and requires immediate attention, as it acts disastrously in several ways. It raises the general tension of the wound, causes separation of the wound walls, and delays wound healing. It provides a favorable environment for the growth and invasion of microorganisms and is readily converted into a collection of pus. As healing progresses, it may become fibrotic with scar tissue formation [27].

Causes of Wound Hemorrhage and Hematoma

Wound hemorrhage occurs most frequently in patients with rebound bleeding following loss of epinephrin effect or patients with hypertension or hemorrhagic disorders. Other frequent contributing causes are drug-induced coagulopathy (aspirin, sodium warfarin), excessive motion, retching, and cough. Massive hematoma is often the result of bleeding from one or more vessels of significant size which have slipped their ties or sloughed their cauterized ends. This form of bleeding usually occurs within the first 2 days after operation. In late developing hematomas bleeding is usually caused by trauma in the form of a blow or bump to the operative site.

Prevention of Wound Hemorrhage and Hematoma

Every effort should be made to obtain complete hemostasis at the time of operation. Blood vessels of large caliber should be ligated with the finest appropriate material or coagulated with fine-pointed forceps and cautery, with as little adjacent tissue as possible. Electrocoagulation may be accomplished by either monopolar or bipolar modes [28]. Dead space should be avoided. Pressure dressing, when properly executed, controls capillary bleeding but does not occlude circulation. The use of drains with or without suction helps to prevent the development of hematoma.

Most hemorrhagic disorders of significance can be suspected from a careful history and physical examination [29]. Particular attention should be directed to episodes of bleeding, such as a complication of previous surgery or injury, hemorrhagic symptoms in other members of the family, and the ingestion of medications known to influence hemostasis adversely [30], including aspirin, oral anticoagulants, phenylbutazone, and indomethacin.

Assessment of the number of circulating platelets should also be included in the routine preoperative evaluation. Examination of a stained blood smear is sufficient for this assessment; six to ten platelets per high-power field are usually visible.

A carefully taken history and physical examination suggest the presence of an underlying bleeding disorder. This suggestion should lead to hematological consultation and precise diagnosis.

Management of Wound Hemorrhage and Hematoma

An expanding wound hematoma must be promptly evacuated. This may necessitate taking down all sutures and reopening the wound under sterile conditions to locate and ligate the bleeding vessel. The blood clot should then be evacuated and irrigated with sterile saline. Unless there is definite proof of infection, wounds from which hematoma have been evacuated should be resutured.

A small hematoma may be evacuated by removing one or two sutures from one end of the incision and inserting a sterile grooved director or hemostat until its tip reaches the center of the hematoma. A firm rolling motion of a sponge direct the blood toward the opening in the incision (Fig. 2). This motion is repeated until all vestiges of liquid or clotted blood are expressed through the newly created tract [31].

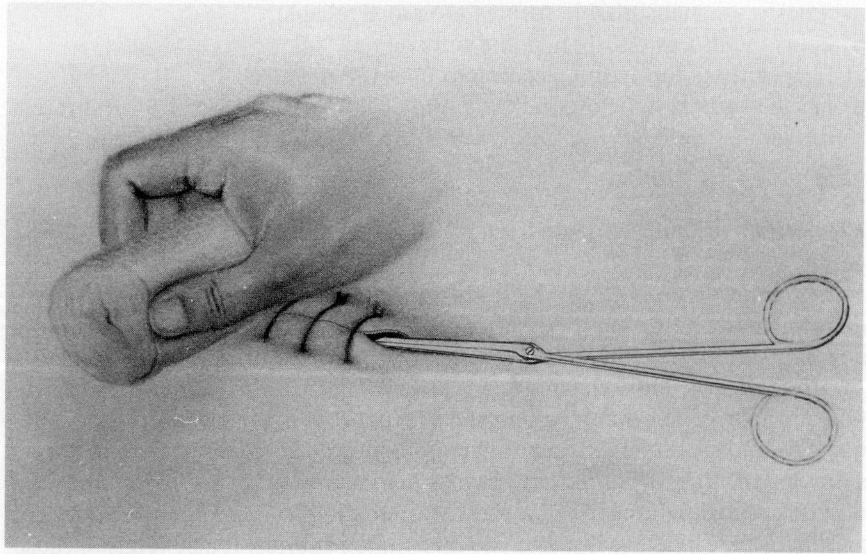

Fig. 2. A sterile hemostat has been inserted until its tip reaches the center of the hematoma. A firm rolling motion of a sponge directs the blood toward the opening in the end of the incision

A valuable alternative method of managing the situation is to await natural liquefaction of the clot, which usually takes about 10 days. A stab wound is made with a number 11 blade, followed by "milking" out of the clot. Such a stab wound should be placed in a relaxed skin tension line.

Wound Dehiscence

Wound dehiscence is a partial or total disruption of the operative wound. It represents failure of the wound to gain sufficient strength to withstand stress placed upon it. Although wound dehiscence may occur at any time following wound closure, it occurs most commonly by the 5th – 8th postoperative days.

Causes of Wound Dehiscence

Systemic risk factors contribute to the development of this complication. It is more common in patients with diabetes mellitus, in obese patients, in elderly debilitated patients with poor nutrition, and in those receiving corticosteroids. Overwhelming force breaks sutures, such as unexpected and uncontrolled movement, for example, coughing, sneezing, vomiting, or a fall.

Local factors predisposing to wound dehiscence are: hemorrhage, infection, and technical errors. The most frequent technical errors leading to dehiscence are:
a) sutures too weak and break, for example, absorbable sutures dissolve too quickly – nonabsorbable sutures are more reliable;
b) knots in sutures poorly tied and unraveling;
c) tying sutures too tightly, leading to pressure necrosis,
d) placing sutures too close to the wound edge so that the sutures cut through the tissue.

Prevention of Wound Dehiscence

Most wound dehiscence results from technical errors. Prevention of this problem includes performing a neat incision, avoiding devitalization of wound edges by careful handling of the tissues during the operation, placing and tying sutures correctly, and selecting the proper suture material. Careful identification and approximation of the skin and subcutaneous layers is essential for adequate wound closure. It is important to obliterate dead space. The use of buried sutures at the time of wound closure may help to prevent dehiscence at the time of suture removal. Interrupted sutures are preferable. A running suture does not approximate skin as accurately as do interrupted sutures. It also tends to cause ischemia of the skin margins and need only break at one point to jeopardize the entire closure. If the suture is too tight, it surely cuts into the tissue more rapidly. The correct tissue tension just avoids blanching the skin held by the suture.

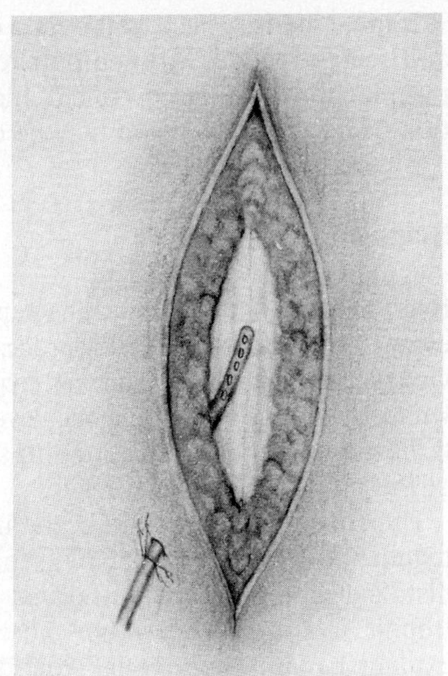

Fig. 3. Drain should be inserted through a separate stab incision so as not to compromise the strength of the main wound

Drains should be brought out through separate stab incisions so as not to compromise the strength of the main wound (Fig. 3). To minimize dehiscence, all wounds are usually supported for 1–2 weeks after suture removal with wound closure tapes.

Extra precautions are necessary to avoid dehiscence in patients with systemic risk factors.

Management of Wound Dehiscence

Wound dehiscence is best managed by prompt elective reclosure of the incision.

If dehiscence of a wound does occur during the first 6 days after closure, assuming there is no infection, it may be safely resutured. Such wound has been shown to gain tensile strength rapidly, as though the wound had not been disrupted [32]. This is thought to be caused by the mobilization of fibroblasts and the production of collagen at the wound edges during the 1st week after wounding.

Trimming or „freshening" of the wound edges may make a slighter neater appearance at first, but the sutures used for resuturing must be left a longer time for adequate healing than if the edges are not trimmed. Trimming of the wound edges abolishes the accelerated increase of tensile strength and is not advisable [33].

Wounds closed after 6 days do not gain tensile strength as rapidly but at about the same rate as if sutured primarily, and the wounds also tend to become infected [34].

If infection is present at the time of dehiscence, it is best to obtain a culture and treat the patient with appropriate antibiotics. Repair should be delayed until the infection has been controlled, and the wound has healed by secondary intention. If necessary, revision may be done at a later time.

Scars and Keloids

Every wound that penetrates the papillary dermis leaves a scar. A scar is the inescapable result of the healing process. It may be a good scar or an ugly scar, obvious or inconspicuous, hairline, hypertrophic, or disabling. A *good scar* is one which is no more than a fine line, level and even with the surrounding surface; it is the same color as the surrounding skin and causes no contracture or distortion of the surrounding structures.

Hypertrophic and keloid scars are two conditions commonly considered together, thus implying that they represent two grades of the same process. The histological appearance on normal microscopy is indeed similar, but hypertrophic scar is limited within the confines of the wound, while keloid scar extends beyond the original wound. Hypertrophic scar seems to stabilize in about 3 months and then gradually softening and tending to regress (Fig. 4), while keloid continues to proliferate for 6 months or more and never regress on its own.

Despite advances in our knowledge of wound healing and advances in surgical techniques, scars remain unpredictable in behavior. Some scars spread, some hypertrophy, and others form keloids.

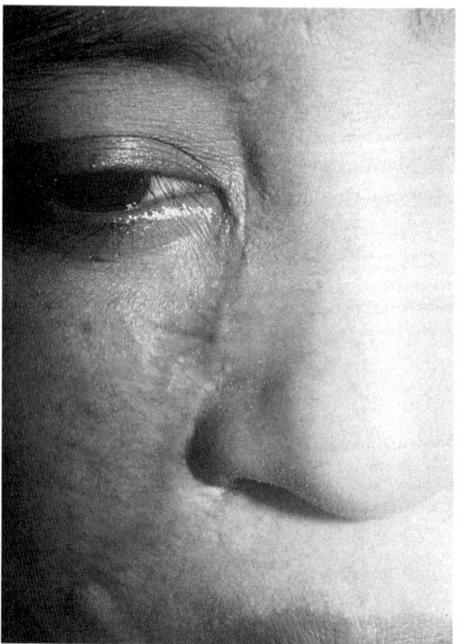

Fig. 4. Hypertrophic facial scar. This gradually softens and regresses

Causes of Unsightly Scars and Keloids

Predisposing Factors

The anatomic sites where unsightly scars most commonly occur are the sternal area, shoulders (deltoid – acromial – scapular), upper back, and chin. Scars in these anatomic regions are apt to spread, as are incisions on the lower extremities. Scars over the lower portion of the nose often become depressed. On the other hand, incisions in the eyelids, penis, scrotum, palms, soles, and mucous membranes leave fine, almost invisible scars [35].

Keloids, although seen most frequently among darkly pigmented races, may be found in susceptible individuals of any race. Older persons tend have less noticeable scars than young adults or children. In children the scars are usually redder and maintain this color longer than comparable scars in elderly patients. This results in poorer looking scars for longer periods of time.

Other Factors

Where relaxed skin tension lines are crossed by incisions, the resulting scars are more prominent and ugly, especially if the joint surface is traversed. A wide and hypertrophic scar may develop in any scar submitted to much skin tension and pull. The farther the scar diverges from the transverse skin tension lines, the greater is its tendency to widen and hypertrophy.

The more oblique the angle of incisions to the skin surface, the greater is the width of the scar on the dermis. The contraction of the dermal scar causes the skin to bulge over it.

The curved or U-shaped incision produces scars notoriously unsightly because it produces the so-called trapdoor deformity.

Surgical technique plays an important role in obtaining the best possible results [36].

Tissue may undergo insults during the wound closure process after being grasped with forceps and closed with tight sutures. Marginal tissues, both skin and subcutaneous, can become anoxic and die, leaving scar tissue in its place.

Failure adequately to close the deeper layers of tissue where a "dead space" may occur can result in the formation of a seroma of hematoma. This is likely to cause wound breakdown (seroma) or organization and fibrosis (hematoma) with scar formation.

Another common mistake is to close a full-thickness wound with only epidermal sutures. After the sutures are removed after the usual 7 days, the wound separates and widens. Excessive tension and ligation of sutures that are too tight increase the risk of a wide scar, as does the use of the larger gauge suture materials. Constriction of the skin by sutures that are too tight causes ischemia and necrosis, with subsequent scar formation and visible suture marks. Sutures which are left in place 14 days caused severe suture marks (Fig. 5).

As discussed above, any infection in the wound results in an unsightly wide scar after healing by second intention.

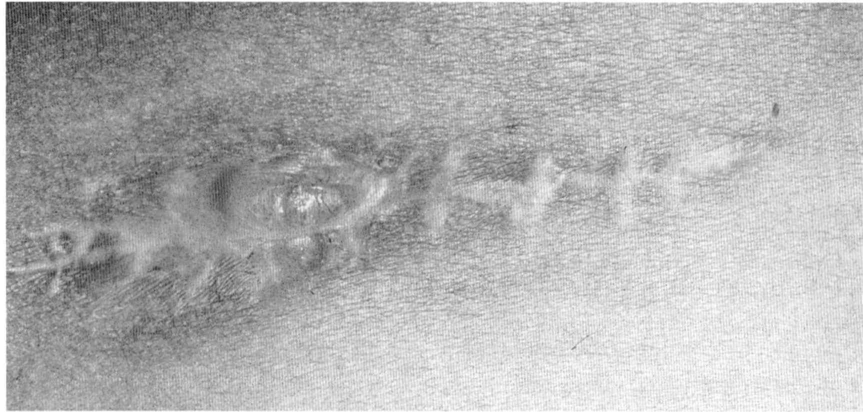

Fig. 5. Constriction of the skin by sutures which are too tight and left in place 14 days caused severe suture marks. A sinus tract forms because buried multifilament nonabsorbable sutures become infected, and the infection works its way to the surface

Prevention of Unsightly Scars and Keloids

The best means of predicting and preventing keloid formation is to determine whether the patient has had previous keloids. Unnecessary or cosmetic surgery on a patient who tends to form keloids should be avoided. A scar that is more unsightly than the lesion is unacceptable. When the patient presents with a malignant lesion, the factor of patient selection becomes less important because the tumor must be removed. After the malignant lesion has been totally removed, careful closure, with the use of skin tapes or subcuticular closure, and early corticosteroid injection are useful.

A clean incised wound heals best, and for many cutaneous lesions a fusiform excision is necessary.

Whenever possible, the incision should be placed in concealed areas of the face, such as the hairline, ear, nasolabial fold or submandibular region. If this is not feasible, the incision should follow the relaxed skin tension lines (Fig. 6). Straight linear wounds that follow the skin tension lines can heal with excellent scars. In the skin region, where the skin tension lines are curved, fusiform excision of tissue should have symmetric skin borders and not be crescent shaped. Fusiform excisions at right angles to the relaxed skin tension lines should be designed in a W-plasty fashion.

Incision perpendicular to the skin surface result in the best scars. The only time that an incision should be oblique or bevel-edged is when the surgeon is attempting to preserve the integrity of hair follicles.

Minimal trauma should be inflicted on the skin edges with instruments, i. e. fine dissecting forceps, avoidance of skin clamps, etc. If necessary a judicious undermining of adjacent tissues should be performed to facilitate wound closure under minimal tension. It is often helpful in deciding where to insert

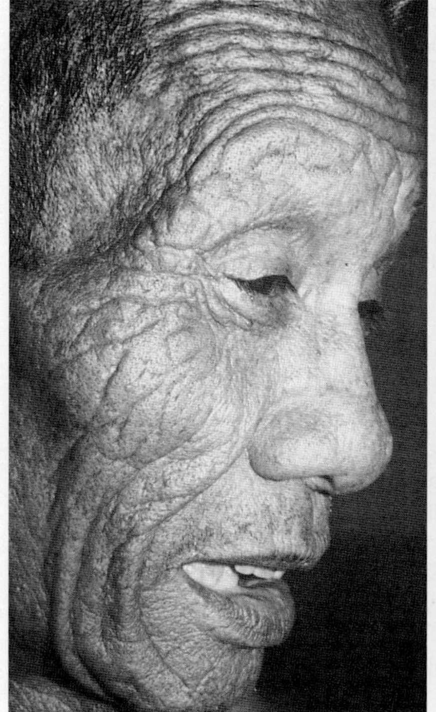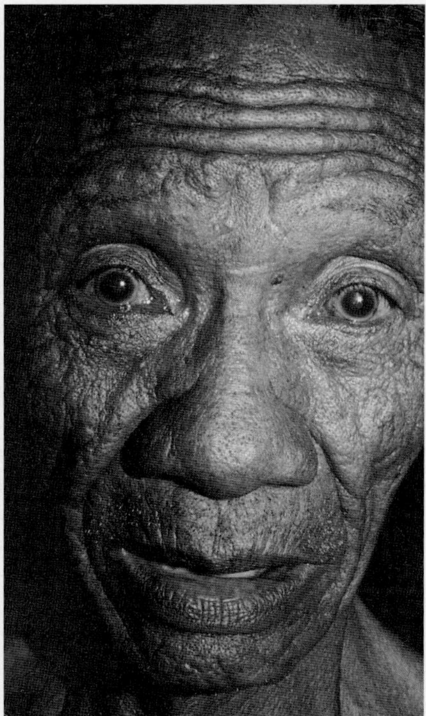

Fig. 6 a, b. The relaxed skin tension lines

sutures in a fusiform wound to place fine hooks at each margin and have them held under slight pressure.

The wound should be carefully approximated in layers, subcutaneous tissue, dermis and epidermis. Dead space should be avoided. To obtain a hairline scar result, subcutaneous fatty tissue or dermis that holds the surface of the skin apart should be trimmed carefully and cleanly with a sharp knife or sharp small scissor to allow the skin edges to fall together neatly and without tension. By firm reapposition of the dermal layer, the wound integrity is preserved, and the epidermis may be gently reapproximated. Thus, when the skin sutures are removed the wound is still approximated by the dermal sutures.

Skin sutures should be of fine gauge 6/0 on the face, and 5/0 to 3/0 elsewhere. Larger sizes (5/0 and 4/0) used on the face and neck wherever greater tensile strength is required. For continuous temporary subcuticular sutures 4/0 is preferred. The material used should be monofilament nylon.

The more loosely the skin sutures can be tied in conformance with good approximation of the cut surfaces, and the earlier they are removed, the smaller is the permanent mark on the skin.

Nonabsorbable sutures should remain in place for as short a time as possible but need to remain long enough for initial healing to avoid wound separation.

No specific time can be set for the removal of sutures. In areas where the skin is flaccid, in the eyelids, for example, the skin sutures may be removed in 3–4 days. In the face and neck, skin sutures may be removed on the 5th – 6th days. In other areas, the sutures should be left in for approximately 10 days. Continuous intradermal sutures may be left 2 weeks or longer. Rigid skin strips with adhesive backing (Steristrips) may be applied across an incision for additional security after suture removal. These strips hold for a few days, and it is necessary to replace them if secure support is to be maintained.

Of course, infection in a wound prohibits proper and prompt healing and should be prevented at all costs.

Management of Unsightly Scars and Keloids

The management of an unsightly or wide scar depends on the site, symptoms, and patient's wishes. It is never wise to rush into corrective surgery. All scars are initially red in color and gradually fade and become less prominent within at least 6 months. Unless the scar is a keloid, this process occurs. Obviously, these scars, when they finally become thoroughly healed, are wide and apparent as compared with the hairline scar achieved by careful surgical wound repair.

The distinction in diagnosis must be made between a hypertrophic scar and a keloid.

Surgical revision alone of hypertrophic scars may be curative when it relieves the causative forces, such as skin infection, skin loss through ischemia, or wound tension. Similar procedures on keloids may result in massive recurrences. For the most part, hypertrophic scars are much easier to treat than are keloids. The treatment of keloids is much more complex than that of hypertrophic scars.

Treatment objectives with keloids may be to alleviate the pain, burning, itching, redness, and bulk of the scar. Treatment of keloids has usually been of four modalities [37, 38], often using a combination of these:
a) corticosteroid intralesionally,
b) application of pressure,
c) surgical excision with intralesional corticosteroid, or
d) surgical excision with radiotherapy.

Triamcinolone acetonide is injected directly into the scar and repeated every 1–2 weeks according to the response. The dosage and administration have been arbitrary. Since clinical responses vary, initial concentrations of triamcinolone acetonide may range from 10 to 40 mg/ml [39]. Care must be taken in using this agent because skin atrophy, telangiectasia, depigmentation, necrosis, ulceration, and cushingoid features may result.

Continuous pressure is particularly suited to scars located over the trunk and extremities. This is difficult to tolerate for scars on the head and neck. Pressure devices have been effective following earlobe keloidectomy [40]. Continuous pressure must be maintained for at least 4–6 months following surgery.

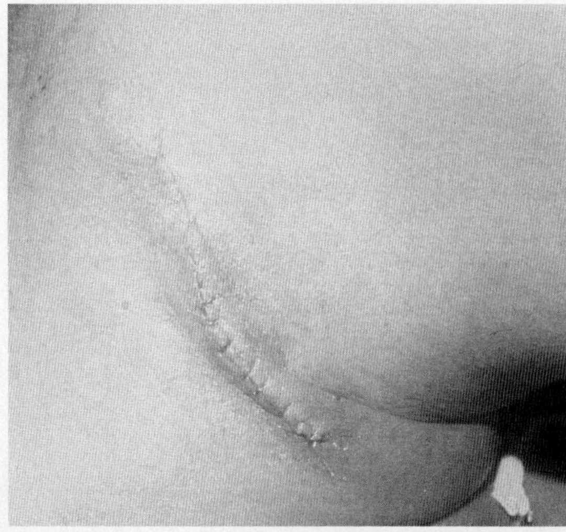

Fig. 7. Hypertrophic scar caused by faulty surgical technique

Excision may be useful to remove the large, bulky, disfiguring keloid, but postoperative intralesional corticosteroid must be used to prevent recurrence.

Radiotherapy after the establishment of the hypertrophic or keloid scar is much less effective alone than together with surgical revision. When used with surgical revision, immediately after surgery is the ideal time for radiotherapy. Although radiation therapy has been used for keloid treatment, a therapy that may promote the formation of skin malignancy should be avoided.

Other modalities have been reported in the literature, such as cryotherapy [41], liquid nitrogen [42], laser surgery [43], intralesional cytotoxic and immunosuppressive medication [44], and topical therapy with retinoic acid [45]. The results must be assessed cautiously. If surgical revision for hypertrophic scar is indicated, there are a number of options. Excision and primary closure are performed, paying particular attention to all the preventable measures described above (Fig. 7). When wound tension is the source, it can frequently be dealt with by the techniques of Z-plasty and W-plasty to alter the lines of force on the wound and to increase the likelihood of sound healing without widening.

Other Complications

Milia

Milia are small epidermal inclusion cysts in or around a scar that appear as small white papules.

Causes of Milia. Small keratinous cysts may be formed where the skin reepidermizes. These may also be seen along sutured incision lines or at suture tract entrance or exit point. These small cysts may form if fragments of the hyperplastic epidermis remain below the skin surface. Remains of transected adnexal

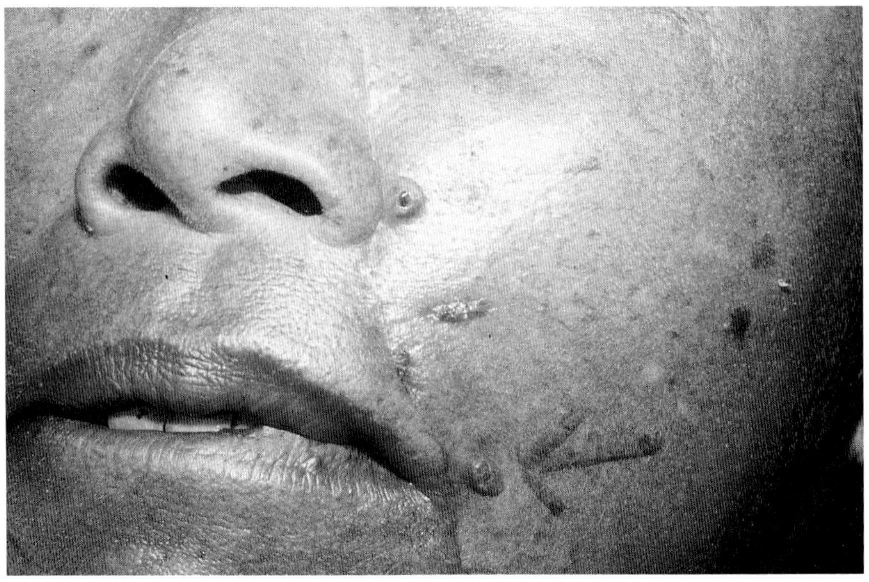

Fig. 8. Nodules (foreign body granulomas) on the right cheek *(arrows)*

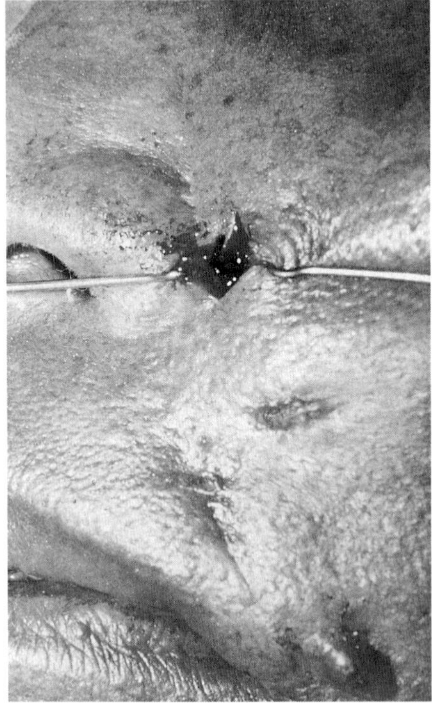

Fig. 9. Incision of the nodule revealed buried black silk sutures

structures such as hair follicles or sweat ducts may also be involved in cyst formation [46, 47].

Management of Milia. These are treated by carefully opening them with a number 11 scalpel blade or sterile needle and expressing the contents with a comedone extractor.

Nodules (Foreign Body Granulomas)

Causes of Nodules. Various foreign bodies such as suture material, or talc (silicate) may form nodules in surgical scars. The successor of talc – starch powder – although an improvement, is not free of problems. Usually nodules are associated with chronic granulomatous reactions to these foreign bodies. A suture granuloma is a painful swelling related to a buried suture of ligature or subcutaneous knots of nonabsorbable suture material (Fig. 8). Talc (silicate) which is still used on most surgical gloves may be transferred to suture material [48]. Many chronic granulomatous reactions may in fact be tissue reactions to talc [49].

Management. As the underlying cause of the nodule is chronic granulomatous reaction to nonabsorbable suture or talc implanted in tissue by means of the sutures, the sutures must be removed (Fig. 9).

References

1. Hunt TK (1979) Disorders of repair and their management. In: Hunt TK, Dunphy JE (eds) Fundamentals of wound management. Appleton-Century-Crofts, New York, pp 68–168
2. Green JP (1965) Steroid therapy and wound healing in surgical patients. Br J Surg 52:523–525
3. Kune GA (1981) The susceptible patient. In: Watts JMK, McDonald PJ, O'Brien P et al. (eds) Infection in surgery. Basic and clinical aspects. Churchill Livingstone, Edinburgh, p 86
4. Taplin D, Zaias N, Rebell G (1967) Skin infections in a military population. Dev Ind Microbiol 8:3
5. Smythe PM, Brereton-Stiles CG, Grace HJ et al. (1971) Thymolymphatic deficiency and depression of cell-mediated immunity in protein – calorie malnutrition. Lancet 2:939–943
6. Bartlett MK, Jones CM, Ryan AW (1942) Vitamin C and wound healing. II. Ascorbic acid content and tensile strength of healing wounds in human beings. N Engl. J Med 226: 474–481
7. Freiman M, Seifter E, Connerton C et al. (1970) Vitamin A deficiency and surgical stress. Surg Forum 21:81
8. Grimmond TR (1981) Skin preparation and surgical handwashing. In: Watts JMK, McDonald PJ, O'Brien PE et al. (eds) Infection in surgery. Basic and clinical aspects. Churchill Livingstone, Edinburgh, p 38
9. Devenish RA, Miles AA (1939) Control of *Staphylococcus aureus* in an operating theatre. Lancet 1:1088–1094

10. Medical Research Council Sub-Committee on Aseptic Methods in Operating Theatres (1968) Aseptic methods in the operating suite. Lancet 1:705-709
11. Evans AJ (1975) The modern treatment of burns. Br J Hosp Med 13:287-298
12. Howard JM et al. (1964) Postoperative wound infections: the influence of ultraviolet irradiation of the operating room and of various other factors. Ann Surg 160 Suppl:1
13. Seropian R, Reynolds BM (1971) Wound infections after preoperative depilatory versus razor preparation. Am Surg 121:251
14. Alexander JW, Fischer JE, Boyajian M et al. (1983) The influence of hair removal methods on wound infections. Arch Surg 118:347-352
15. Stokes EJ, Waterworth PM, Franks V et al. (1974) Short-term routine antibiotic prophylaxis in surgery. Br J Surg 61:739-742
16. Williams REO (1959) Epidemic staphylococci. Lancet 1:190-195
17. Lindblom G, Laurell G (1967) Studies on the epidemiology of staphylococcal infections. Acta Pathol Microbiol 69:237-245
18. Dineen P (1981) Prevention and treatment of deep wound infections. In: Dineen P (ed) The surgical wound. Lea and Febiger, Philadelphia, pp 146-149
19. Sebben JE (1982) Avoiding infection in office surgery. J Dermatol Surg Oncol 8:455-458
20. Gross DJ, Jamison Y, Martin KHT et al. (1989) Surgical glove perforation in dermatologic surgery. J Dermatol Surg Oncol 15:1226-1228
21. Dodds RDA, Guy PJ, Peacock AM et al. (1988) Surgical glove perforation. Br J Surg 75:966-968
22. Brough SJ, Hunt TM, Barrie WW (1988) Surgical glove perforation. Br J Surg 75:317
23. Hruza GJ, Snow SN (1989) Basal cell carcinoma in a patient with acquired immunodeficiency syndrome: treatment with Mohs micrographic surgery fixed-tissue technique. J Dermatol Surg Oncol 15:545-551
24. Borges AF (1985) Basic techniques. In: Harahap M (ed) Skin surgery. Green, St Louis, p 89
25. Winton GB, Salasche SJ (1985) Wound dressings for dermatologic surgery. J Am Acad Dermatol 13:1026-1044
26. Altemeier WA, Burke JF, Pruitt BA et al. (1984) Manual on control of infection in surgical patients, American College of Surgeons, 2 edn. Lippincott, Philadelphia, pp 173-189
27. Sebben JE (1988) Hematoma. In: Harahap M (ed) Principles of dermatologic plastic surgery. PMA, New York, pp 57-65
28. Blankenship ML (1985) Electrosurgery, electrocautery and electrolysis. In: Harahap M (ed) Skin surgery. Warren, St Louis, pp 823-840
29. Salasche SJ (1986) Acute surgical complications: cause, prevention, and treatment. J Am Acad Dermatol 15:1163-1185
30. Hicks PD, Stromber BV (1985) Hemostasis in plastic surgical patients. Clin Plast Surg 12:17-23
31. Winton GB, Salasche SJ (1985) Wound dressings for dermatologic surgery. J Am Acad Dermatol 13:1026-1044
32. Douglas DM (1959) Acceleration of wound healing produced by preliminary wounding. Br J Surg 46:401
33. Dunphy JE, Jackson DS (1962) Practical applications of experimental studies in the care of primarily closed wounds. Am J surg 104:273-281
34. Shepard GH (1971) The healing of wounds after delayed primary closure: an experimental study. Plast Reconstr Surg 48:358
35. Datubo-Brown DD (1990) Keloids: a review of the literature. Br J Plast Surg 43:70-77
36. Bernstein G (1988) Factors in obstaining a hairline scar: choice of site, and methods of incision. In: Harahap M (ed) Principles of dermatologic plastic surgery. PMA, New York, pp 3-24
37. Pollack SV (1988) Keloids and hypertrophic scars. In: Harahap M (ed) Principles of dermatologic plastic surgery. PMA, New York, pp 79-87

38. Grossman JA (1984) Minor injuries and disorders – surgical and medical care. Lippincott, Philadelphia, pp 101–102
39. Murray JC, Pollack SV, Pinnell SR (1984) Keloids and hypertrophic scars. Clin Dermatol 2:121–133
40. Brent B (1978) The role of pressure therapy in management of earlobe keloids: preliminary report of a controlled study. Ann Plast Reconstr Surg 1:579–581
41. Shephard JP, Dawber RPR (1982) the response of keloid scars to cryosurgery. Plast Reconstr Surg 70:677–682
42. Ceilley RI, Babin RW (1979) The combined use of cryosurgery and intralesional injections of suspensions of fluorinated adrenocorticosteroids for reducing keloids and hypertrophic scars. J Dermatol Surg Oncol 5:54–56
43. Kantor GR, Wheeland RG, Bailin PL et al. (1985) Treatment of earlobe keloid with carbon dioxide laser excision: a report of 16 cases. J. Dermatol Surg Oncol 11:1063–1067
44. Oluwasanmi JO (1974) Keloids in the African. Clin Plast Surg 1:179–195
45. De Limpens J (1980) The local treatment of hypertrophic scars and keloids with topical retinoic acid. Br J Dermatol 103:319–323
46. Ordman LJ, Gillman T (1966) Studies in the healing of cutaneous wounds. I. The healing of incisions through the skin of pigs. Arch Surg 93:857
47. Ordman LJ, Gillman T (1966) Studies in the healing of cutaneous wounds. II. the healing of epidermal, appendageal, and dermal injuries inflicted by suture needle and by the suture material. Arch Surg 93:883
48. Khan MA, Brown JL, Logan KV et al. (1983) Suture contamination by surface powders on surgical gloves. Arch Surg 118:738–739
49. Perou ML (1973) Iatrogenic foreign body granulomas: a study of selected cases with the polarizing microscope. Int Surg 58:676

Hair Transplantation and Alopecia Reduction

Walter P. Unger

Complications of Hair Transplantation

For discussion purposes complications that may occur in relation to hair transplanting can be divided into two general categories: (a) surgical complications and (b) aesthetic complications. Aesthetic complications are further subdivided into those that are due to errors of technique and those that are the result of planning errors. The approximate incidence of each of the complications is noted where applicable, and suggestions on how they may be avoided are made. Lastly, the treatment or correction of the problem is discussed.

Surgical Complications

Persistent Pruritus

While a small amount of pruritus is not unusual, occasionally a patient complains of persistent or marked pruritus post-operatively in either the donor or recipient area. The aetiology may be as simple as severed or injured nerves, an irritant or allergic reaction to the alcohol, povidone iodine, or other preparation solutions used during the time of surgery or, less commonly, varying degrees of folliculitis. If this complication arises during the first 2–3 weeks post-operatively a combination of a corticosteroid cream and antibiotic such as Valisone G (Garamycin) cream three times daily (or more often if necessary) is recommended. After the 2- to 3-week period a simple corticosteroid cream such as Lidex cream .05% three times or more per day may be used. In all instances when folliculitis is noted it is wise to take a sample of exudate for culture and sensitivity and start a wide-spectrum antibiotic for a period of 7–10 days (see also "Infection" below).

Persistent Pain

Discomfort is limited to the first 24 h in most patients and is either minimal, requiring no analgesics, or can be completely eliminated with acetaminophen with 30 mg codeine, propoxyphene napsylate (100 mg every 4–6 h) or meperidine (25–100 mg every 4–6 h). Occasionally it lasts several days to 1 week.

A very small number of patients (0.2% or fewer) have discomfort of variable degrees over a longer period, rarely extending to several months. The pain is almost always limited to the donor area and is most often spasmodic. Most patients describe intermittent short sharp "twinges" lasting one to several seconds occurring separately or in small groups. Sometimes a discrete site of tenderness rather than intermittent pain is the primary concern of the patient. Most often such areas are associated with elevated scars. No specific aetiology is known, but most of these individuals seem to be relieved by the local infiltration of a combination of triamcinolone acetonide 10 mg/cm^3 and lidocaine 1% with 1/100 000 epinephrine into the general area of pain or tenderness. The usual concentration that I use is 3.33 mg/cm^3. The injection is repeated 2 and 4 weeks later if necessary. The neurologist who first utilized this treatment on one of the patients whom I had sent him with this complaint suggested that the cause might be an injured nerve that had not been completely severed but had been "nicked" or otherwise injured during the transplanting process. A subsequent inflammatory response to this injury is settled by the infiltrations of local corticosteroid. Whether or not this is the mechanism behind the complaint remains a matter of conjecture, however. If two or three infiltrations do not produce relief, excision of the area is nearly always curative.

An even smaller number of patients, perhaps 1 in 2000, have noted more frequent, though otherwise normal headaches for 3–18 months post-operatively. This complaint is so unusual that it is not possible to be certain of a causal relationship to the hair transplanting. Analgesics generally used for headaches are effective. Sometimes these headaches are associated with small tender nodules which can be palpated in the donor area. In over 20 000 cases I have encountered palpable tender nodules in only two individuals. Once again, a combination of lidocaine with triamcinolone acetonide to a strength of 3.33 mg/cm^3 may produce relief after one to three treatments. If these fail to resolve the problem, excision is usually curative.

Arteriovenous Fistulae

Arteriovenous fistulae occur in approximately 1 in 500 cases and present as a slowly enlarging mass which on palpation pulsates. Nearly always they are first noted within 1–3 weeks of the surgery and have a reddish-blue colour. After enlarging for several weeks they pass through a non-pulsating cystic stage followed by a firm nodular stage and then usually disappear spontaneously in 2–3 months. Tromovitch et al. [1] prefer treatment to waiting for the lesion to resolve spontaneously. They identify the arterial inflow by finger palpation and place a large percutaneous suture around the artery. Alternatively, they dissect out the AV fistulae. This approach is far simpler if it is deferred until pulsations have stopped as intraoperative bleeding is reduced substantially. The author has always simply reassured the patient and waited for spontaneous resolution of the problem.

Severe Oedema

Significant post-operative oedema virtually always occurs with the first session if more than 50 grafts are transplanted. With a smaller number of grafts the amount of oedema becomes progressively less. In addition, for reasons still unknown, oedema usually decreases with subsequent sessions unless intervals of 12 or more months between operations are used.

It is likely that an important component in oedema formation, aside from the surgery itself, is the anaesthetic used. If one produces a line of anaesthesia using 1% lidocaine with epinephrine along a proposed frontal hairline, oedema forms anterior to that line, regardless of whether any surgical procedure is carried out. Lidocaine is slightly hypertonic and has an osmotic effect on intravascular fluids. In addition, by affecting permeability directly, it has been shown to have a specific effect on the balance of sodium and potassium ions within and outside the cytoplasm of peripheral nerves. It may therefore have a similar effect in producing ionic imbalance between intravascular and extravascular fluids. Local anaesthetics also have varying degrees of protein-binding and vasodilating characteristics [2]. If the anterior scalp is the recipient area, oedema begins on the forehead usually within 48–96 h, gradually increases, drops to the bridge of the nose, periorbital tissues and then the cheeks. When it is severe, rupturing of small blood vessels can produce ecchymoses and "black eyes", but this is quite uncommon if patients follow post-operative instructions carefully. The most important of these instructions are staying erect or lying with the head at a 45° angle for the first 4 days and applying ice packs to the forehead or any other areas of oedema formation for as much time as possible. Operating on recipient areas posterior to the frontal portion of the scalp results in oedema which drops posterior to the ears or onto the nape of the neck, where it is far less noticeable and minimally disconcerting. The possibility of reducing oedema with corticosteroids, proteolytic enzymes, non-steroidal anti-inflammatory medication such as ibuprofen (Motrin) or vitamin E has never been investigated in a double-blind controlled study. A majority of practitioners, however, now are empirically convinced that systemic corticosteroids (for example, 40 mg intramuscular triamcinolone acetonide or 60 mg methylprednisolone preoperatively) or ibuprofen, significantly diminishes the amount of post-operative oedema in most cases, and routinely employ them [3].

Some physicians feel that preventing or minimizing oedema may be important for more than cosmetic reasons. It is possible that circulation to the hair matrices could be reduced enough in some individuals to produce smaller hair yields per graft. The decreased circulation might be secondary to the oedema itself or to precipitation of protein and increased fibrosis.

Significant ecchymoses occurs during the first session in approximately 1 in 50 patients. Cold compresses (15 min on, 15 min off) staying at a 45° angle or more, and finger pressure to massage oedema away from the periorbital area and onto the temples are all helpful in reducing and alleviating the problem.

Scarring

Scarring in the *recipient* area is almost always the result of improper technique, and this is discussed under "Aesthetic Complications". The only exception to this general rule is true keloidal healing, which is a rare problem. In virtually all cases it can be avoided by careful pre-operative screening of patients on the basis of history and an examination of previous injuries to head, neck, arms and upper trunk. If there is any doubt, a single test graft should be performed at the edge of the area of alopecia at least 3 months prior to the scheduled surgery. Using these simple rules of avoidance, I have not encountered a single case of keloidal scarring.

Scarring in the *donor* area can be divided into an over-depletion of the donor area hair through over-zealous harvesting of grafts at any given site and scarring secondary to infection or local arterial damage. Over-depletion of the donor area can be avoided by simply recognizing that the sparser, finer textured and darker coloured the hair, the wider the intact rows of hair between harvested rows should be. Alternatively, if total excision of the donor area is employed [4] – that is, no intact rows of hair are left between harvested rows – the same factors would suggest less aggressive harvesting.

Scarring due to arterial interruption occurs primarily if the post-auricular or occipital artery is severed, if a significant branch of the superficial temporal artery is cut, or if there is excessive tension at sites of closure. An example of the latter is a situation where an alopecia reduction has been carried out within 1–14 days prior to transplanting.

If any vessel of significant size is severed during the course of harvesting, a single wide and deep suture should be employed to stop the bleeding rather than multiple sutures going in varying directions. Alternatively, the blood vessel may be cauterized. In the temporal area it is wise not to take any more than two rows of grafts during any one session. In addition, unless patients come from very distant areas, we try to avoid carrying out transplantion for preferably 3 weeks after an alopecia reduction to allow some tissue laxity to return to the scalp. If this is not practical, or if donor rows are being taken superior to multiple previous donor rows, we prefer to use total excision of donor sites rather than leaving intact rows of hair between the donor rows (Fig. 1). This avoids the possibility of the intact row necrosing post-operatively because of inadequate blood supply. This is in fact a good general rule to follow whenever suturing in donor sites appears to result in excessive suture line tension.

Post-operative Bleeding

Post-operative bleeding virtually never occurs in patients whose donor areas are sutured routinely, as appropriate suturing of the donor area prevents bleeding at that site. Bleeding in the recipient area, when the grafts have been properly placed into each site, also virtually never occurs. The exception is if there is a bleeding diathesis as a result of a genetic defect or the ingestion of substances which increase the tendency to bleeding. An incidence of post-operative bleeding of 1 in 1000 would be high given the above parameters. Some physicians routinely use a Gelfoam powder sprinkled over the entire donor area prior to putting a pressure dressing in place. The haemostatic effect of Gelfoam is well established. In addition, it mixes with the patient's serum to form a continuous semi-solid layer that is relatively easy to peel off completely when the bandage is removed the next day.

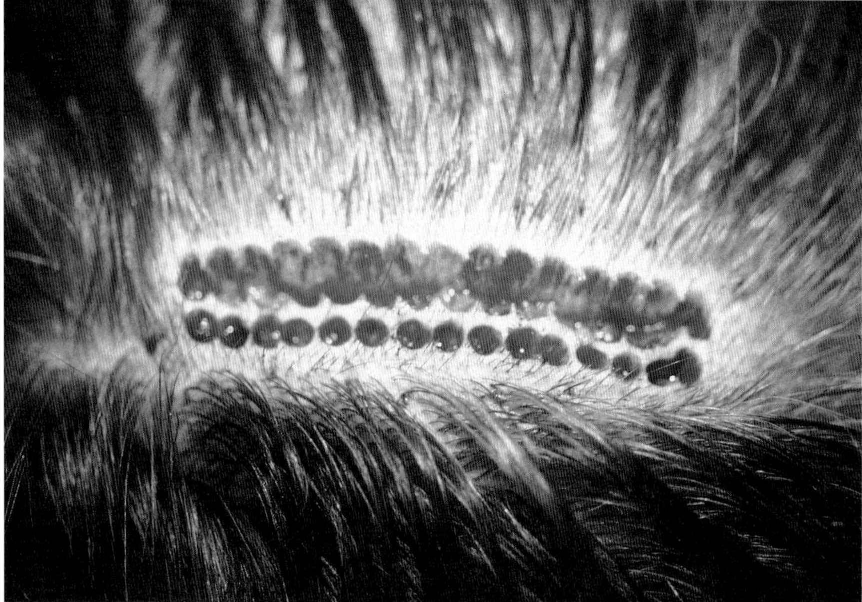

a

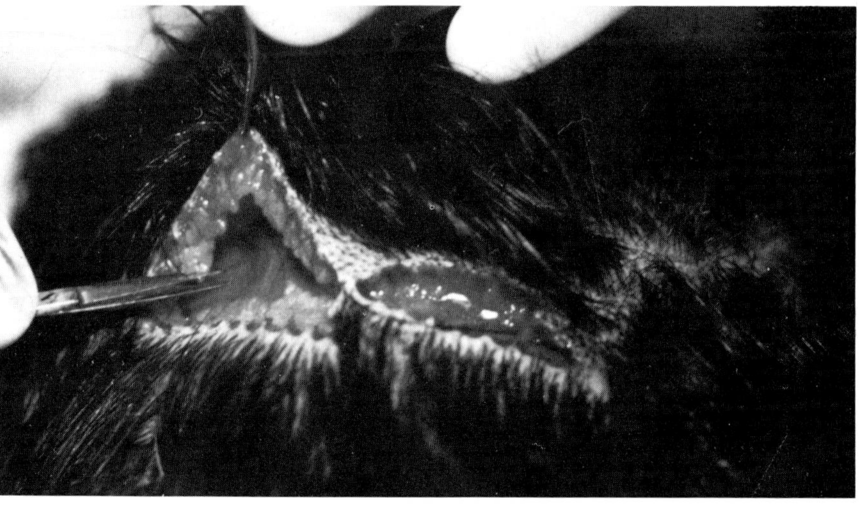

b

Fig. 1 a–d. Total excision of the donor area. **a** Two rows of donor grafts have been cut and removed. The grafts on each row are almost touching while an intact band of hair-bearing skin approximately 2 mm wide is left between the rows. **b** The intact row has been excised (and will be used for obtaining unigrafts, micrografts or "slit" grafts) and the area is being undermined. **c** A running single layer suture is used to close the wound. If any significant tension were present, galeal sutures would have also been employed. The donor site is easily and totally covered by surrounding hair. **c** One week after. **d** The sutures have been removed and only a fine scar line is present

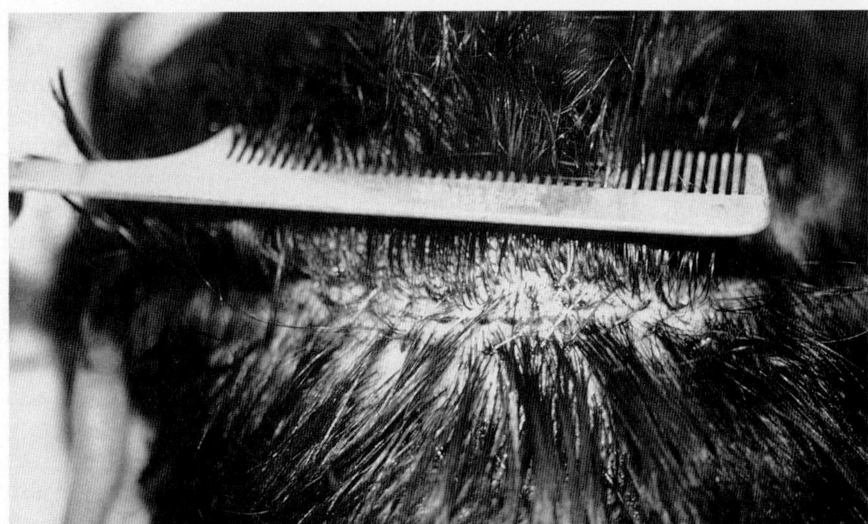

Fig. 1 c

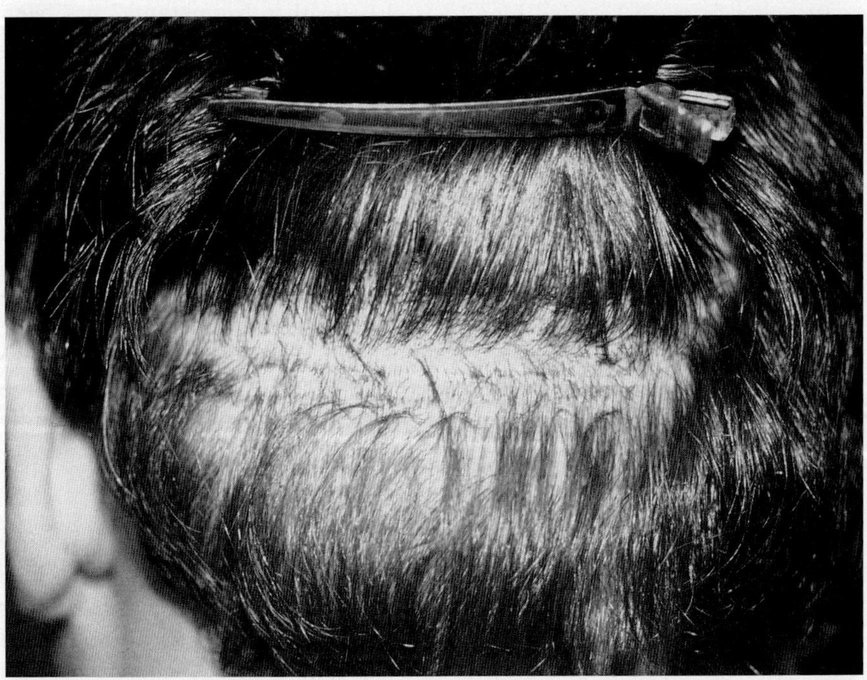

**Fig. 1 d

Genetic defects which cause excessive bleeding nearly always can be ascertained by a proper personal and family history being taken. For many years a routine clotting and bleeding screen was ordered pre-operatively. After over 20 years of doing this, however, without a single case of an unreported bleeding diathesis being discovered, we discontinued pre-operative bleeding and clotting screnes.

Patients are advised not to take acetylsalicylic acid for at least 1 week and preferably 2 weeks prior to surgery, and vitamin E for 3 weeks prior to surgery [5]. They are also given a list of food and medications which contain vitamin E or acetylsalicylic acid. These include nuts, whole grain cereals, peanut butter, wheat germ, leafy green vegetables, sweet potatoes, egg yolk, milk, organ meats, mayonaise, and molasses for vitamin E, and ascriptin, citrocarbonate, Bufferin, and various cold remedies for acetylsalicylic acid. Patients are also asked to abstain from alcohol for 48 h before surgery and for 24 h post-operatively.

Those few patients who tend to bleed excessively during the operation also sometimes bleed in the recipient area in a minor fashion intermittently over a period of several days after each procedure. In such individuals it can be advantageous to put a new pressure bandage on, similar to the one used post-operatively, for an additional 24–48 h. This has been necessary in the author's practice in approximately 1 case per 2000. Since routine suturing of donor sites has been instituted, bleeding from the donor area in such individuals has been greatly reduced.

Bleeding from an "eroded blood vessel beneath a haematoma" has been reported as occurring 2 weeks after surgery, but this must be extremely rare, as it has not been reported before or since.

Haematoma

Haematomas are extremely unusual after the first 48 h post-surgery and should be virtually completely preventable at any time. Advising patients to avoid those activites which may predispose to bleeding during the first 48 h (e. g. strenuous exercise, alcohol, acetylsalicylic acid, bending over) should reduce their incidence. I have never encountered a haematoma post-operatively in any of the individuals on whom I have operated. If the patient notices an area beginning to elevate, steady local manual pressure for 10–15 min usually can abort the haematoma. Those that do form can be emptied via a small incision and gentle pressure.

Alteration of Hair Texture and/or Colour

Approximately 5% of patients notice a temporary alteration in the texture of the transplanted hair consisting of an increased "kinkiness" or curl. The cause of this change in texture is almost certainly trauma to the hair follicles at the time of their removal, cleaning and transfer to the recipient site. As this occurs in a minority of patients, it also suggests an increased sensitivity to handling of the hair follicle in these individuals. The texture changes are temporary and last between 6 and 24 months [6].

This change in texture should be distinguished from differences in texture that occur as the result of having taken donor hair from areas with a different texture than originally present in the recipient site. Quite frequently, for example, the hair in the inferior temporal area or inferior occipital area is slightly more wirey or "kinky" than that which originally existed in the recipient site. If grafts are taken form these areas, the "altered" texture is permanent. In most cases the patient is not unhappy with this alteration because it adds fullness and body to the transplanted area. However, patients should be forewarned if significant differences in texture are noted at the time of the original examination.

Similarly, hair colour may vary substantially from the anterior frontal scalp to that seen in the temporal and occipital areas. Often the hair colour is darker in those latter sites, especially in blond or "dirty blond" coloured individuals. Once the hair has been transferred to the new recipient site, time may gradually cause the hair to change to the colour of the original hair at that site. Bleaching or hydrogen peroxide may be used to accelarate this process or camouflage it until it occurs.

The author nearly always takes some grafts from the temporal area during each transplanting session. There are two purposes for this. The first is that the texture and density of hair tends to be finer and lower in the temporal area, and these grafts are often useful in producing a more subtle and natural-looking hairline than denser grafts with coarser hair. The second, however, relates to hair colour changes which occur as the individual ages. Often the temporal hair greys well before hair from the parietal and occipital area. Unless one takes some grafts from the temporal area to transplant into the frontal area, when the individual begins greying he may develop quite grey temples and remain with a rather dark coloured frontal area. This produces an artificial or almost hairpiece-looking result. If, on the other hand, some temporal hair has been scattered in the frontal area during transplanting sessions, the grey comes into that area very naturally at the same time as it does in the temporal sites.

Skin Discoloration

Twenty-four hours after the operation, some grafts appear paler than their original colour, others slightly erythematous, while still others are erythro-violaceous. The skin in the donor area, however, has been protected from the ageing effects of the sun and environment and is nearly always paler than skin in the anterior recipient site. This colour difference tends to accentuate the new hairline against the adjacent aged forehead skin. Gradually the grafts "age" and blend more naturally with the colour of the forehead. In the interval, appropriate water-based make-up or tanning agents can be used by the fastidious patient. Patients are also advised to pull their hair back to expose the hairline whenever they are sunbathing and use sun-screening agents on their face and foreheads but not on the skin of their hairline grafts. This allows the grafts to sunburn slightly and speeds up the ageing process. Lastly, they are encouraged to let their hairline hair fall slightly anteriorly so that the colour difference is not obvious. Tattooing the grafts has been advised by some operators, but I have never recommended this as it often becomes problematic as the hair greys with age.

Infection

Our infection rate is less than 1%, and although no recent surveys have been conducted, the author suspects this is the approximate rate of infection experienced by most transplant surgeons. In 1973 Norwood[7] reported the results of a survey which indicated 38% of hair transplant physicians had infection rates of approximately 1% or higher. This figure has probably been reduced with the more prevalent use of peri-operative prophylactic antibiotics. In our office 330 mg PCE three times daily is started the night before surgery and continued for 5 days post-operatively.

For the first few days the recipient site often looks somewhat oedematous and erythrovialaceous. There should, however, be no local pain, tenderness, purulent discharge or pustules present, and the patient should be requested to report any such symptoms or signs immediately. Occasionally after several weeks or months one or more small pustules develop adjacent to or on the surface of one or more of the grafts. This usually represents a sterile rejection phenomenon where, for example, a small spicule of hair which was inadvertently left on the side of a graft is being extruded. Despite this, patients should be asked to report all pustules, and swabs for culture and sensitivity should be performed. A local antibiotic applied three times daily is adequate until the results of the culture are known. If there are any signs of true infection such as peripheral erythema, tenderness or pain, systemic antibiotics should also be added while awaiting the results of the laboratory tests. The penicillinase-resistant penicillins are the author's antibiotics of choice.

If the infection has occured in the donor area prior to the removal of sutures, those sutures in the immediate vicinity of the infection should also be removed as soon is practical.

In approximately 0.05% of patients a mild chronic folliculitis occurs in the recipient sites. Usually a 10- to 14-day full-dose course of tetracycline or erythromycin eliminates it. Occasionally, however, other antibiotics such as 100 mg minocycline twice daily, or 250 mg cloxacillin four times daily may be necessary. Sometimes low-dose antibiotics must be continued for a period of several additional weeks or months, for example, 250 mg tetracycline twice daily, 333 mg PCE twice daily, or 100 mg minocycline daily. Often the cultures in such individuals show only common bacterial flora thought to be non-pathogenic. If a more persistent low-grade folliculitis develops, it is wise to check the patient for an underlying predisposition to infection, such as diabetes mellitus.

Aesthetic Complications

Technical Errors

Poor Growth. There are many reasons for poor growth, but fortunately all are essentially avoidable. The main causes are (a) improper cutting of grafts, (b) improper handling and over-zealous cleaning of the grafts, (c) drying out of grafts due to insufficient saline or Ringer's solution in the cleaning dish, (d) sessions which are too large in relation to the pattern used, (e) too short intervals between sessions, (f) grafts that are too large or too close together, and (g) untreated infection.

The most important factors which result in the proper cutting of grafts include sufficient experience by the surgeon, razor-sharp instruments, and repeated injections of saline into the donor area during the cutting of grafts to keep the donor tissue hard [8]. Relative novices in transplanting should check their grafts to confirm that they are angling the punch properly after each five grafts have been cut. The punches themselves should be sharpened after each patient use. In our office the sharpening is done with a "Honing Machine" that is readily available (Trans Canada Dental, Oakville, Ontario, Canada). Grafts should be handled as little as possible, and undercleaning is preferable to over-zealous débriding and removal of fat. Ideally approximately 1 mm fat should be left beneath the deepest hair follicle.

One should always keep the blood supply to the recipient area in mind when patterns and sizes of sessions are being decided upon. If a U-shaped pattern is being utilized, four rows of standard round grafts may be very safely employed and whether completion of these four rows requires 80, 90, 100 or 115 grafts is relatively unimportant [9]. Intervals between sessions should never be less than 5–6 weeks if the recipient site is the same. If on the other hand, one is operating on the left side on one occasion and the right side of the scalp on another one, or the anterior scalp on one occasion and the posterior scalp on another, these sessions can be as close as one day apart – again keeping in mind that the pattern employed should not result in embarrassment of the blood supply to the recipient areas [9].

We employ very few 5-mm grafts because of a tendency for hair not to grow in the central portion of these grafts. The occasional use of a 5-mm graft to fill a larger than expected bare area, however, is not problematic. In addition grafts should ideally not be any closer than one graft apart from each other [9].

The only corrective measure for poor hair growth is additional good punch transplanting.

Cobblestoning. Elevation of grafts above the surrounding recipient site is uncommon if the grafts have been properly cleaned and trimmed, and if there is a proper ratio of graft size to recipient site hole size (see below). Graft elevation however does occur in some grafts in some individuals as a result of excessive post-operative bleeding beneath the grafts. This occurs in fewer than 0.5% of patients. Moderate, steady, manual pressure for a sufficient period of time to stop bleeding prior to bandaging the patients minimizes its occurence.

If the grafts are slightly elevated, often in 6–12 months they will flatten out spontaneously. Those that fail to do so may be flattened with, for example, superficial cautery with a Bovie electrocautery machine set at 25–50 and unipolar delivery, dermabrasion, or occasionally "shaving" with a sharp scalpel. The final result can and should be a smooth surface.

Peripheral Scarring. A ring of scar tissue may occur around the periphery of grafts if an improper ratio of donor graft size and recipient site hole size is employed. In general grafts obtained with a 5-, 4.5- and 4.0-mm punch fit nicely into recipient sites made with 4.0-, 3.5- and 3.25-mm punches, respectively. At the time recipient sites are being cut, however, it is wise to prepare one test hole with the smallest sized punch considered appropriate and then to try the graft in the hole to make sure that it fits snugly without a peripheral empty zone being present around it, or at the other extreme without the graft bulging above the surrounding surfaces. If either occurs, the size of the recipient site punch should be altered appropriately [9].

Scarring around the graft should be avoided not only for cosmetic reasons but also because as the scar contracts the blood supply to the graft and subsequent hair growth may be altered. Cosmetically significant peripheral scarring is entirely avoidable if the above precautions are respected.

Incorrect Hair Direction. This technical error should also never occur. There is virtually always some hair left in the recipient area whether it be the odd terminal hair or small vellus hairs which indicate the original hair direction at that location. The recipient site punch should be angled in a similar direction when the recipient hole is being cut so that when the transplanting is completed the hair lies as it did originally. Some transplant surgeons prefer to alter hair direction so that it grows at a more acute angle to the scalp, producing a more pronounced overlapping or shingling effect on the hair and an appearance of denser hair [10]. One can do this as long as (a) the hair changes its direction in a sufficiently gradual and organized fashion that it looks natural, (b) one waits long enough between sessions to see the altered direction of the transplanted hair, and (c) there is relatively little of the original hair present in the recipient sites. Changing the angle of the recipient site holes from the original hair direction results in the destruction of any original hair surrounding the recipient site hole as well as, of course, the removal of hair in the recipient site plug.

Planning Errors

Hairline Too Low or Too High. The lateral ends of the transplanted hairline are chosen by fate rather than the physician or patient. Both the beginning and the end of the hairline is the *ultimate* anterior-superior most point of the permanent rim of hair in the temporal area. It is important at the time that the hairline is planned to make as accurate as possible an estimate of where those points will be in the long run.

The mid-point of the hairline, however, is chosen by the patient and the physician. It should be anterior enough that the hairline itself will have a smooth oval shape, but one should bear in mind that the hair will fall forward 0.5–1 in. after transplanting is completed, and that this will be the individual's hairline when he is aged in his 80s as well as at the time of surgery. If future alopecia reductions are contemplated, any proposed hairline is made longer looking and more oval shaped by the subsequent alopecia reductions, and this too should be considered. On the other hand, the mid-point of the hairline should not be so far posterior as to result in a "flat" or almost straight hairline. Once more, subsequent alopecia reductions tend to take the flatness out of such a line.

If the operater has placed the hairline too far posteriorly, correction of this problem is relatively simple, as long as there are sufficient donor grafts remaining to move the hairline more anteriorly and to improve its shape. The only "trick" to master is that if the lateral points of the hairline have been properly chosen, one must use smaller grafts laterally and enlarge them as well as add more rows as one moves towards the mid-line. Proper spacing and sizes of grafts requires careful consideration and experience. If the hairline has been placed too far anteriorly, it presents more of a problem. Sometimes it can be moved more posteriorly with the use of an alopecia reduction posterior to the frontal hair. On other occasions grafts that are placed too far anteriorly may be excised, and the sites sutured or electrolysis may be used to destroy the hair in such grafts. In either of the latter two circumstances the cosmetic result is improved but still compromised by the original work (Fig. 2).

Incorrect Filling Of Fronto-parietal Recessions. In most men, as they age, the frontal hair recedes medially at the same time as the anterior border of the temporal hair recedes posteriorly, resulting in the production of a triangle referred to as the fronto-temporal triangle (Fig. 3). In a very small percentage of adult men this does not occur, and they maintain an almost female-like hairline. Such hairlines always draw attention to themselves because they are so unusual. The hairline of former American president Ronald Reagan, for example, is a prominent example. One of the most common errors in planning is bridging of these fronto-temporal triangles. Good cosmetic surgery generally does not draw attention to itself, and any patient who asks for this type of hairline is asking for the majority of people to stare at his hairline for the rest of his life.

If the ideal texture, density, and colour of donor hair is available and properly selected (fine, low, light, respectively), and enough micro-grafting is carried out, *sometimes* these hairlines can look very natural. The operater, however, must be extremely skilled. (In brief, unless all factors are very good to exellent the result looks unnatural).

If transplanting in the fronto-temporal triangle has been done improperly, even extensive corrective surgery may not produce a good hairline. One of the main reasons for this is that hair in the frontal triangle, when present naturally, is quite sparse and fine, and often such donor material is not available, so that one is working with a major disadvantage from the start.

There are, however, several approaches that can be used to improve results if the fronto-temporal triangle has been transplanted.

a) If not too many grafts have been placed into the fronto-temporal triangle these can be excised and sutured leaving tiny scars that are far less noticeable than the grafts themselves (Fig. 2).

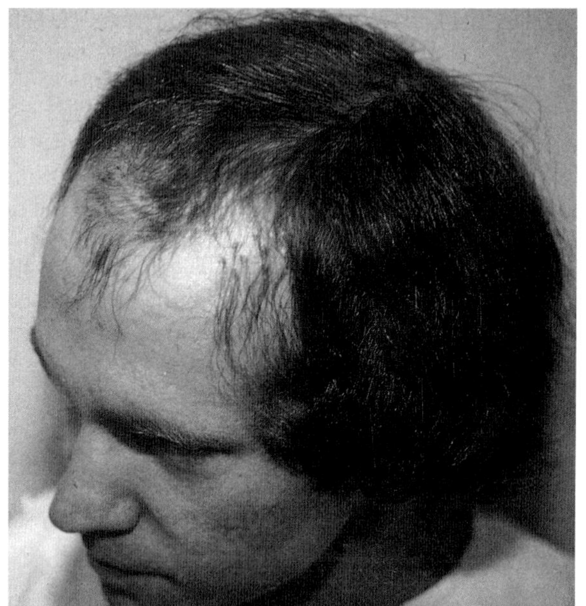

a

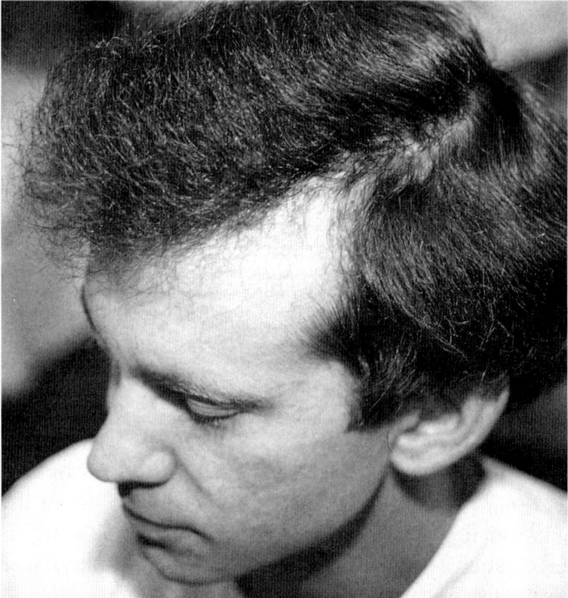

b

Fig. 2 a, b. This patient had been operated on by another physician. a Grafts have been placed too inferiorly and anteriorly in the Fronto-temporal triangle producing an unnatural hairline design. b The incorrectly placed grafts were excised and sutured, one to three grafts at a time, during subsequent hair transplanting sessions in a manner that would not interfere with the blood supply to the recipient area. Some scattered hair in poor growing grafts was also removed with electrolysis. The results of correction and additional punch transplanting are demonstrated.

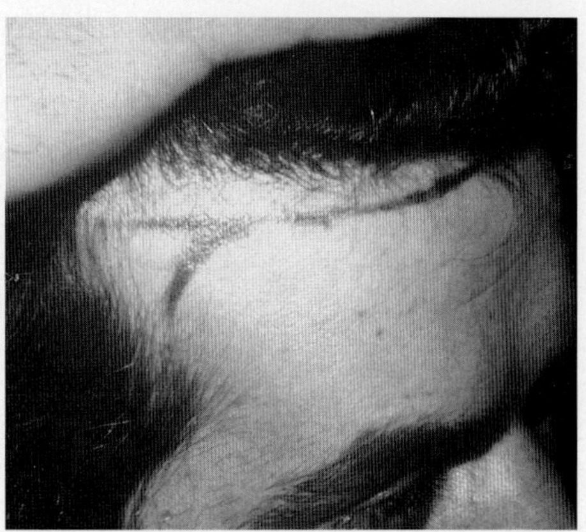

Fig. 3. A young adult man showing a posteriorly receded temporal hairline and a medially receded frontal hairline producing a "fronto-temporal triangle" of alopecia. Two potential new hairlines have been drawn with a grease pencil. The superior line is the more natural of the two. The inferior line requires more extensive filling of the fronto-temporal triangle and will always draw attention to itself because of its relative rarity in adult men

b) If the grafts are well blended to surrounding skin, electrolysis may be used to remove hair from the grafts.

c) The fronto-temporal triangle can be filled in with grafts of various sizes to produce a more diffuse growth of hair, with an added new and sparser anterior margin of hair. The use of micro-grafts, slit grafts and 2-mm or smaller round grafts may improve results considerably.

d) Poorly placed grafts can be excised, and the resultant hole filled with a non-hair-bearing, appropriately sized graft.

Insufficient Numbers of Grafts To Complete Properly What Has Been Started. Another all too common complication in transplanting occurs in individuals in whom transplanting was started at the anterior as well as posterior aspects of the scalp when they were quite young, without an accurate assessment having been made of how large their ultimate bald area would be (or how large the permanent hair-bearing donor area would be). In these patients a toothbrush-like appearance is present in areas where an inadequate number of grafts have been transplanted to produce proper density. The following approaches may improve matters considerably.

1. Employ alopecia reductions to excise the areas of lesser density and at the same time move any grafts from the strips that are excised and place them into areas that will remain and should be thickened. A second transfer of grafts can often be accomplished without any significant damage to that graft. This technique allows one simultaneously to remove areas that would otherwise require grafts which are not available and to provide grafts that can be used to thicken remaining areas. Alopecia reduction is particularly useful on the lateral aspects of transplanted areas when the alopecia has extended farther inferiorly than was initially anticipated.

2. "Mini-reductions" can often be carried out in areas where larger reductions would remove too many good grafts. In this approach one simply punches out holes, using an ordinary trephine, wherever one would normally put a

graft and then sutures the holes closed (Fig. 4) [11]. Almost any configuration of these lines of punched out holes can be used as long as the blood supply to the transplanted area is not compromised. The holes should correspond to the size of the bare areas that one is dealing with. For example, in one place one may require a 3-mm trephine to punch out the bare area and in another place a 4-mm and still another a 4.5-mm trephine, etc. Often one or more lines containing 20 or more holes each can be closed with simple running sutures. In such cases, areas of alopecia that would have required 20–30 grafts (or 40–60 grafts if two or more lines are punched out) is removed without the "expenditure" of any grafts.

3. Previously harvested donor areas should be carefully searched for grafts that can still be removed from them. Often these occur in small groupings of five to ten grafts scattered here and there. On other occasions a large number of grafts can be obtained in temporal areas that have not been harvested because many inexperienced punch transplant surgeons do nut use this area for donors. The temporal areas of the scalp are actually good donor sites if one is looking for grafts that are not too dense, have finer hair, and are due to grey earlier than hair elsewhere on the scalp. The author frequently makes extensive use of such grafts for hairlines simply because these characteristics are ideal for hairlines. Naturally one must be sure not to go into areas that can reasonably be expected to lose their hair or become overly sparse in the future.

4. Often a single long line of potential donor grafts can be removed from just superior to the most superior previously harvested rows. A single row encircling the hair-bearing scalp, for example, can yield 40–50 grafts in many individuals without encroaching on areas that will be lost in the future.

5. One can often cut out some rows of intact hair left between previously harvested rows. The scars superior and inferior to each newly harvested row are excised after the donors are removed, and the whole area is closed with a single or double layer of sutures depending on the tension of closure. This in effect is an alopecia reduction in reverse, and there is a limit to how much can be removed from any individual depending on his hair density, texture, and colour. However, often 50–100 or more grafts can be salvaged using this technique. If the distance between intact rows left between previously harvested rows is less than 4 mm (as it often is) a 3.0- to 3.75-mm punch can be used to harvest it. The grafts may then be bisected and inserted into slits made with a scalpel blade in the recipient area or used as smaller than usual round grafts.

As usual, "an ounce of prevention is worth a pound of cure," and physicians should be very wary of treating both the anterior and posterior aspects of the scalp in younger individuals unless they have considered one or more alopecia reductions and a very careful family history as well as physical examination. Patients in their early 20s in particular should be advised to save their grafts for the anterior half of their head so as to frame their face and to transplant that properly before attempting to transplant the posterior aspects of the scalp. Sometimes it is difficult to convince a patient of the wisdom of doing this, especially if

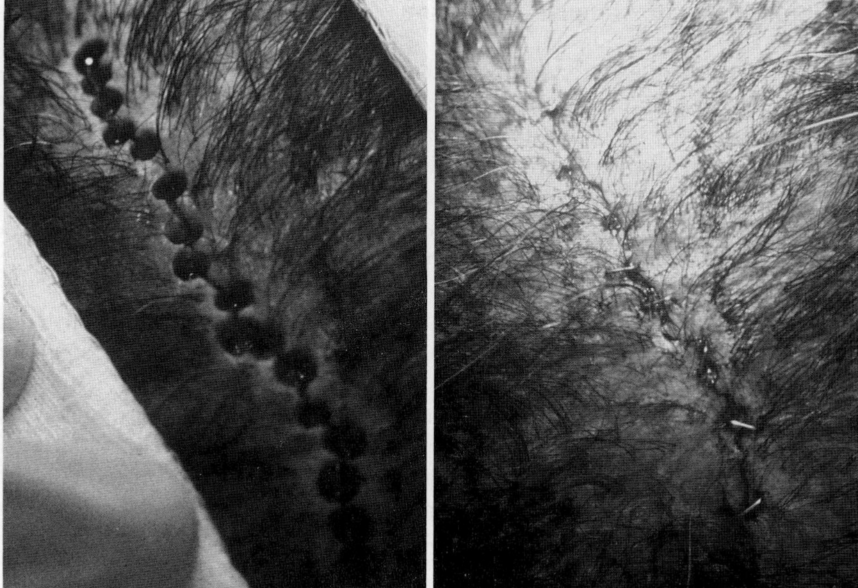

Fig. 4. a. A flattened S-shaped row of potential recipient sites varying from 3 to 4 mm in size (according to the size of the hairless areas) has been prepared and the bridges of skin between them incised. The pattern can be linear, T-shaped, Z-shaped, S-shaped, etc., conforming to the empty sites as long as the blood supply to the rest of the area is not compromised. Most often this is done concomitantly with punch transplanting into the same general area. **b** Instead of grafts being inserted into the potential recipient sites the defect has been sutured with tooth-shaped edges apposed to concave edges wherever possible. The sutures were removed 7–10 days later. Hairless spaces have thereby been eliminated without the expenditure of any grafts. This technique is referred to as "mini-reduction" and is used extensively by the author during corrective punch transplanting

the major area of thinning is occurring first in the vertex area. However, the long-term problem of perhaps having enough grafts to transplant the posterior one-half or two-thirds of the eventual bald area but not enough grafts for the cosmetically more important anterior portion should be emphasized to the patient.

Conclusion

It is worthwhile emphasizing that punch transplanting when carried out by even minimally experienced physicians is remarkably free of significant complications, with the exception of those aesthetic complications due to planning errors. (In addition, those surgical complications which do occur are usually rapidly controllable and easily connected). Planning errors, however, can lead to cosmetically disastrous and psychologically devastating results.

Complications of Alopecia Reduction

In general, the complications associated with alopecia reductions overlap extensively with those that may occur in punch transplantation, and their avoidance and treatment are identical in each case. These overlapping complications include operative and post-operative bleeding, post-operative haematomas, infection, nerve damage, hypertrophic and keloidal scarring, and post-operative facial oedema. Several other complications, however are, unique to alopecia reductions as contrasted to punch transplantation. These include:

a) suture reaction,
b) poor scars (wider scars than the usual fine line, grooving or indentation of the scar itself, unsightly scarring in the persistent hairy fringe – most often in the occipital area),
c) complications due to embarrassment of blood supply (temporary hair loss associated with the trauma of surgery, permanent hair loss associated with more extensive decrease in circulation, wound dehiscence, necrosis of part of the flap), and
d) post-reduction "stretchback".

Suture Reaction

Suture reaction may occur with either the superficial sutures utilized for the skin or the deeper sutures placed in the galeal layer. The former can be virtually entirely eliminated by removal of sutures 7 days after sugery rather than, for example, leaving self-dissolving sutures in place until they dissolve on their own. Galeal sutures are usually chromic catgut, vicryl, or dexon. When chromic catgut is used, such reactions occur in approximately 10% of patients. Dexon produces a substantially lower rate of suture reaction, and to date we have had no suture reactions with the use of vicryl. When it does occur, normally there is little or no apparent reaction for 2–3 weeks post-operatively. Then an area of erythema associated with a small pustule develops over the suture, with eventual necrosis of the overlying skin and finally "spitting" of the suture material sometime later. Treatment consists of removing the sutures as quickly as practical and hot compresses three times per day, followed by topical antibiotics until the opening heals. The author usually uses simple saline compresses, and the antibiotic most often employed is bacitracin ointment. Any unsightly resultant scars may be excised or removed at the time of punch transplanting over the scars.

Poor Scars

Scars that are wider than the usual fine line may occur in some individuals, either because galeal sutures were not tight enough, or the patient's healing is intrinsically poor. Such scars occur in fewer than 1% of patients. If a subsequent alopecia reduction is planned, they should be left and included in

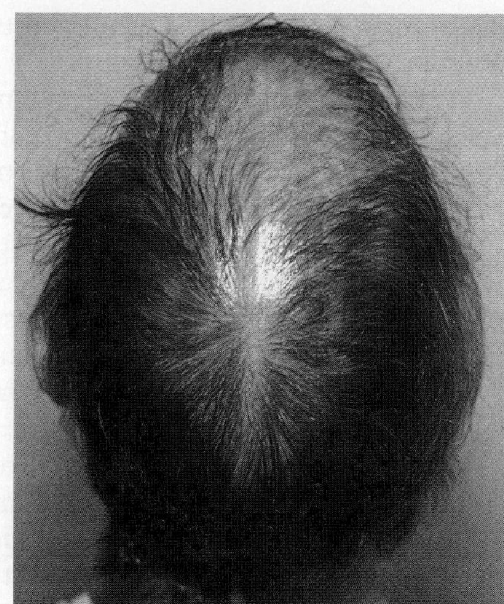

Fig. 5. An "axe-like" scar in the superior occipital fringe subsequent to an alopecia reduction. Such scars can be minimized by curving the posterior end of the incision to the right or left

the excised tissue. If no further alopecia reductions are contemplated, the scar may be excised once healing is completed, in the form of a "mini-reduction" using a punch and interdigitating the apposing skin edges [11] or as a simple scalpel excision. In view of a history of poor healing, two levels of sutures should be used even if minimal tension is present. Grooving or indentation of the scar line should occur in fewer than 0.1% of cases. It is due to the same factors as noted above for wider than usual scars and can be repaired in most cases with the same procedures outlined for that complication. When it is noted in our practice, the patient nearly always has a thicker than usual scalp (although this does not occur in the majority of patients with thick scalp tissue).

Unsightly scarring in the persistent hairy fringe usually takes the form of an "axe-like" scar extending into the occipital hair (Fig. 5). Such scars can be greatly minimized by

a) not extending excisions beyond the most inferior point the fringe is expected to reach in the future and/or
b) curving the posterior end of the scar slightly to the right or left (corresponding to the hair direction in that area), thereby avoiding a linear vertical scar and changing it into one that is more easily camouflaged [12].

Impaired Blood Supply

Complications due to decreased blood supply most commonly consist of temporary hair loss adjacent to the suture line and are associated with the trauma of the surgery. This "telogen effluvium" occurs in approximately 20% of patients, and because it is temporary, it requires no particular treatment. On the other hand, all patients in whom there is some persistent hair in the area of the alopecia reduction should be pre-warned that it may occur so that they are not alarmed if it does.

Permanent hair loss may also occur in the area adjacent to the suture line if an undue amount of tension has been employed at the time of the closure, undermining has been too superficial, one or more major blood vessels have been severed, or post-operative infection occurs. The incidence of this complication in our practice is virtually nil and consists of perhaps two or three cases in the last dozen years. Because we rarely extend alopecia reductions into areas which we do not intend to punch transplant subsequently, any defect is corrected at that time. If the individual decides not to transplant that area either temporarily or in the long term, any iatrogenic alopecia may be excised with a subsequent alopecia reduction.

Wound dehiscence has never occurred in our practice. This is caused by the factors noted above for permanent hair loss or by failing to use galeal sutures. Alopecia reductions should never be performed without these deeper sutures being employed. By far the commonest cause for wound dehiscence is an overzealous excision of tissue resulting in undue tension at the suture line. One should never lose sight of the fact that this is a cosmetic procedure, and that it is best to err slightly on the side of taking a little less tissue than one optimally could than a little more. If undue tension is noted when one attempts to close the wound, galeal incisions can be made parallel to the excision line ("galeal scoring") to ease the tension at the suture line. If dehiscence does occur, saline compresses or compresses employing an antibacterial solution should be used three times daily, associated with appropriate topical and/or antibiotics until the wound heals. One may then attempt to excise the area or punch transplant it.

Necrosis of part of the flap is caused by the same factors as noted above for wound dehiscence and can be avoided and treated by the same means.

Stretchback

Post-reduction "stretchback" occurs with all alopecia reductions and perhaps should not be listed as a complication but rather as an expected sequela. It may be considered a complication if there is more than 30% stretchback post-operatively in that it is probably avoidable in most cases by better operative technique or a less aggressive approach. Unger has recommended that one attempt during alopecia reductions to remove redundant skin rather than trying to remove as much as possible and closing under excessive tension [12]. Those surgeons who aim to remove the most possible skin produce marked tension on the remaining scalp tissue and therefore note an increased amount of stretchback as opposed to those whose aim is to remove redundant skin and close with minimal tension. Stretchback is therefore a function of surgical technique as well as of the inherent healing of the individual. Unger, for example, has reported an average stretchback of less than 15% in his patients while Nordstrom has reported stretchback of 10%–50% depending on how many prior reductions were performed [13].

"Major" Reductions

All of the above relates to the complications that may be encountered subsequent to regular and modified major alopecia reductions. Brandy [14] and others, however, have described various types of alopecia reductions carried out after extensive undermining involving the severing of occipital, post-auricular and posterior branches of the superficial temporal arteries. These may be referred to as major alopecia reductions, bilateral occipital parietal flaps or bilateral temporal flaps. Complications secondary to embarrassment of blood supply occur more frequently and in a more severe form in these types of reductions.

The exact incidence of temporary hair loss (telogen effluvium) and permanent hair loss is difficult to ascertain. Previous writers have tended to minimize the reporting of their occurrences. In particular, large areas of permanent hair loss may occur in occipital and parietal areas, and I have seen at least one dozen such cases for corrective surgery. The author and his brother M. Unger, who performs large numbers of alopecia reductions, believe that until improvements in technique and frank reporting indicate an extremely low incidence of this complication, the potential benefit from the procedure is not sufficient to outweigh the potential disadvantages. Brandy [15] has described two possible routes of minimizing circulatory embarrassment. The first is tying off occipital arteries bilaterally 3 weeks prior to the reduction to allow for the development of a collateral circulation, and the second is severing of only one occipital artery at the time of the reduction instead of the usual two. Until several operators have tried this and reported a *very* low incidence of permanent hair

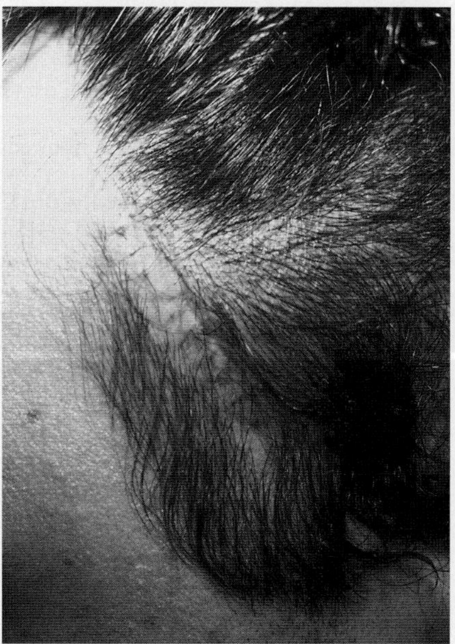

Fig. 6. Temporal scar secondary to a "major reduction"

loss in the hair-bearing rim, I would not recommend the procedure for my patients.

A second problem with major reductions is the presence of a vertical scar in the temporal area, which may be difficult to conceal post-operatively (Fig. 6). It is especially likely if the scar is wider than usual, or if temporal hair is or will be sparse. As long as patients are forewarned of the possibility of this "complication", it should be seen as part of the cost of achieving the extensive gains that are possible with these major alopecia reductions. The scar may be treated with punch grafts, slit grafts, of micro-grafting to improve it if it should become a cosmetic embarrassment.

References

1. Tromovitch T et al. (1988) Sequelea and complications of hair transplantation. In: Unger WP, Nordstrom RE (eds) Hair transplantation, 2nd edn. Dekker, New York, pp 399–408
2. Covino BG (1972) Local anesthesia. N Engl J Med 286:875, 1035
3. Pinski JB (1988) Hair transplantation. In: Unger WP, Nordstrom RE (eds) Hair transplantation, 2nd edn., Postoperative Course: usual course, Dekker, New York, p 385-390
4. Hill TG (1980) Closure of the donor site in hair transplantation by a cluster technique. J Dermatol Surg Oncol 6:190
5. Unger WP (1989) In: Orfanos CE, Happle R (eds) Hair and hair diseases. Surgical Treatment of Androgenetic Alopecia, Springer, Berlin Heidelberg New York, pp 1001–1030
6. Tromovitch T et al. (1988) In: Unger WP, Nordstrom RE (eds) Hair transplantation, Sequelae and Complications of Hair Transplantation, Dekker, New York, pp 399–408
7. Norwood OT (1973) Personal Communication
8. Alt T (1988) The donor site. In: Unger WP, Nordstrom RE (eds) Hair transplantation. Dekker, New York, pp 145–209
9. Unger WP (1988) The recipient area. In: Unger WP, Nordstrom RE (eds) Hair transplantation. Dekker, New York, pp 211–272
10. Stegman S, Tromovitch T (1984) Cosmetic dermatologic surgery. Year Book Medical Publishers, Chicago, pp 87–92
11. Unger WP (1983) Concomitant minireductions and punch transplanting. J Dermatol Surg Oncol 9(5):388–392
12. Unger M (1988) Alopecia reduction. In: Unger WP, Nordstrom RE (eds) Hair transplantation. Dekker, New York, pp 435–496
13. Nordstrom REA (1984) Scalp kinetics in scalp reductions for male pattern bladness. Ann Chir Plast Esthet 29:292–296
14. Brandy DA (1986) The Brandy bitemporal flap. Cosmet Surg, pp 11
15. Brandy DA (1986) The bilateral occipito-parietal flap. J Dermatol Surg Oncol 12(10): 1062–1066

Skin Grafts

Ann F. Haas and Ronald G. Wheeland

Introduction

While skin grafts have been used for centuries to provide coverage for a number
of different types of defects, there are complications that can be encountered
with their use. Since the technique appears to be deceptively easy to perform, an
awareness of the potential pitfalls that can compromise or complicate skin grafting is vital in order for it to be a valuable tool for the dermatologic surgeon. This
chapter summarizes the various types of skin grafts and how they are used, as
well as the complications associated with both the donor sites for the various
types of grafts and complications related to the recipient areas.

Types of Skin Grafts

There are essentially four major types of skin grafts: the split-thickness skin graft
(STSG), the full-thickness skin graft (FTSG), the composite skin graft, and a
new graft technique using autologous skin grown in culture. Each of these types
of skin grafts have different indications and different complications associated
with their use.

Split-Thickness Skin Grafts

The STSG consists of a sheet of epidermis and a variable amount of the underlying dermis. Depending upon the amount of tissue that is harvested, STSGs
can be described as thin (0.008–0.012 in.) medium (0.012–0.018 in.), or thick
(0.018–0.030 in.). Each of these different thicknesses of STSGs have different
indications for use.

In general, STSGs are used for the repair of defects that cannot be successfully reconstructed using local or regional flaps or FTSGs because of their large
size. Thin STSGs are used to allow better evaluation for possible recurrences
following skin cancer surgery. Medium STSGs are sometimes used to provide
temporary coverage for a wound when definitive reconstruction is planned at a
later date. STSGs can be used to provide a backing for a local flap which is used
to repair a through-and-through defect of the nose or ear. Medium on thick

STSGs are used to provide coverage of wounds where a ful thickness skin graft would not likely survive.

The choice of thickness for a STSG has largely to do with the potential for survival. For example, a thin STSG has a greater potential for survival than a thick graft because of the finer capillary network which is exposed on the cut under surface of the graft to permit better absorption of nutrients from the wound bed. Since the total volume of tissue in a thin STSG is less than that of a thick STSG, there is a reduction in the metabolic requirements of the graft itself. For this reason, a thin STSG is ideal for a wound which has some degree of vascular compromise. However, in other cases where there may be excessive pressure or repeated trauma, a thicker STSG may be used to provide better protection and preserve as much normal function as possible. There are exceptions to this rule, however, since is has been shown that STSGs can provide comparable function without increasing the operative procedure necessary for reconstruction of the palmar surface following release of burn scar contractures in a pediatric population [1].

Full-Thickness Skin Grafts

The FTSG consists of epidermis and the full thickness of dermis. These types of grafts are generally used to reconstruct optimally a wound when there is insufficient local tissue to repair the defect successfully with a local random pattern or axial pattern flap. Because they offer a better cosmetic result over STSGs, these types of grafts are chosen more frequently when the best cosmetic result is desirable. FTSGs are frequently used in the treatment of children because they tend to grow as the child grows, unlike STSGs. Another important indication for FTSGs is in the reduction of wound contraction. If, for example, wounds on the lower eyelid, nasal ala, supraorbital area, or lip were allowed to contract due to placement of a STSG, distortion of the normal anatomic features might result in disfigurement or deformity.

Composite Skin Grafts

A composite skin graft is one composed of both skin and some adjacent complex tissue, typically cartilage. Hair transplantation plugs, used for the correction of male-pattern alopecia, are also sometimes considered a type of composite graft.-Composite grafts, composed of skin and the underlying cartilage, are typically taken from the ascending helix of the ear and used to repair a large defect on the opposite ear or to reconstruct the alar rim.

Autologous Skin Grafts

Autologous skin grafts are the most recent addition to the regimens used to replace lost skin. In this technique, a small piece of tissue is harvested from the patient, and using established laboratory techniques, the donor tissue is expanded many times over in a tissue culture laboratory to provide large amounts of tissue which are eventually returned to the patient. Autologous skin grafts have been used primarily in the treatment of severe burn wounds, but they have also been employed to provide coverage for decubitis and venous stasis leg ulcers, to provide coverage of large defects that results from removal of giant congenital nevi, and to cover STSG donor sites [2–5]. More recently, research has shown that these types of grafts may be beneficial in reducing recurrences following removal of hypertrophic scars or keloids [6].

General Criteria in Assessing Patient Risk Factors

An assessment of the risk factors involved in skin grafting can be exceedingly important in predicting the likely outcome of a skin graft procedure. There are many factors that can act alone or in combination to compromise the result and cause graft failure, regardless of the type of graft employed. It is often helpful to anticipate these problems and modify the procedure accordingly.

Local Factors

The most frequent cause of graft failure is inadequate preparation of the graft bed. If there is insufficient vascularity to support the metabolic demands of the graft, failure is inevitable. Unrelated problems can play a role in vascular impairment, including previous irradiation of the recipient site and prior surgery that may have induced formation of excessive fibrosis at the base of the defect. Both of these processes can reduce the amount of vascular supply available. Exposed bone that lacks its periosteum, exposed cartilage without its attached perichondrium, or exposed tendon that lacks its peritenon, will not likely support a graft as well because of reduced blood supply. If the base of the wound has a large amount of nonviable tissue, or if there are foreign bodies or crushed material present, there will be interference with survival of the graft. Other local problems that can be important in the success in skin grafting are the presence of bacterial colonization or overt infection and the presence of excess granulation tissue. While a normal degree of vascularity is required for a skin graft to survive, if excess granulation tissue is present in the bed of a wound, the graft often fails. This frequently can be reduced by the application of topical medications, such as saline or silver nitrate, prior to performing skin grafting.

Systemic Factors

There are a host of systemic medical conditions that can also compromise graft survival. Arterial or venous insufficiency and sickle cell disease are associated with vascular compromise and may inadvertently impact negatively on graft survival. Other systemic illnesses can also compromise vascularity at the recipient site, including rheumatoid arthritis, systemic lupus erythematosus, and other immunologic diseases. Also, diabetes, hematologic disorders, use of systemic steroids, and vascular constriction induced by nicotine can also result in inadequate vascular supply and subsequent graft failure.

Among the most compromised wounds found on the body are lower leg ulcers. The combination of dependent position, underlying vascular insufficiency, and bacterial contamination make treatment with skin grafts much more difficult and the risk of graft failure substantially higher. The major risk factors that should be evaluated prior to grafting leg ulcers include: ischemic heart disease or cerebrovascular disease; a history of multiple hospital admissions; use of multiple medications; difficulties with mobility, arthritis, or a history of multiple falls; local leg problems including ischemia or previous deep vein thrombosis; a history of leg ulceration of greater than 5 years' duration; and whether the patient lives alone. A recent study has demonstrated that patients who receiving STSGs for the treatment of venous ulcers who had four or more of these risk factors suffered a much higher frequency of ulcer breakdown and a higher mortality from natural causes than others [7].

An adequate history and physical examination should reveal many of the potential problems that could compromise the results of skin graft surgery. Medical management of unrelated systemic disorders and general surgical treatment of underlying arterial or venous insufficiency may be necessary before skin grafting should be performed. In addition, the elimination of smoking preoperatively in patients who are to receive a skin graft should be strongly encouraged.

Complications Related to Split-Thickness Skin Graft Donor Sites

In general, selection of a STSG donor site should take into account the potential cosmetic disfigurement that results from the scar following removal of tissue. In addition, the practicality involved with wound care and the type of instrumentation to be used for the harvest of a STSG should also be taken into consideration. For STSGs to be applied to facial defects, the donor sites should be placed above the normal blush line. This allows the graft most closely to match the adjacent normal tissue because of the intrinsic physiologic properties of blushing that occurs only in this distribution. For this reason, donor sites for STSGs on the face are typically chosen from the supraclavicular areas, lateral neck, preauricular area, and scalp. The scalp can be an excellent source for multiple STSGs since the grafts are cut superficially and the regrown hair camouflages the graft scar without affecting the hair growth [8–12]. In children, however, excessive blood loss secondary to the large surface area of the scalp may preclude its use as a suitable STSG donor site [11]. In addition, pale individuals may find scalp skin to be too hyperpigmented to permit a good color match at the recipient area [13].

For defects found on the trunk or extremity, STSG donor sites are often utilized in hidden areas including the pubic area, lower abdomen, buttocks, and thighs. Some consideration should also be given to the potential problems that are associated with the postoperative care required for the STSG donor site. For elderly or debilitated patients, the anterolateral thigh might be the best choice for a donor site since the ability of the patient to care for a wound in this area might be improved over a similar wound made on the buttocks or lower back. Since the cosmetic result may be less important than the function of the patient during the postoperative period, this is an important factor to take into consideration.

STSG donor defects are often the source of a great deal of postoperative pain and may be more problematic for the patient than is the recipient site. Other primary problems associated with the donor area include bleeding, drainage of serous fluid, and infection. With the development of synthetic surgical dressings, the amount of pain that the patients suffer during the postoperative period at STSG donor sites has been substantially reduced. The most commonly used donor site dressing is the polyurethane membrane (PUM). The occlusive nature of PUMs reduces the discomfort almost immediately after placement and also has the hidden benefit of speeding the rate of reepithelialization. Unfortunately, one problem associated this type of dressing is that the serosanguineous material that drains from the wound surface accumulates beneath the dressing and often results in leakage. For this reason, application of a strip of tape around the perimeter of the dressing and the use of a bulky gauze pad positioned at the dependent border to collect any leakage of serum is often necessary [14].

The PUMs can be left in place as long as the accumulated fluid which collects beneath the dressing is relatively limited in amount. If excess fluid accumulates, this can be drained by puncturing the dressing with a sterile needle, aspirating the fluid, and then patching the puncture hole with another small piece of PUM. Although infection is a potential problem associated with the occlusion of any wound, it is not a common occurrence at STSG donor sites. However, if infection does occur, it may result in the creation of a full-thickness wound. Infection should be treated with appropriate antibiotics, débridement as necessary, and topical measures to remove the exudate [15].

One acute problem associated with the harvesting of STSGs relates to the accidental cutting of the graft too deeply, resulting in a full-thickness wound. This can occur if the dermatome adjustment is not properly checked prior to initiating the procedure, or if consideration is not given to the relatively thin skin found in young children, geriatric patients, and chronically ill individuals. This can also be the result of sudden changes in surface tension on the skin due to unequal skin traction by the surgeon or the assistant. If a full-thickness defect is created, this should be closed by suturing, if possible, or if the area is large, a STSG may be applied. On occasion, a STSG may be of irregular shape and inadvertent button-holing may occur. This results in an unsatisfactory graft with subsequent poor healing, and additional tissue may be required to cover the recipient site satisfactorily.

In the chronic phase of healing of the STSG donor site other unique problems can be encountered. First, hypertrophic scars or keloids may develop at the donor site, especially in susceptible patients. This complication can be successfully managed in many patients with the use of intralesional steroids delivered at the time of graft harvesting to reduce the tendency for hypertrophic scars to form [8, 15]. In addition, a permanent textural scar is virtually inevitable whenever STSGs are harvested.

A more common complication seen at the donor site of STSG harvesting is temporary or permanent pigmentary changes. Donor sites may develop irregular pigmentation after harvesting, which is typically darker than normal color [12]. If thick STSGs are utilized, the donor site may become lighter than the normal surrounding skin [15]. Adequate psychological preparation of the patient and appropriate selection of the donor site may help to minimize the potential cosmetic problems that results from this procedure.

Complications Related to Full-Thickness Skin Graft Donor Sites

Although less commonly, complications may also occur at FTSG donor sites. Probably one of the more common problems that is encountered is the removal of excessive tissue so as to prevent easy closure of the donor site area. If this occurs, the wound may be closed with undue tension, resulting in ischemia, wound dehiscence, or pain at the donor site. Since only limited tissue is available for FTSGs, only a limited number of donor sites are available for this purpose. One site used for facial defects is the preauricular area. If excess tissue is harvested from this area, the sideburn hair found in men tends to be moved posteriorly and may be closer to the ear than is normal. This may result in a visible cosmetic asymmetry. The postauricular area is another common site to obtain FTSGs. In situations where excess tissue is removed from this area there may be some retraction of the ear, making its appearance more flat on the harvested side than on the normal side. While this may not be readily visible, it may cause problems in individuals who wear glasses since the arm of their glasses may rub either on the ear or the scalp.

As with all wounds, some consideration should be given to the orientation of the final scar that will be required for the surgical reconstruction. Since the supraclavicular area is a common site for FTSG donor tissue, it is important to recognize that in women who wear dresses with low-cut necklines, a scar in this area may be visible; thus another site should perhaps be chosen. Since most FTSG donor sites are closed primarily, a common complication at the donor site is the spreading of the scar. This is usually a function of the location or amount of wound tension, which should be largely anticipated in advance and avoided if appropriate support of the site is provided with subcutaneous suture materials or topical measures postoperatively.

As with all cutaneous surgical procedures, a possible complication is that of pain, but this can generally be minimized by proper selection of the donor site and avoiding tension during wound closure. Hematoma or seroma formation may also occur, especially if the tissue is being harvested from a thin anatomic site such as the lateral neck. This complication can frequently be avoided with proper dressing materials.

Complications Related to Split-Thickness Skin Graft Recipient Sites

Most skin graft failures can be ascribed to flaws in the recipient site rather than to technical defects in the skin graft procedure itself [8]. A major graft bed problem is inadequate local blood supply. If an STSG is applied to an area with limited blood supply, such as on denuded bone, cartilage, or tendon, the graft is unlikely to survive. These tissues should either be covered with a local or regional flap or given time to develop sufficient granulation tissue so that graft survival is likely. A general rule of thumb is that a graft placed over an avascular defect which is less than 1 cm in size may survive due to a bridging effect where nutritional supply comes from the random graft vessels connecting with the adjacent vascularized tissues, a phenomenon known as inosculation.

One technique that has been utilized to provide a more suitable graft bed over exposed cranial bone is to débride the outer table of the skull either with a chisel, burr, or carbon dioxide laser to allow granulation tissue to form from the diploë which spans the exposed bone and provides a vascular supply for the graft. On the ear a similar technique can be performed, where a small series of punch biopsies are removed from the center of the defect through the cartilage to the tissue on the opposite side of the ear [9]. This allows granulation tissue to grow from the opposite side through the holes that have been cut in the cartilage and provide a well-vascularized bed for the subsequent graft procedure.

If excessive granulation tissue develops at the skin graft recipient site, it must be trimmed or flattened to improve the potential for graft survival. This can be accomplished with simple scissor removal or application of dressings containing hypertonic saline or with silver nitrate sticks.

All efforts should be made to reduce the risk of infection at the recipient site, for if it is infected, graft loss is inevitable. The number and type of bacteria that are present determine whether success or failure occurs. Although all wound are essentially contaminated to one degree or another, true infection occurs only in wounds in which the local defense mechanisms are overwhelmed by a large amount of bacteria or by the virulence of the bacteria that are present. It has been suggested that the presence of more than 100 000 organisms per gram of tissue usually leads to graft loss [8, 12, 13, 15]. Streptococcal infection can lead to total loss of the graft. In addition *Pseudomonas* produces a great amount of exudate which can cause the graft to float off the recipient bed of the wound before healing is accomplished. Topical agents that are effective in controlling wound bacteria include silvadene, sulfamylon cream, and solutions of acetic acid and sodium hypochlorite. In addition, enzymatic débriding agents such as Debrisan, Elase, and Travase are also effective, but these are not as good as repeated sharp excision of the wound to prepare it for the graft. Should the graft become infected, the infected area should be débrided so that as much of the graft can be salvaged as possible.

Graft failure can also result from bleeding or oozing that occurs at the recipient bed because the hematoma separates the graft from its nutritional supply. Hemostasis can be accomplished in most cases with ligation, cautery, or pressure. Use of hemostatic agents such as Oxycel or Gelfoam are contraindicated for FTSGs and STSGs. If bleeding seems to be excessive, the graft procedure should probably be deferred until a later time.

Technical errors are a common cause of graft failure. Although it seems unlikely, a common technical error that occurs in STSGs is the placement of the graft upside down with the donor epidermis applied on the base of the wound. Obviously, for survival to occur the dermal side of the graft must be placed directly onto the recipient bed. It is usually quite obvious which side of the graft is the dermal side, since the graft always curls downward toward the dermal side. One recommendation that has been made in the past is to use a PUM on the donor site prior to split-thickness grafting [16]. This adds only about 0.003 in. in thickness to the graft, but greatly aids in harvesting. The PUM remains on the donor site both during the harvesting procedure and after it has been sutured into the recipient site. This technique prevents the graft from curling onto itself and rapidly allows proper orientation. This technique also facilitates trimming an irregular perimeter, making the shaping of the graft much easier. The graft is then attached to the wound in traditional fashion with the PUM remaining in place, which separates on its own in about 1 week.

Another complication that may occur with STSGs, especially in a wound that has been allowed partially to reepithelialize, are epithelial cysts or milia that develop beneath the graft from residual islands of epithelial tissue below the graft [15]. Milia may also form from buried sweat glands below the graft [8, 12]. If milia form, they should be opened and expressed individually. Recently, a "sponge deformity" has been described following STSGs of burn wounds. In this situation multiple small epithelial remnants that are retained begin partially to reepithelialize the wound before the graft had been positioned. This results in the development of small pocklike bridging and scars, which causes both a functional and cosmetic deformity [17]. This problem can be prevented by excising the wound to a greater depth or by applying a thinner graft. If this occurs, the areas of abnormality can be treated with simple excision and closure.

The most common problem associated with STSG recipient sites is poor color match. This may be a function of a lack of blushing that occurs in normal facial skin but not in the grafted tissue or of the hyperpigmentation that commonly develops. Another common complication is the lack of hair at the recipient site, which is exspecially important in the STSG treatment of the bearded portions of a male patient's face. Less commonly, typically with larger grafts, there may be a complaint of xerosis. This is presumably due to a lack of glandular tissue in the STSG tissue. In addition, there may temporarily be a lack of sensation or a different sensation af the graft site. This usually improves with time. STSGs tend to tolerate friction poorly and as a consequence are somewhat fragile. Because of this, they are not usually indicated for areas where pressure or tension is likely to occur. Despite this fact bullae have been reported at STSG sites, presumably due to friction.

Another common complication that is intrinsic to STSGs is contraction deformity. If a STSG is placed on an area where there is a free margin, especially the upper lip or eyelid, there may be contraction of the underlying structure resulting in impair function. In a similar way, since STSGs typically fail to grow proportionally in children, they tend to become more obvious with time.

On occasion, an STSG is meshed with small expandable slits that provide additional tissue for covering a large wound where only a limited amount of donor tissue exists. Meshed grafts are often associated with significant contraction since the expanded slit areas that have been cut into the graft must heal by second intention. While useful in the treatment of irregular or concave areas in which surface exudates are likely to accumulate, especially in large burn wounds, they should not be used on cosmetically important areas because the overall period of time required for healing is lengthened and the cosmetic results are inferior.

Complications at Full-Thickness Skin Graft Recipient Sites

The most important consideration for FTSGs is the selection of a donor site that most closely resembles the recipient area. However, this is not always possible. Ideally, for facial defects the donor site should be above the blush line; for treatment of defects in hair-bearing areas the quality and texture of hair should be evaluated; conversely, if a defect occurs in an area that does not contain hair, it would be inappropriate to select an FTSG from a hair-bearing area.

Since FTSGs retain most of the color and textural qualities of the donor site, careful choices must be made in evaluating the tissue at the time of surgery to prevent problems from occurring. For facial defects, most FTSGs are taken from the pre- or postauricular area, lateral neck, upper eyelid, supraclavicular area, or occasionally the nasolabial fold. One potential problem with some of these areas is that the skin is often protected from the sun compared to the sun-exposed face, so that the match may not be ideal. The supraclavicular tissue may be thinner or more sun damaged than the face, and therefore the match may not be of high quality. If the nasolabial fold is chosen as a donor site for the nose, excising tissue from one fold may result in an asymmetry with the opposite side, requiring a second excision to be performed on the opposite side at a later date.

An accurate measurement of the defect to be repaired with an FTSG is of absolute importance. Inaccuracies in measurements are uncommon on flat surfaces but considerable difficulty may occur when dealing with convex or concave surfaces. The vertical component of the defect must be considered when measuring the overall size of the defect. Templates using a sterile gauze, Telfa, or sterile aluminum foil can be used to measure defects on these contoured surfaces. By creating an appropriate pattern, a template can be created which approximates the size and shape of the wound itself [9]. This can then be transferred to the donor site with an appropriate increase of 10%–20% to account for contraction that occurs after removal, using a surgical marking device. The exact amount of tissue can be excised and then transferred to the recipient site without distortion. If, despite these maneuvers, the graft is too small and must be stretched to accommodate the defect, it is probably better to use two grafts rather than to compromise the results by stretching a solitary graft which is of insufficient size. The tension on a graft decreases its survival and increases the chance for failure.

A common cause of FTSG failure is a result of not removing all subcutaneous tissue from the base of the graft. If the subcutaneous fat is not removed, because it is poorly vascularized, the graft's dermal vessels are not in contact with the recipient bed. This results in insufficient vascularization and subsequent failure of the graft itself.

In all cases, if there is complete hemostasis in the recipient bed at the time that the graft is placed, bleeding in the graft bed will disrupt the graft and cause it to be lost. The graft bed should always be completely dry before the graft is placed. If bleeding is profuse, grafting should be delayed for several days to allow appropriate control of bleeding prior to application of the graft. Bleeding can typically be controlled with electrocautery, ligation, or simple external pressure. One good technique to use prior to the final application of a dressing for a FTSG is to flush any debris, clots, or material from beneath the graft using chilled normal saline. Slits cut into the FTSG also help to prevent accumulation of fluid which could disrupt the graft from the wound bed.

To prevent the formation of hematomas or seromas several different techniques can be utilized. First, the perimeter of the graft should be secured with sutures or staples. Second, the graft is immobilized with several long interrupted sutures placed at various points around the perimeter to be used to tie over the surface of a bulky dressing. In addition, a running basting stitch to secure the central portion of the graft has been described, which not only holds the graft to the bed but loculates any hematoma/seroma which may form, thus limiting fluid dissection between graft and bed [16]. Using the closed technique, the success of the graft procedure is not evaluated for a period of 1 week.

A second technique that has been used is the simple, or open, technique, in which a minimal wound dressing is applied to permit daily observation of the healing wound. The greatest problem associated with this technique is that this requires large amounts of wound care. It is for this reason that the tie-over dressing or bolster method is the most popular one used today. By providing even pressure of a constant nature on the graft, immobilization and maximum revascularization can occur.

One problem that occurs with this technique is that at the time of bolster removal, adherence between the graft and the dressing causes the graft to be inadvertently pulled off when the dressing is removed. This complication can be minimized by the use of a new monofilament plastic dressing, known as N-terface. This dressing permits the exudate from the graft to pass through the dressing without adhering to it. This minimizes disruption of the graft during dressing changes.

An occasional problem that occurs with some FTSGs is hypertrophic or keloidal scar formation that may occur in susceptible individuals. An abnormal scar may also be seen primarily in children at the junction of the normal skin and the graft. This problem can be minimized by carefully fitting the graft into the bed of the wound and orienting the scar so that it is not at right angles to the direction of skin folds. Segmental interposition of the skin graft edges can be used to break up the scar line around the edge of the graft and decrease tension. In areas such as the axilla scarring is reduced if the grafts are oriented horizontally. Avoiding graft tension by using as large a graft as necessary to permit tensionless placement may also be beneficial. The use of large graft sheets is also recommended since the junctional scars often occur at the edges of smaller skin grafts which are placed into a large wound [15]. If this type of scarring does develop, intralesional steroids and compression dressings provide improvement.

FTSGs generally assume the sensation characteristics of the recipient wound, not of the donor site. Although innervation is abnormal in virtually all grafts, the sensation generally returns to normal more quickly in FTSGs than in STSGs.

There are special problems that can arise when a FTSG is placed on the lower extremity. The first is that the new blood vessels that form are often disrupted if the affected limb is held in a dependent position. This may result in the formation of small blisters on the grafted skin surface, an indication of excessive hydrostatic pressure. For that reason, lower extremity wounds should be kept elevated for approximately 2–3 weeks after FTSGs have been applied. Thereafter, to insure greatest success, external elastic compression is recommended when the leg is held in a dependent position to facilitate lymphatic drainage and prevent congestion in the graft. Despite all of these precautions there are occasions when grafts fail. Minimizing vascular congestion, reducing the risk of infection, and immobilizing the graft in its recipient bed without tension enhance the probability of graft survival. However, in virtually all circumstances the risk of graft failure should be evaluated for the patient in advance.

Many complications of FTSGs are the result of abnormal healing or inappropriate selection of graft material. It is imperative that many factors be evaluated to provide the patient with the best functional and cosmetic result. To minimize as many problems as possible, ideal graft selection, preparation of the recipient bed, and good surgical technique are required. A number of anticipated problems can be dealt with in advance to reduce some of these types of complications. It is well known that STSGs contract much more than FTSGs, up to 70% in some cases. However, even FTSGs can be expected to contract somewhat. In areas where contraction might produce some anatomic distortion, such as near the vermilion order of the lip, the nasal ala, or the lower eyelid, this fact must be taken into consideration. As a consequence, FTSGs are usually cut between 150% and 200% larger than the eyelid defect to compensate for the potential contraction that will occur. For other sites only a 20%–25% increase in size of the FTSG is required.

The graft may develop a trapdoor deformity or pin cushioning, which is secondary to wound contraction. This complication is usually unpredictable but can be minimized by undermining beyond the borders of the defect. In some cases a true hypertrophic scar can also form, resulting in an abnormally appearing graft. This scar can be expected to soften and flatten with time, but the use of intralesional steroid injections into the fibrous tissue below the graft may speed this process. On occasion, it may be necessary to debulk the graft by incising one edge of it and removing the excess fibrous scar tissue that has formed beneath [9].

Pigmentary changes may also be a source of cosmetic disfigurement with FTSGs. This may be the result of selecting an inappropriate donor site or because the patient exposed the graft to ultraviolet light during the acute healing phase. It is generally recommended that the patient use sun protection in the form of a topical sun screen with an sun-protection factor of at least 15 for a minimum of 6 months after skin grafting [15]. In some cases an entire anatomic unit may be grafted to make the anticipated resultant pigmentary changes and textural differences less noticeable.

Although FTSGs are less fragile than STSGs, they may also be susceptible to traumatic injuries, especially when used for the treatment of ulcers on the lower legs, decubitus ulcers, or defects overlying cartilage or bone. These risks can generally be minimized by limiting postoperative motion and elevating the extremity to protect it from any inadvertent trauma that might induce graft breakdown.

While textural problems are infrequent with FTSGs because they retain most of the qualities of the donor site, contour deformities may be a problem. Any irregularities in the surface contours can be expected to improve spontaneously with time. However, significant differences between the thickness of the graft and the depth of the defect can cause a permanent deformity. If a very large defect is present, and it is anticipated that a FTSG will not provide sufficient volume to fill it in, a technique known as delayed grafting may permit sufficient granulation tissue to fill in the bed of the defect to achieve a better result than by simple placement of an FTSG. It should be remembered, however, that if reepithelialization has begun by the time an FTSG is applied, the new epithelium must be removed, otherwise milia or cysts will form. If there are minor elevation differences between the graft and the surrounding skin, focal dermabrasion can often substantially improve the cosmetic result [18]. In addition, the carbon dioxide laser has been used in a technique known as laser-abrasion to even out the irregularities in the surface [19]. This technique is especially beneficial in the treatment of smaller grafts where the anatomic location or the small size of the graft would not permit performance of normal dermabrasion. Another advantage is the precision with which the laser energy can be delivered and the uniformity of ablation that is possible. Lastly, with the laser there is usually complete hemostasis, which improves visibility to reduce the risk of removing excess tissue.

Complications Associated with Autologous Grafts

This relatively new technique has been effectively utilized in the treatment of large recipient defects, especially following excision of congenital giant melanocytic nevi and burn injuries. As this technique has evolved, it has become apparent that the same complications exist for it as for both STSGs and FTSGs. The susceptibility to infection, hematoma, shearing, and loss because of improper preparation of the graft bed are idential to the other types of grafts. Autologous grafts are used primarily to provide a functional, not a cosmetic result and their indications are therefore somewhat different.

Complications of Composite Grafts

The most common situation in which composite grafts are utilized for cutaneous surgery is in reconstruction of the nasal ala which is lost due to trauma or extirpation of malignancy. The donor site is usually the ascending auricular rim of the ear. For grafts larger than 2 cm in diameter the risk of failure is substantial. All of the potential problems seen with STSGs and FTSGs apply with composite grafts as well. However, there is the added disadvantage that the vascular requirements for a composite graft is greater than for any of the other types of grafts. As a consequence of this, larger defects cannot be adequately treated in this fashion. Meticulous technique must be used to provide the greatest possibility of a good cosmetic result.

Conclusion

Although the technique of skin grafting has been used for nearly 3000 years, in order to treat patients most satisfactorily with a variety of cutaneous defects the dermatologic surgeon must understand the requirements of both the graft and the recipient site to achieve the best results and the highest level of success. While complications can be encountered, these are typically a function of improper selection of the donor tissue or improper preparation of the recipient site. With meticulous technique and care to prevent secondary infection and bleeding, a good functional and cosmetic result can be obtained in most cases. The future for utilizing autologous skin graft material is especially exciting, and additional developments are certain to appear in the near future.

References

1. Pensler JM, Steward R, Lewis SR, Herndon DN (1988) Reconstruction of the burned palm: full-thickness versus split-thickness skin grafts-long term follow-up. Plast Reconstr Surg 81(1):46–49
2. Philips TJ, Kehinde O, Green H, Gilchrest PA (1989) Treatment of skin ulcers with cultured epidermal allografts. J Am Acad Dermatol 21(2/1):191–199
3. Moi MA, Nanninga PB, van Gendenburg JP, Westerhof W, Mekkes JR, VanGinkel CJ (1991) Grafting of venous leg ulcers. An intraindividual comparison between cultured skin equivalents and full-thickness skin punch grafts. J Am Acad Dermatol 24(1): 77–82
4. Gallico GG III, O'Connor NE, Compton CC, Remensnyder JP, Kehinde O, Green H (1989) Cultured epithelial autografts for giant congenital nevi. Plast Reconstr Surg 84(1):1–9

5. Kumagai N, Nishina H, Tanabe H, Hosaka T, Ishilda H, Ogino Y (1988) Clinical application of autologous cultured epithelia for the treatment of burn wounds and burn scars. Plast Reconstr Surg 82(1):99–110
6. O'Connor NE, Gallico GG, Compton CC (1990) Modification of hypertrophic scars and keloids with cultured epithelial autografts. Proc Am Burn Assoc 22:7
7. Harrison PV (1988) Split-skin grafting of varicose leg ulcers – a survey and the importance of assessment of risk factors in predicting outcome from the procedure. Clin Exp Dermatol 13:4–6
8. Rudolph R, Ballantyne DL (1990) Skin grafts. In: McCarthy JG (ed) General principles. Saunders, Philadelphia, (Plastic surgery, vol 1), pp 221–274
9. Skouge JW (1991) Skin grafting. Churchill Livingstone, New York
10. Zingaro EA, Capozzi A, Pennisi VR (1988) The scalp as a donor site in burns. Arch Surg 123:652–653
11. Lesesne CB, Rosenthal R (1986) A review of scalp split-thickness skin grafts and potential complications. Plast Reconstr Surg 77(5):757–758
12. Fisher JC (1987) Skin grafting. In: Georgiade NG, Georgiade GS, Riefkohl R, Barwick WJ (ed) Essential of plastic, maxillofacial and reconstructive surgery. Williams and Wilkins, Baltimore, pp 23–32
13. Scheflan M (1984) Complications of skin grafting. In: Greenfield LJ (ed) Complications in surgery and trauma. Lippincott, Philadelphia, pp 35–39
14. Skouge JW (1987) Techniques for split-thickness skin grafting. J Dermatol Surg Oncol 13(8):841–849
15. Rudolph R (1984) Skin grafting. In: Goldwyn RM (ed) The unfavorable result in plastic surgery-avoidance and treatment, 2nd edn. Little, Brown, Boston, pp 143–149
16. Glogau RG, Stegman SJ, Tromovich TA (1987) Refinements in split-thickness skin grafting technique. J Dermatol Surg Oncol 13(8):853–858
17. Engrav LH, Gottliev JR, Wlakinshae MD, Hermbach DM, Grube B (1989) The "sponge deformity" after tangential excision and grafting of burns. Plast Reconstr Surg 83(3):468–470
18. Robinson JK (1987) Improvement in the appearance of full-thickness skin grafts with dermabrasion. Arch Dermatol 123:1340–1343
19. Wheeland RG (1988) Revision of full-thickness skin grafts using the carbon dioxide laser. J Dermatol Surg Oncol 14(2):130–134

Skin Flaps

NICHOLAS R. TELFER, ANNA TONG and RONALD L. MOY

Introduction

The incidence of flap complications is a direct reflection of the widespread use of a variety of cutaneous flaps in dermatologic surgical practice. Basically, a skin flap is a segment of tissue incorporating its own blood vessels that is moved in one or more steps to a recipient area leaving the flap base attached. The indications for using a flap to repair a defect are multiple (defects that cannot be closed primarily, deep defects requiring bulk to repair, and wounds containing exposed bone, tendon, or cartilage which would not support a skin graft), and in general a flap, which moves neighboring skin into a defect, provides a better color and texture match and thus a preferable cosmetic result than a skin graft. Due to its self-nourishing quality, a flap is less likely to necrose or "fail" than a graft.

Skin flaps may be classified according to the distribution of their blood supply; axial-pattern flaps receive a blood supply from defined cutaneous vessels and anastomoses, and random-pattern flaps (which are not based upon defined vessels), are nourished by dermal and subdermal plexi, which in turn are fed by deeper perforating musculocutaneous vessels [1]. In general dermatologic surgical practice axial pattern flaps are rarely used, with the notable exception of the midline forehead flap [2]. The rich arterial supply of facial skin allows the dermatologic surgeon to design and create a wide variety of well-vascularized random-pattern flaps.

As with all types of surgery, complications may arise when skin flap surgery is performed. These include problems common to all types of surgery (bleeding, infection, etc.) and complications more specific to flaps (dehiscence, tip necrosis, etc.). In many instances, both extrinsic and intrinsic factors are involved in the etiology of flap complications. Extrinsic factors relate to the systemic condition of the patient (cigarette smoking [3], immunocompetence, malnutrition) and intrinsic factors relate to problems with the design and execution of the flap (excessive tension, kinking of pedicle, compression [4]. Some complications predispose to the development of further problems; for example, hematoma formation predisposes to infection, dehiscence, and necrosis of a flap.

Necrosis

The most serious complication in flap surgery is the death of tissue due to insufficient or compromised blood supply [Fig. 1]. Depending upon the degree of vascular compromise, necrosis may range from a superficial epidermal slough of the tip of the flap to a full-thickness loss of the entire flap. In either situation healing will proceed by secondary intention, in the former by epithelialization and in the latter by wound contraction, reepithelialization, and scar formation. Compromised flap perfusion is frequently related to poor surgical planning and rough tissue handling. Other factors include excessive tension on the flap combined with postoperative edema, which further increases tension at the suture lines. Similarly, a flap which has been undermined too superficially is at increased risk of necrosis, and this risk is increased still further by the compressive forces of a pressure dressing. The design of flaps should always include an assessment of the length of the flap related to the width of its base, as both animal experiments [4] and clinical experience suggest that the creation of an overly long flap (length to width ratio greater than 3:1) almost inevitably leads to the necrosis of distal flap due to arterial insufficiency.

Many flaps appear pale at the completion of surgery; this is physiologic and often related to vasospasm and reversible epinephrine-induced vasoconstriction. However, if a flap remains persistently pale the possibility of flap ischemia and potential necrosis must be considered. Factors such as a persistent vaso-

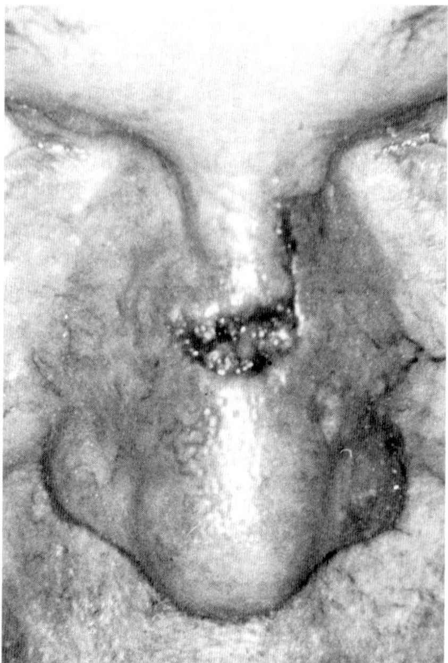

Fig. 1. Full-thickness necrosis of the tip of a rhombic flap on the nasal bridge

constrictive effect of epinephrine, excessive tension, and an excessive length to width ratio must be considered. Management is directed towards identifying any reversible underlying causes; for example, tension due to hematoma formation is relieved by evacuation of the blood clot and the control of all bleeding points, and tension created by an overly stretched flap with tight sutures is managed by release of the sutures and reorientation to minimize wound tension. In extreme situations, some surgeons would manage a poorly designed or overly long flap by removing all sutures and allowing the flap to fall back into its original bed in an attempt to avoid full-thickness flap necrosis. When flap necrosis is already evident, many favor a conservative approach and allow spontaneous demarcation of the eschar to progress unimpaired. Debridement should be avoided or at least delayed until the eschar is ready to separate, as early and excessive debridement may not only damage underlying and neighboring healthy skin but also interfere with healing beneath the eschar.

The most effective way to avoid excessive flap tension and minimize the risk of necrosis is appropriate surgical planning. Principles of flap design dictate that the length to width ratio of a flap may be varied, with relatively long flaps surviving well on the face, but not elsewhere on the body, that the removal of dog ears should not involve narrowing of the pedicle (thereby increasing the risk of ischemia), and that tension within the flap can be minimized by adequate undermining of the flap and adjacent areas. Once the flap is created, emphasis is placed on gentle tissue handling and the careful positioning of sutures, which allows tension to be distributed throughout the flap and to be minimized at the wound edges. Flap positioning commonly involves the use of subcuticular stitches, particularly at areas of greatest tension (for example, in closing the secondary defect of a rhombic flap). Skin sutures must be tied snugly to evert skin edges but not so tight that postoperative edema will result in excessive tension. Proper suturing techniques also include placement of knots away from the flap surface and the accurate alignment of all corners and angles, using either corner stitches or simple, small-bite, interrupted sutures. Certain suture materials are extensible and will elongate as the wound edges swell (e. g., monofilament polypropylene and nylon).

As skin flaps can tolerate only a limited period of ischemia before irreversible tissue damage ensues (5), early detection of circulatory compromise is imperative to the preservation of the flap. Parameters such as capillary refill, tissue turgor, and flap color may all be used to assess the adequacy of blood flow.

Infection

Pathogenic organisms may cause both direct and indirect damage to a flap; these effects are produced by inflammatory and immune responses and the release of destructive proteolytic enzymes which disrupt both wound healing and subcuticular sutures. Infection is more likely to develop in wounds containing large amounts of devitalized tissue (excessive electrocautery), foreign material (sutures), and any hematoma. Inflammatory edema also increases wound tension, which may contribute to the development of ischemia and possibly flap necrosis.

Infection may lead to flap dehiscence, particularly if buried sutures are disrupted. The risk of flap dehiscence may be limited by the use of adhesive surface strips (e. g., Steri-Strips). When a flap shows signs of infection, it is often reasonable to remove alternate sutures in order to facilitate drainage and minimize both constriction and ischemia of the wound edges.

The early signs of infection (edema, erythema, etc.) are similar to those of normal wound healing, and consequently many infections only become clinically apparent between the 4th and 7th postoperative days. Delayed hemorrhage, increasing edema, erythema, tenderness, and purulent exudation from suture lines are all features suspicious of infection (Fig. 2). Management should include taking swabs for microbiologic study and the commencement of oral antibiotic therapy. As most wound infections are due to *Staphylococcus* or *Streptococcus* species, good initial choices include a penicillinase-resistant penicillin, cephalosporin, or erythromycin. Further oral antibiotic therapy is guided by the results of laboratory culture and sensitivity tests. A notable exception involves wounds on the ear, especially where cartilage has been exposed. In this setting, *Pseudomonas aeruginosa* infection is not uncommon and requires treatment with an antibiotic such as ciprofloxacin. Severe wound infections with abscess formation will necessitate opening the flap, drainage, and irrigation with sterile saline.

Infections may occur as a combination of both wound contamination and lowering of natural host defenses, and consequently specific measures can be directed to the prevention of infection. In combination with the use of a scrupul-

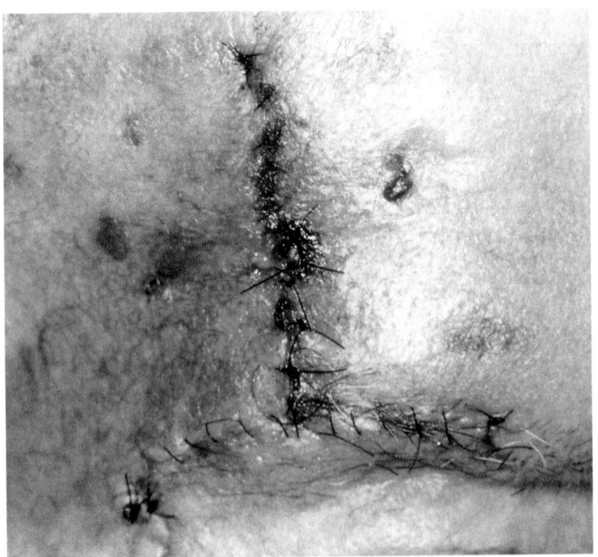

Fig. 2. Purulent exudate from A-to-T advancement flap above the eyebrow noted on the 4th post-operative day. Culture grew *Staphylococcus aureus*

ous sterile technique [6], antibiotic prophylaxis may be helpful in certain circumstances. The antibiotic should be directed against the most likely infecting organisms and, again, a cephalosporin, penicillin, or erythromycin are commonly selected because of their qualities of broad-spectrum efficacy, relative safety, and excellent tissue penetration. Antibiotic prophylaxis may be considered in patients with anticipated long procedures during which the wound remains exposed (e. g., multiple-stage Mohs micrographic surgery), in normally heavily colonized anatomic sites (such as the ear, axilla, and groin), and in patients at increased risk of infection, for example, diabetic and immunocompromised patients. The healing of clean and uncomplicated surgical wounds, by contrast, has been shown *not* to benefit from the use of prophylactic antibiotic therapy [7].

The timing of antibiotic administration is important; antibiotics commenced too early may increase the risk of development of resistant microbial strains, and antibiotics commenced more than 3 h postoperatively may be less effective as the wound coagulum may tend to protect trapped bacteria and interfere with penetration of antibiotics into the tissue [7]. Consequently, to achieve maximal benefit, prophylactic antibiotic therapy, where indicated, should be commenced 24–48 h orally or no less than 2 h intravenously prior to surgery so that therapeutic levels of antibiotic agents can accumulate in the tissues [7]. Postoperatively, antibiotics may be continued for 1–2 days to minimize bacterial contamination that may occur before epithelial migration seals off the suture lines and needle puncture sites. Prolonged postoperative administration of antibiotics (more than 48 h) tends not to increase protection and increases the potential risks of drug toxicity and the development of antibiotic-resistant bacterial strains [7].

With good surgical technique and the gentle handling of tissue, most wounds on the head and neck can withstand minimal bacterial contamination without becoming infected.

Hematoma

Hematoma formation may range in severity from a minor, self-limiting problem to an acute postoperative emergency, or to a progressive chain of complications leading to ischemia, infection, and wound dehiscence. Initially, an amorphous gel-like mass of clot forms, which can be readily expressed from the wound. Several days postoperatively, the clot begins to organize and form an adherent, rubbery mass which may only be removed by opening the flap. From the 7th to 14th days, fibrinolytic activity progressively liquefies the hematoma, which at this stage may be aspirated, avoiding the need for opening the wound. After 14 days, most hematomas have been totally reabsorbed [8].

The most common causes of hematoma formation are inadequate intraoperative hemostasis and coagulopathies. It is a principle of all cutaneous surgery, and in particular of flap surgery, that intraoperative hemostasis be meticulous, with all bleeding points cauterized or tied off. Preoperatively, all patients should be asked about personal and family histories of increased bleeding, for example after dental procedures. In may cases, coagulopathy is medication-related, with salicylates being the most common and unnoticed culprits. Many cold remedies (Alka-Seltzer, Anacin, etc.) contain aspirin, which irreversibly inhibits the cyclooxygenase pathway of platelet aggregation, thus prolonging the bleeding time. Other nonsteroidal antiinflammatory drugs such as ibuprofen (Motrin, Advil, etc.) produce a reversible inhibition of the same pathway. Patients with liver disease, in poor nutritional state, or taking anticoagulant therapy are all at increased risk for hematoma formation. To prevent bleeding complications during elective flap surgery, aspirin should be withheld for 2 weeks prior to surgery and for 1 week thereafter. In general, elective flap surgery should be avoided in patients taking anticoagulants [9]. However, when this is not possible, careful titration of Coumadin dosage to produce prothrombin times as close to 1.2 as possible or temporary conversion to heparin therapy (because of its short half-life and more responsive short-term control) has been suggested [10].

A rapidly developing and large hematoma is an emergency. It usually manifests with sudden pain beneath the dressing and bluish, tender swelling at the site of the wound (Fig. 3). This is managed by the removal of a section of cutaneous and subcutaneous sutures, giving access to the hematoma, relieving wound tension, and preventing further strangulation of the flap. The area is secured by digital compression while a local anesthetic is injected and the wound cleaned. The clot is evacuated and the wound irrigated with sterile saline. All bleeding points are sought, tied off, or electrocauterized, and the flap resutured in position. Antibiotic therapy, if not already started, should be commenced.

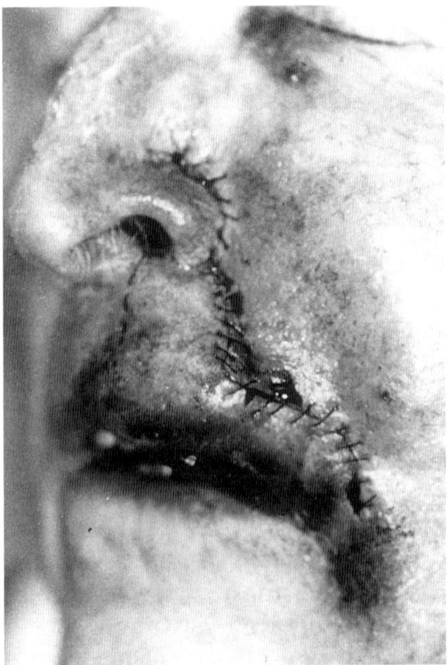

Fig. 3. Painful, expanding hematoma beneath cheek advancement flap presenting 24 h after surgery

Fortunately, the majority of hematomas which form beneath flaps are small and self-limiting. They tend to go undiscovered or are left untreated, and eventually liquefy and are reabsorbed.

Dehiscence

With the exception of premature suture removal, dehiscence of a flap is seldom a primary event, and is usually a consequence of infection or hematoma formation. Within a few days following surgery, there is active fibroplasia at the wound margins and tensile strength begins to develop very slowly; at 2 weeks the wound possesses only 3%–5% of the strength of normal skin [8]. In facial surgery, most cutaneous sutures are removed after 1 week, or sometimes even earlier, making flaps vulnerable to dehiscence. At this time, the flap is held in place by buried sutures, coapted epithelial bridges, fibrinous coagulum gapping the dermal wound, and blood vessels crossing from one side of the wound to the other. Cross-linking of newly formed collagen progressively increases wound strength, which reaches a maximum of 80% of the tensile strength of normal skin several months after surgery [8]. Considerable mechanical support may be supplied by the use of wound closure tapes applied across the suture lines at the time of suture removal, especially if the tapes are secured in place with a liquid tissue adhesive [11].

The management of flap dehiscence depends upon the etiology; where infection or hematoma are involved, these must be dealt with appropriately. The next decision will be whether or not to resuture the flap in place. In most cases this will be appropriate unless the flap is clearly nonviable. If dehiscence occurs several days postoperatively, the flap can be resutured without freshening of the wound edges because, at this stage, active fibroblasts are present in the wound margin and trimming may delay rather than enhance healing. Antibiotic therapy is indicated in nearly all cases of flap dehiscence.

"Pincushioning"

"Pincushioning" also called "trapdooring", is the development of an elevated bulging deformity of a flap, which has a U-, C-, or V-shaped cross section [12]. This complication may affect many types of flaps, but appears to be a particular problem with some, for example, nasolabial transposition and island pedicle flaps (Fig. 4). Although no definite etiology has been identified, many possibilities have been postulated, including lymphatic and venous obstruction, hypertrophy or contracture of the scar, overly thick or fatty flaps, and inadequate undermining of the flap and the area peripheral to the surgical defect [12].

Management depends on the severity of the deformity, which will often slowly improve with time. Intralesional injections of triamcinolone acetonide, 20–40 mg/ml, are commonly used, repeated every 4–6 weeks as necessary. More severely deformed flaps may require surgical revision, thinning, defatting and

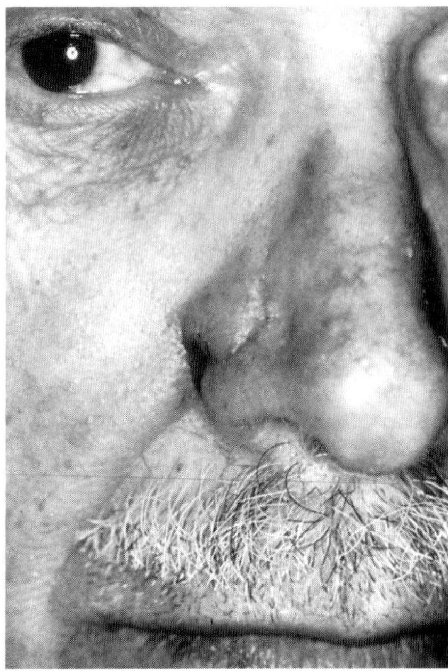

Fig. 4. Prominent "pincushion" deformity of a nasolabial transposition flap seen 4 weeks after surgery

the use of z-plasties to break up and elongate the scar lines. Excision of redundant skin and subcutaneous tissue and replacement with a full-thickness graft harvested from the postauricular region has also been described [13].

Scarring

Scarring may occur unexpectedly, but it is most often a sequela of other complications such as necrosis, dehiscence, and infection. Treatment depends upon the functional and cosmetic result and should probably be deferred until several weeks after surgery. In many cases, scarring will mature and become less evident with time; however, improvement may be facilitated by the use of intralesional steroid injections at 4- to 6-week intervals. Surgical revision procedures include excision of splayed scars, and focal dermabrasion ("scarabrasion"), which is particularly useful for uneven scars and for the "blending in" of prominent suture lines [14].

Conclusion

The essential factor in the prevention of complications in cutaneous flap surgery is careful planning and good surgical technique. As most dermatologic flap surgery is elective, a thorough preoperative evaluation is necessary to identify those patients at increased risk of infection, bleeding, or poor wound healing.

Intraoperatively, the principles of meticulous hemostasis, gentle tissue handling, obliteration of dead space, and avoidance of excessive wound tension are of paramount importance. Postoperatively, patients should receive clear verbal and written instructions on what to do and not to do with their wounds and dressings. It is a sound practice for dermatologic surgeons to remove the sutures from their own flaps, thereby ensuring an examination for signs of complications. Some flap complications may be unavoidable, but many can be minimized or entirely resolved by prompt and adequate therapy. When flap complications do arise, the cause of each should be sought and remedied in an attempt to maximize the cosmetic outcome and minimize any future surgical revision.

References

1. Jurkiewicz MJ, Vasconez H. In: Clinical Surgery, concepts and processes (Davis JH et al., eds. 1987) Mosby, St Louis. pp 3129–3170
2. Shumrick KA, Smith TL (1992) The anatomic basis for the design of forehead flaps in nasal reconstruction. Arch Otolaryngol Head Neck Surg 118:373–379
3. Goldminz D, Bennett RG (1991) Cigarette smoking and flap and full-thickness graft necrosis. Arch Dermatol 127:1012–1015
4. Kerrigan CL (1983) Skin flap failure: pathophysiology. Plast Reconstr Surg 72:766–774
5. Campbell SP, Moss ML, Hugo NE (1992) When does a random flap die? Plast Reconstr Surg 89:718–721
6. Sebben JE (1988) Sterile technique and the prevention of wound infection in office surgery – Part I. J. Dermatol Surg Oncol 14:1364–1371
7. Sebben JE (1985) Prophylactic antibiotics in cutaneous surgery. J Dermatol Surg Oncol 11:901–906
8. Salasche SJ (1986) Acute surgical complications: cause, prevention, and treatment. J Am Acad Dermatol 15:1163–1185
9. Fisher HW (1977) Surgery on patients receiving anticoagulants. J Dermatol Surg Oncol 3:210–212
10. Borman RJ, Danby D, Turner RC (1991) Management of the anticoagulated patient for elective surgery. J Foot Surg 30:308–309
11. Moy RL, Quan MB (1991) An evaluation of wound closure tapes. J Dermatol Surg Oncol 16:721–723
12. Koranda FC, Webster RC (1985) Trapdoor effect in nasolabial flaps. Arch Otolaryngol 111:421–424
13. Walkinshaw MD, Caffee HW (1982) The nasolabial flap: a problem and its correction. Plast Reconstr Surg 69:30–34
14. Katz BE, Oca AG (1991) A controlled study of the effectiveness of spot dermabrasion ("scarabrasion") on the appearance of surgical scars. J Am Acad Dermatol 24:462–466

Liposuction

William P. Coleman III

After 10 years of extensive worldwide use liposuction remains one of the safest cosmetic surgical procedures. Numerous retrospective clinical studies have revealed that major complications are extremely rare, but there is a small incidence of minor ones [1-3].

Minor Complications

Skin Irregularities

In the first few years of worldwide use of liposuction, dents, depressions, and other contour abnormalities were quite common. It became apparent that tunneling with large cannulas increases the potential for noticeable changes on the surface skin (Fig. 1). Cannulas of 8 mm or larger were gradually abandoned for instruments in the range of 3-6 mm. Although more tunnels are required to remove the same amount of fat than with larger instruments, the potential for contour abnormalities is dramatically reduced.

Liposuction surgeons have also learned to maintain the cannula at a depth of at least 1 cm below the dermis. More superficial liposuction removes the superficial layer of fat which provides a buffer zone that hides the liposuction work.

Often when cannulas are used through an incision at a great distance from the adiposity, the surgeon inadvertently directs the tip of the cannula too superficially. Using the contralateral hand to constantly monitor the depth of the cannula is an important principle of good liposuction technique. Sometimes dents occur secondary to hematoma formation, becoming apparent only when the blood is removed or reabsorbed.

The best treatment for contour depressions after liposuction is to fill them in with fat transplanted from neighboring tissues. This ordinarily involves removal of a small amount of fat around the periphery of the dent to decrease the volume differential followed by reinjecting this aspirated material into the concavity. Fat transplantation used in this way gives excellent results and the take is much more consistent than when fat is transferred to distant areas of the body. This is probably due to the similar blood supply and physiology of both the donor and recipient areas [4].

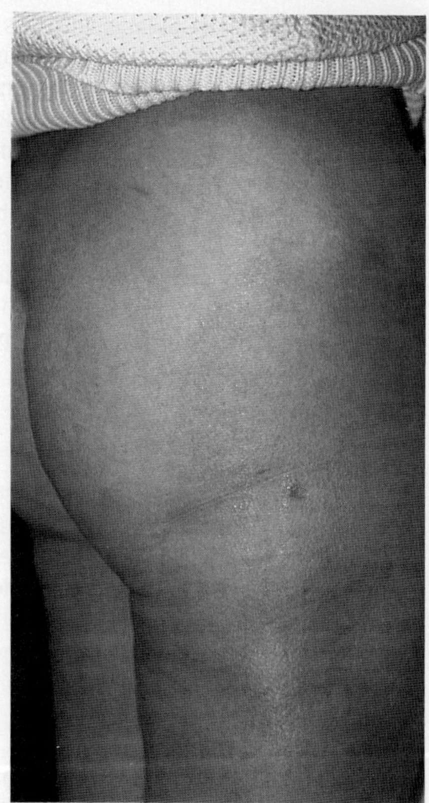

Fig. 1. A severe dimple of the thigh after liposuction

Waviness of the skin overlying the areas of liposuction is usually due to a horizontal tunneling pattern. When the liposuction cannula is directed across the body instead of in a cephalocaudal direction, the force of gravity may cause the healing tunnels to collapse over each other like the folds of a curtain. This defect is very difficult to correct, but a secondary liposuction with the tunnels directed in the right direction may be of some help.

Hematomas

Although hematomas were quite common in liposuction during its earliest years, this complication is quite rare now. Because this procedure involves creating numerous cavities throughout the fat, bleeding into these cavities can collect as a hematoma. Good preoperative hematologic evaluation helps to eliminate potential patients with bleeding disorders. Also. careful patient instruction on preoperative avoidance of alcohol, aspirin, and other anticoagulant substances help to minimize bleeding during liposuction.

The most important factor in minimizing liposuction bleeding, however, is the proper use of epinephrine in the surgical site. The tumescent technique, which involves the use of large volumes of very dilute solutions of lidocaine and epinephrine, has become the standard approach to dermatologic liposuction [5]. This technique has been shown dramatically to decrease the potential for intraoperative bleeding, probably due to the thorough penetration of the anesthetic solution throughout the surgical site [6].

Treatment of hematomas is not required in most cases. If these collections are smaller than 2 cm, they usually reabsorb spontaneously. If they do not reabsorb within 2 weeks postoperatively, and if they are larger than 2 cm, drainage is necessary. This can usually be accomplished using a large-bore needle and merely aspirating collected blood. Occasionally hematomas become infected, and it is useful to cover the patient with appropriate antibiotics, especially if aspiration is required.

Seromas

Seromas are accumulations of serum. These may appear after liposuction and require drainage just as with hemotomas. Seromas are relatively uncommon with the modern use of smaller instruments and less aggressive technique.

Hyperpigmentation

Some individuals, especially those with darker colored skin, are prone to hyperpigmentation after any skin injury. This change may appear in the overlying skin, especially if there has been bruising. Sun exposure of the treated area during the 1st month postoperatively also contributes to the development of hyperpigmentation. This discoloration usually resolves spontaneously and requires no treatment. However, patients may be interested in hydroquinone bleaching agents to accelerate this process.

Scars

The incision sites for liposuction are usually 5 mm or less in diameter so that only very small incisions result. In many cases these entry sites can be hidden in the pubic hair, the fold of the umbilicus, or in areas covered by bathing suits or clothing. However, some liposuction entry sites do require visible scars. As with all surgical healing, there is a great variation in the appearance of these scars depending on the scarring ability of the patient's skin. Surgeons should be sure to make the closure as cosmetically acceptable as possible, especially in conspicuous locations. Scar erythema and hyper- or hypopigmentation are quite common and usually fade with time. Keloids or hypertrophic scars may require intralesional injections of triamcinolone or even reexcision in unusual cases.

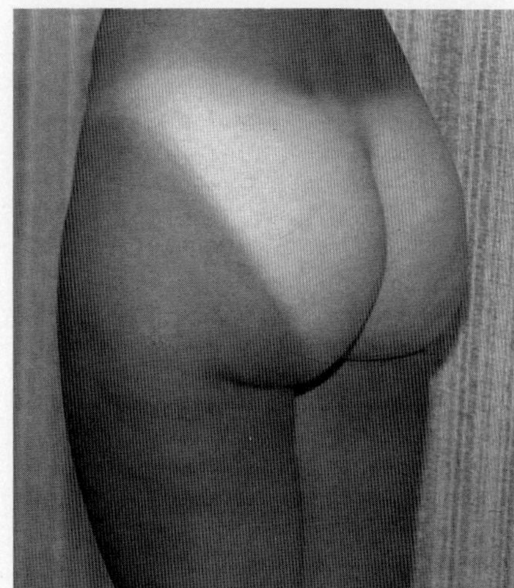

Fig. 2. Ptosis of the buttocks after liposuction

Ptotic Buttocks

The fat of the upper thigh may act as the buttress lending support to the overlying buttocks. If progressive liposuction is performed near the infragluteal fold, loss of some of this fat may lead to ptosis of the buttocks [7]. This is commonly seen in aging individuals and is considered unattractive (Fig. 2). For this reason liposuction should be used very sparingly around the infragluteal fold. Surgeons should never attempt to deepen this fold by horizontal liposuctioning. Once buttock ptosis occurs, there is no real treatment for it.

Banana Folds Of The Thigh

Often after liposuction of the thigh area a prominent collection of fat becomes more apparent below the infragluteal fold, usually in the shape of a banana (Fig. 3). Patients and physicians often did not notice that this was present preoperatively. This deformity may result from suction of the lateral thigh fat, revealing this previously present excess on the posterior thigh which was formerly disguised by the lateral adiposity. This problem can be addressed by feathering the liposuction into the posterior thigh at the time of the lateral thigh surgery. If the banana fold does appear, however, a revision liposuction may be required to smooth it out. This should be done carefully without disturbing the infragluteal fold and adding to ptosis of the buttocks.

Loose Skin

In those individuals with nonelastic skin overlying the area of liposuction, some redundancy may remain after removal of the underlying fat. Even in elderly in-

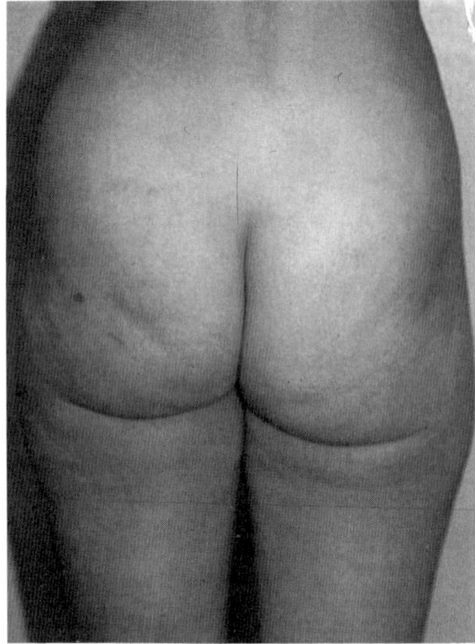

Fig. 3. Banana folds remain below the buttocks after liposuction

dividuals the skin usually tightens up in time. However, if it does not, skin excision may be required. This is particularly true for the lower abdomen. Multigravidae with extensive striae may have poor quality skin which does not contract well after liposuction.

Patients need to be instructed preoperatively to expect skin excision if it will be necessary. If the surgeon is relatively sure that this will be required, it can be done at the time of surgery. If the patient has a chance of avoiding the long scar associated with such procedures, one can prepare the patient for this possibility and plan to perform the excision if required. Generally it is a good idea to allow the operative site at least 6 months before, assuming that the skin will not contract. Such procedures on the abdomen should not be confused with abdominoplasty, which requires repair of the rectus muscles and often relocation of the umbilicus. Many patients assume that there is only one type of "tummy tuck," but often liposuction alone solves the problem if there is not excessive overlying skin, and the muscles are in reasonable shape.

Asymmetry

In some cases of liposuction, after the swelling has subsided, it becomes apparent that more fat remains on one side of the body than the other, resulting in an obvious asymmetry. This must be differentiated from cases in which the patient's bony skeleton and/or muscle development is asymmetrical. When asymmetry is due to excess fat on one side more than the other, a revision liposuction usually helps to make the sides more even. However, all patients should

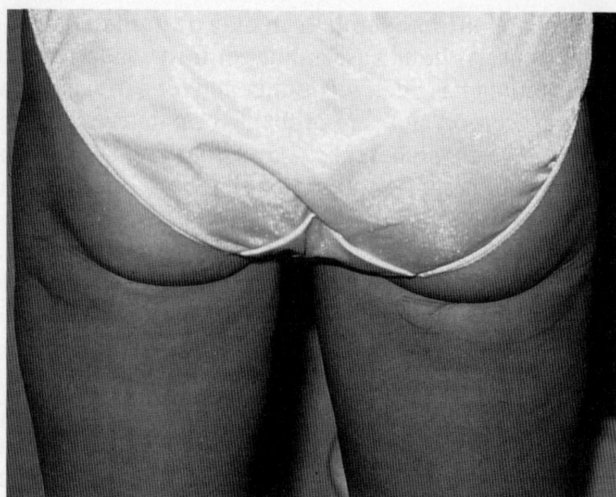

Fig. 4. Obvious assymetry
remains in spite
of liposuction

be warned in advance that most humans are asymmetrical to begin with, and
liposuction can only be used to remove fat; thus perfect symmetry cannot be
expected postoperatively (Fig. 4).

Major Complications

Although live-threatening complications of liposuction are quite rare, there are
a number of infrequent occurrences after liposuction which both the patient and
the physician must be prepared for. Retrospective surveys of liposuction
patients have revealed that the risks of these complications are all far less than
1% [1–3].

Thromboembolic Problems

Pulmonary embolism is a dreaded complication of any surgical procedure, and
liposuction is not immune to this potential disaster. Most of the deaths that
result from emboli are the result of preexisting deep vein thrombosis, a problem
which is usually asymptomatic [8]. Older patients, obese individuals, and those
with a prior history of thrombophlebitis are at higher risk for this complication.
Women, especially those taking estrogens, are more susceptible to thrombo-
embolic phenomena.

In the few deaths from thromboembolism following liposuction many of
these patients had combined procedures, most commonly abdominoplasty, at
the same time as liposuction. Abdominoplasty alone presents a much higher
risk of thromboembolism than liposuction, and combining these procedures
increases the risk [9].

Evolving thromboembolism may be hard to detect as there may be no early symptoms. Although ascending contrast venography and ^{125}I-labeled fibrinogen leg scanning has been recommended for early diagnosis of deep vein thrombosis, these blood clots are probably best detected by Doppler ultrasound or impedance plethysmography. Profusion lung scanning and ventilation scanning are used to diagnose pulmonary emboli, but pulmonary angiography may be more sensitive [10].

Although some recommend anticoagulant therapy in high-risk patients, it is best to avoid performing liposuction in these individuals all together. All patients should be mobilized within 24 h after surgery and continued on an increasing exercise schedule to decrease the potential for blood clot formation.

If symptoms of pulmonary embolism do occur, death may be rapid so that treatment should be instituted as rapidly as possible. Cardiopulmonary specialists should be consulted as rapidly as possible to institute treatment such as anticoagulants and fibrinolytic agents such as streptokinase or urokinase. Surgical intervention is rarely successful.

Infection

Although the incision for liposuction is small, the wound is large and infection of so much tissue is a feared complication of this procedure. Infection is rare in liposuction and can be minimized with the proper attention to sterile technique and patient prepping. The operating room should be maintained and cleaned in an appropriate fashion. Dirty cases should be performed elsewhere. Instruments must be properly sterilized and maintained. Thorough patient preparation with chlorhexidine or similar agents is important. In the few cases of reported death from infection after liposuction, there was a strong indication of a lack of basic principles of antisepsis.

Although the need for prophylactic antibiotics has been debated for all areas of surgery, their use has become quite common in liposuction. An oral cephalosporin given early enough so that blood levels are present at the time of surgery is adequate. The antibiotic should be continued for several days after surgery. Alternatively, parenteral antibiotics may be employed with a follow-up dose of oral agents. The use of sterile gowns and masks is sometimes debated for liposuction; however, these inexpensive materials provide better protection against contamination then sterile gloves alone.

Accidental Deep Cannula Penetration

Although the liposuction cannula is blunt, in rare cases it has found its way into the abdominal cavity or other submuscular locations. This is usually due to excessive force and loss of control of the location of the cannula tip. The liposuction surgeon should strive for a gentle technique and constant monitoring of the location of the cannula. The contralateral hand should grasp for the tip at all times so that its location is constantly known [11]. If excessive force is required to pass a cannula through a difficult area, it should be withdrawn and another tunnel sought. Force may result in the cannula penetrating deeper then intended.

A gentle technique also results in less bruising and a quicker patient recovery. Bleeding is also reduced by a gentle technique. If the surgeon has difficulty passing larger cannulas on the first try, small instruments should be substituted. If necessary, larger instruments can be used after the tunnels have been well defined.

Excessive Bleeding

In the early years of liposuction it was assumed that a 25% or more of the aspirate was blood [12]. Indeed, the typical liposuction procedure at this time was quite bloody. The development of the tumescent anesthetic has significantly decreased the potential for bleeding in liposuction [6]. It is estimated now that in most cases more blood is lost in the preoperative blood testing then during the procedure itself. The typical aspirate is yellow, with at worst a slightly pink color. If blood is encountered, the instrument should be relocated to another tunnel.

The only reason for excessive bleeding during liposuction today, with the use of the tumescent technique, is the patient's having a coagulation defect. This may be due to intrinsic or extrinsic factors. All patients should be told to discontinue anticoagulant substances including aspirin and alcohol well before the time of surgery. Patients requiring anticoagulants for other medical conditions should be rejected for liposuction until the conditions are no longer present. It is appropriate to perform proper preoperative blood testing including a CBC with platelet count, a PT, and a PTT to determine an intact coagulation system. Patients with marginal results should be referred to a hematologist for consultation before proceeding with the liposuction.

With breakthroughs in thorough epinephrine saturation of the liposuction site through the tumescent technique, larger procedures can now be performed without the risk of significant blood loss. Autologous blood transfusion is largely unneccessary in liposuction patients today. The volume of the liposuction procedure, however, is directly limited by the amount of blood loss. The *Guidelines for Liposuction* published by the American Academy of Dermatology recommend 2000 cm^3 aspirate exclusive of the infranate as the suggested maximum volume removal during one liposuction procedure [13]. If the patient needs significantly more fat removed, it should probably be done during two or more separate serial liposuctions.

Anesthetic Complications

The more profound the anesthetic agent employed, the greater is the risk of complications. For this reason, it is best to perform liposuction using the least sedation possible. The tumescent anesthetic technique has made it possible to perform liposuction entirely without sedation. However, some patients are anxious and do require tranquilizers such as Valium or Halcion. Mild narcotics such as Demerol are also useful in allaying anxiety. If the surgeon choses to employ intravenous sedation or general anesthesia, the assistance of a nurse anesthesist or anesthesiologist is recommended.

Even when potent intravenous sedatives or general anesthetic agents are not employed, it is important to monitor all liposuction patients for blood pressure, pulse, and respiration. If agents with potential for respiratory depression are used, a pulse oximeter is highly recommended. As with all outpatient surgical procedures, an appropriate crash cart kept up to date should be available in the operating room.

Conclusion

Liposuction is one of the safest of all the cosmetic surgical procedures. Recent advances in instrumentation and anesthetic techniques have made it extremely safe and easy on the patient. However, some major and minor complications do occasionally occur. The wise liposuction surgeon is acquainted with these and does everything possible to avoid them. However, he should remain vigilant to their appearance and be prepared to treat them if they occur.

References

1. ASPRS Ad Hoc Committee on New Procedure (1987) Five year updated evaluation of suction assisted lipectomy. American Society of Plastic and Reconstructive Surgeons, Chicago
2. Bernstein G, Hanke CW (1988) Safety of liposuction. A review of 9478 cases performed by dermatologists. J Dermatol Surg Oncol 14:1112
3. Newman J, Dolsky R (1984) Evaluation of 5,458 cases of liposuction surgery. Am J Cosmet Surg 1:27
4. Fournier P (1987) Body sculpturing through syringe liposuction and autologous fat reinjection. Rolf, Los Angeles, CA, USA
5. Klein J (1990) The tumescent technique. Anesthesia and modified liposuction technique. Dermatol Clin 8:425
6. Lillis PJ (1988) Liposuction surgery under local anesthesia: limited blood loss and minimal lidocaine absorption. J Dermatol Surg Oncol 14:1145
7. Fischer G (1991) Liposculpture. J Dermatol Surg Oncol 17:984
8. Moylan J (1989) Current treatment of embolic disease. Clin Plast Surg 16:381–384
9. Teimourian B (1989) Complications associated with suction lipectomy. Clin Plast Surg 16:385-394
10. Hull RD, Raskob GE, Hirsch J (1986) The diagnosis of clinically suspected pulmonary embolism: practical approaches. Chest 89:417S
11. Collins P (1990) The methodology of liposuction surgery. Dermatol Clin 8:395
12. Chrisman B, Coleman WP III (1988) Determining safe limits for untransfused outpatient liposuction: personal experience and review of the literature. J Dermatol Surg Oncol 14:1095
13. American Academy of Dermatology (1990) Guidelines of care for liposuction, revised. American Academy of Dermatology, Evanston, IL, USA

Skin Expansion

Brian B. Burkey and Michael J. Sullivan

Introduction

As medicine and surgery progress, many patients are surviving radical tumor resections and serious disfiguring trauma that before were often fatal. The need to deal with these resultant large wounds has led to the development of a wide array of pedicled flaps and, more recently, free tissue transfer. These advanced surgical techniques transfer tissue from a distant body site to the defect. The distant tissue, which often has a different color and texture, may not provide an optimal cosmetic result.

The idea of expanding local tissue and advancing it to close large defects was first described in a single case of ear reconstruction by Neumann [16]. This technique of tissue expansion, primarily skin expansion, was not advanced and popularized, however, until the work of two separate investigators, Radovan [20] and Austad [4], in the late 1970s. In the last decade, however, there has been a widespread acceptance of the technique, and a number of applications have been described. Enthusiasm for its use remains great despite high initial complication rates primarily because of results which are unattainable with other methods.

This chapter deals almost solely with the most commonly used method of tissue expansion, i. e., chronic skin expansion. We describe the technique briefly and explore the complications associated with it, as well as their cause and recommended treatment. A separate section focuses on methods to avoid the complications incurred with skin expansion. Rapid skin expansion is a relatively new technique which is not well understood and is mentioned only for completeness.

Technique

Successful tissue expansion depends on preoperative planning. The primary goal of tissue expansion is to expand and relocate healthy, well-vascularized tissue to an adjacent defect. Planning the appropriate expander size, its placement in relation to the defect, and the placement of incisions used for implantation are all equally important in eventually attaining an adequate amount of well-vascularized tissue for reconstruction.

Several expansion protheses are commercially available. The expander type commonly used by the authors consists of two parts: an inflatable silastic bag

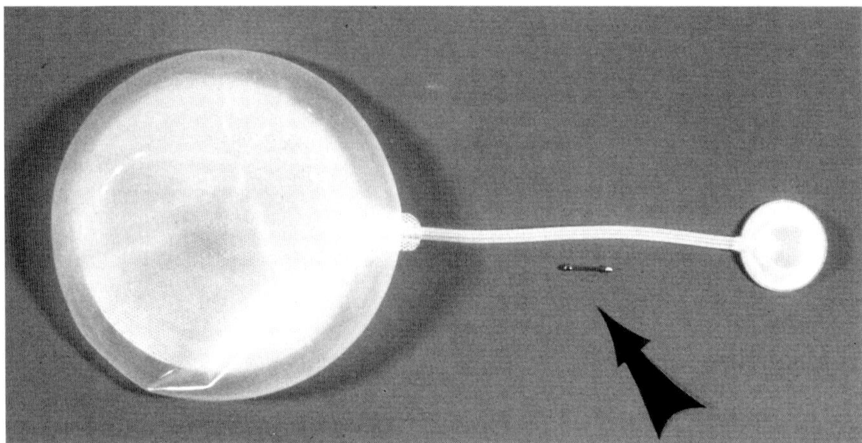

Fig. 1. Sample expander. The connector tubing can be shortened if necessary by inserting a metal connection (arrow)

and an injection port (Fig. 1). These are joined by connector tubing, the length of which can be easily adjusted. The injection port contains a gel-filled valve that prevents leakage of injected fluid. Self-expanding implants which are filled with hypertonic saline and expanded by osmosis are available. However, they are not widely used because of the inability to control the rate of inflation and the possible health hazard associated with inadvertent rupture [13].

The expander is usually placed adjacent to the defect. The incision used for implantation should be as short as possible. If possible, the incision is planned so as to be eliminated with the advancement of the flap, at the time of reconstruction. The incision should be parallel to the blood supply of the tissue to be expanded so as not to jeopardize its vascularity.

A pocket large enough for the expander to be placed without bending is created in a subcutaneous, subfascial, or submuscular plane, depending on the tissues to be expanded. Meticulous hemostasis is exercised. All pockets should be irrigated with antibiotic solution prior to placing the prosthesis and prior to closure. A separate pocket should be created for the injection port, which is kept distant from the expander and in a readily accessible spot. The pockets should be closed with an absorbable, buried suture and the overlying skin closed with permanent, nonreactive suture. Careful closure is necessary to avoid inadvertent injury to the prothesis. Perioperative antibiotics to cover skin organisms are employed, as is a light pressure dressing.

Expansion begins at the time of surgery. Normal saline is injected with a 23-gauge butterfly needle so as to just obliterate any dead space created during the expander implantation. Wound drains are avoided using this technique, but care must be taken to minimize tension on the closure. Expansion is individualized, but it usually resumes in 7–10 days and is continued on an outpatient basis every 3–7 days. At each expansion, the skin over the injection port is sterilized and normal saline injected until the patient reports discomfort, or until the overlying skin loses its capillary refill. A small amount of saline can be withdrawn to restore patient comfort or ensure skin perfusion. Selected, motivated patients may proceed with expansion at home after instruction. Skin sutures are kept in place during expansion.

The endpoint of expansion occurs when adequate tissue for the reconstruction is achieved. This is variable but usually requires 3–6 weeks of expansion. The degree of expansion can be estimated by subtracting the width of the expander base from the distance over the expander, from one edge to the other. For rectangular or crescentic expanders, the expander used should have a base 2.5 times as large as the defect to be closed for enough tissue to be gained at the expander's capacity [22].

At the time of reconstruction, the expander can be overinflated before removal to gain additional expansion, and removed. The skin flap is then advanced to close the defect. The capsule should be kept intact, as this is the site of a rich vascular network which supports the flap's viability. This capsule does slightly restrict the mobility of the flap but has been shown to resorb with time [13, 19].

Complications

Complication rates associated with skin expansion were initially reported to be as high as 50% [18], but more recent series have stressed that complication rates are generally lower and vary depending on the experience of the operator and the site and status of the tissue to be expanded [1, 2, 12].

The most reliable area for expansion is the chest, which may explain the early growth of tissue expansion for the purpose of breast reconstruction. The head and neck is regarded as the most difficult area to expand, with complication rates reported as high as 40%–60% [1, 6, 9]. This is believed to be secondary to the irregular contours of the scalp, forehead, cheek, and neck. Unfortunately, it is precisely this area where tissue expansion may play a major role for the patient and physician because of a paucity of suitable, available tissue for reconstruction at these sites [8].

Most authors also acknowledge the increased complication rates associated with expansion of burned and irradiated skin. This is most probably due to the decreased elasticity and vascularity evident in these tissues. Still, in situations where no other reconstructive options exist, burned and irradiated skin can be expanded safely if appropriate precautions are taken [15]. Likewise, with appropriate preoperative planning several series have supported the safety of tissue expansion in children [9, 18].

Untoward sequelae accompanying skin expansion can be divided into minor and major complications. Minor complications usually do not significantly impact upon the course of skin expansion or its overall result but do inconvenience the patient. Major complications, on the other hand, invariably alter the eventual outcome of the expansion and reconstruction.

Minor complications include cosmetic deformity, transient pain, skin discoloration, and seroma. The cosmetic deformity associated with skin expansion relates to the temporarily altered contour of the skin overlying the expander secondary to the increased subcutaneous volume. This is more of a problem in the latter stages of the expansion and in expansion of conspicuous areas, such as the head and neck. All patients find this bothersome, and dissatisfaction can best be avoided by counseling the patient preoperatively concerning this expected sequela. Careful patient selection can identify those patients with a psychological intolerance to the distorted body image [4].

Pain associated with the inflation of the expander is usually the limiting factor in the rate of expansion. This pain is usually transient, lasting approximately 4–6 h after the expansion and should be controlled by oral analgesics. This pain is a more prominent factor in expanding the scalp and forehead and the distal extremities [1, 12, 13]. Pain with scalp expansion may be lessened by performing galeotomies at the time of expander placement.

Discoloration of the skin overlying the expander may occur and is believed to be due to the increased vascularity of the capsule combined with the thinning of the dermis. The red or blue discoloration is not an indication of cyanosis or infection and is reversible after removal of the expander [6].

Finally, small seromas are not infrequently observed near the expander or the injection port. This may be a result of the implantation or a small leak from the gel-filled valve in the injection port. Seromas require no specific treatment and rarely interfere with the expansion process.

The most common major complication with tissue expansion is exposure of the expander resulting from erosion or dehiscence of overlying skin. This occurs in 8%-21% of expansion cases [1, 15, 18] and can be caused by either incisional dehiscence, inadequate tissue cover, or pressure necrosis of the skin overlying a fold in the inflatable bag. Fortunately, exposure of the implant is usually noted near the completion of skin expansion but almost invariably prevents further expansion (Figs. 2, 3). Conservative wound care, the use of prophylactic antibiotics and a slowing of the expansion schedule *may* allow the physician to gain adequate tissue for reconstruction without further complications. Early implant exposure from wound dehiscence or inadequate tissue cover, however, is best treated by removal of the implant and reimplantation after adequate healing [4, 13].

Occasionally, a fold in the expander bag is identified only after several expansions. The fold creates unequal tissue pressures and eventuates in tissue necrosis and exposure. Although this situation is not always correctable, some authors advocate deflation and reinflation of the expander with external manipulation as a method of repair. Whether correctable or not, expansion should then proceed at a slower rate than one normally would employ [6, 12, 14].

Infection surrounding the implant site is an uncommon complication of skin expansion, but one that requires aggressive treatment when detected. This complicates between 0%–10% of all tissue expansions and averages 5% in the larger reported series [1, 15, 18, 20]. Predisposing factors to infection include failure to adhere to sterile technique during implantation or expansion and later implant exposure. Infection is usually caused by *Staphylococcus* or *Pseudomonas* organisms [12, 15]. Treatment involves the drainage of purulent material and the institution of intravenous antibiotics. If the infection responds to these measures,

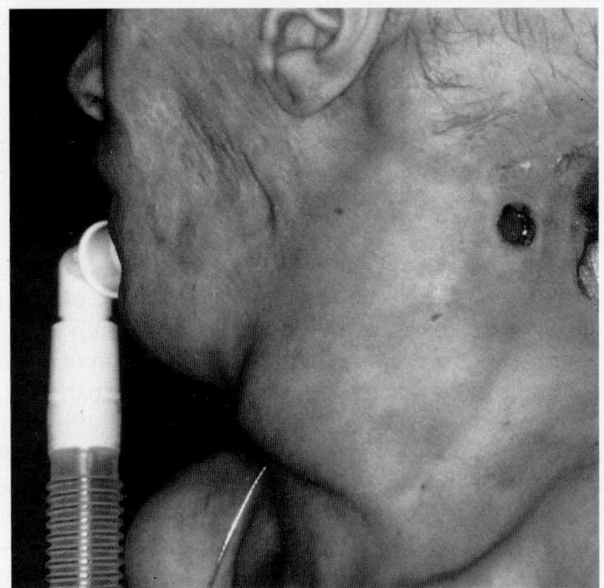

Fig. 2. Expander placed in an irradiated field. Atrophy of skin on the posterior aspect of the neck with exposure of the expander is apparent

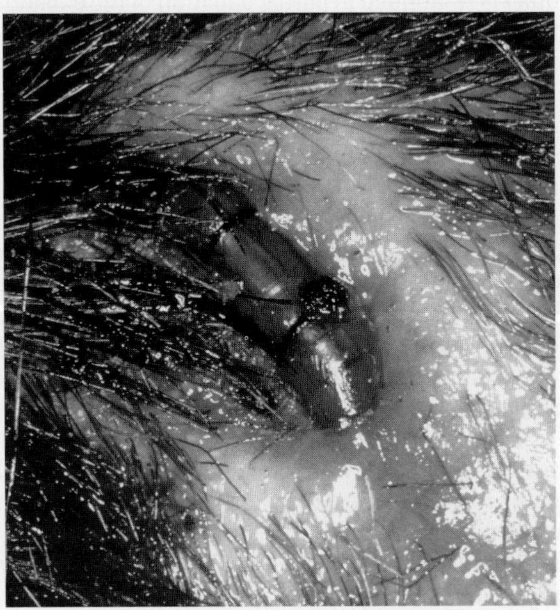

Fig. 3. Connector tubing overriding the expander with pressure necrosis of the skin

expansion can be resumed slowly; but if the infection worsens, it is advisable to remove the implant and replace it at a later date [4, 13].

Mechanical failure leading to deflation or rupture of the expander is a very uncommon occurrence, accounting for difficulties in about 2% of expansions [1, 12]. These failures are rarely due to defects in the expander and are usually secondary to an error in the assembly or an inadvertent puncture of the implants resulting in leaks. Once such an event is recognized, the only option is to replace the expander.

Intractable pain which prevents further expansion has been reported anecdotally. These cases probably represent a failure of proper patient selection and counseling. All cases eventually required removal of the implant.

Hematomas resulting from the implantation of expanders are extremely uncommon, occurring in less than 1% of skin expansions. All authors emphasize meticulous hemostasis during the placement of the implant, although there is division over whether to use suction drainage of the wound or light pressure dressings postoperatively [1, 4, 11, 21]. Once recognized, hematomas are best treated by a careful reexploration of the wound using strict sterile technique. One report of a delayed hematoma noted 2 months into a scalp expansion was thought secondary to erosion of the occipital artery and was treated with removal of the implant and control of the hemorrhage with partial reconstruction [3].

Despite the placement of expanders directly over the course of major nerves, neuropraxia has uncommonly been reported as a sequela of tissue expansion [1, 15]. It may arise as a result of direct compression of a neural bundle or as a result of neural traction secondary to restrictive anatomy. The sural, radial, and facial nerves have been involved in two large series, and in every case the neuropraxia quickly responded to partial deflation of the expander. Expansion was then continued at a slower rate. This is the expected outcome as long as treatment is initiated before the onset of demyelination [13].

Resorption of bone adjacent to a tissue expander has been noted as a complication of skin expansion in the head and neck [1, 17]. The reported cases involved expansion of the forehead and scalp and most often resulted in erosion of the outer table of calvarial bone. Full-thickness erosion of the skull has rarely occurred [17]. The expander applies constant pressure in all three dimensions, and although bone is the tissue most resistant to expansion, it is not difficult to understand how this complication might occur on occasion. If bone resorption is evident during the removal of the implant, no specific treatment is required unless a cosmetic deformity exists. Recontouring of the defect or placement of a tissue substitute (e. g., methylmethacrelate) provides better cosmesis in this situation.

Substantial migration of the implant is rarely a problem during tissue expansion, although it has been reported [6, 9]. It presents a problem only if the movement results in the expansion of inappropriate tissue or the development of excessive pressure on overlying tissue. If this occurs, the expander should be repositioned and secured and expansion continued after adequate healing. This problem is better avoided than treated.

Flap necrosis after a reconstruction with expanded skin occurs rarely [4, 12]. In fact, expanded skin flaps have been shown to have an increased survival length compared to both acutely raised flaps and traditionally delayed skin flaps [7]. Treatment, when it occurs, involves conservative management of the wound with débridement and closure by secondary intention.

Scarring is as prevalent in surgery utilizing skin expansion as in any other type of surgery. Every effort should be made to minimize scars by utilizing atraumatic technique and placing expanders through incisions that will eventually be excised during the flap rotation and reconstruction. Adequate expansion to ensure a tension-free closure also helps to avoid hypertrophic or widened scars. Still, standing cones and conspicuous scars occur occasionally. These should be allowed to mature to at least 6 months before committing the patient to revision surgery. Many standing cones flatten with time and may not require revision. If revision surgery is indicated, this can usually be performed under local anesthesia, and the routine principles of scar camouflaging should be followed.

Avoidance of Complications

Complications are always better avoided than treated; some sequelae, however, may be unavoidable. Good judgement and surgical technique assures the physician the best results with a minimum of personal frustration and patient dissatisfaction. These issues are discussed below.

Implant exposure is potentially the most easily avoided complication. This problem results from the necrosis or dehiscence of skin overlying the expander. To prevent this outcome, the physician must be attentive to detail throughout the expansion process. In the preoperative planning it is best to avoid attempts to expand burned or irradiated skin, unless absolutely necessary. As mentioned, these tissues have higher associated complication rates, and if normal skin is available near a defect, it is the better choice to expand. It is also wise to avoid expansion near a skin graft, as this thin skin provides the path of least resistance for implant expansion and exposure. During the implantation, once a pocket of adequate size to prevent folding of the implant is created and the implant is placed, the two-layer closure described above should be employed. If possible, it is best to include muscle and/or fascia between the skin and the expander, as these provide an additional barrier to erosion by the implant [1].

When acutely expanding the silastic bag, it is important to assure adequate circulation to the overlying skin. This requires experienced judgement as there is no instrument for assessing perfusion that is currently available to the clinician. The best assurance of good flow is the presence of brisk capillary refill, as described above. This test may be difficult to evaluate. When in doubt, it is always best to expand over a longer period than to risk skin breakdown. Recently, investigations were carried out to find a good correlate of tissue perfusion by measuring oxygen tensions transcutaneously. These relationships varied from patient to patient, and thus no critical criteria were established; however, it was noted that in any one patient pain *always* preceded the development of tissue anoxia [10]. Careful observation of the expanded site during the process also warns the physician of impending exposure and allows corrective action to be initiated, as outlined above.

Infection of the implant site is best avoided at the time of implantation through the use of perioperative prophylactic antibiotics, the adherence to sterile technique, and the atraumatic handling of tissue. One author also advocates soaking the implants in gentamicin solution prior to inserting them [6]. Again, during the expansions, care must be taken to sterilize the skin prior to manipulating the injection port.

The likelihood of mechanical failure of the expander unit can be lessened by several methods throughout the expansion process. It is advisable to avoid expander placement in psychotic patients where trauma to the implant is a high risk. Intraoperatively, the physician should be meticulous in assembling and securing the prothesis, as well as in closing the wound, to avoid leaks and punctures in the implant. Strategic location of the injection port avoid later accidental punctures of the silastic bag during the expansions.

Averting hematomas related to expander implantation is accomplished by assuring adequate intraoperative hemostasis, by obliterating all dead space around the expander through suturing or partial inflation of the expander, and by using light pressure dressings postoperatively. Manders et al. [12] also caution against the use of expanders near hemangiomas. Likewise, expanders should not be placed near large vessels where erosion could lead to catastrophic bleeding.

In a similar way, the physician should anticipate the effect of expander inflation on the course of adjacent named nerves in an effort to avoid neuropraxia. This is especially true when expanding the face or distal extremities.

The effect of scalp expanders on the underlying skull is difficult to predict, as mentioned earlier, but experienced reconstructive surgeons do advise delaying elective scalp expansion in children until there is complete closure of the fontanelles [17]. Tissue expansion of the head and neck is also complicated by migration of the expanders due to gravity. This can be prevented by securing the expanders in their tissue bed with slowly resorbing absorbable sutures [6].

Avoiding necrosis of the expanded and transposed flap at the conclusion of the expansion process is perhaps the most vital step in the technique of skin expansion. Loss of some or all of the flap may undo all the preceding work and cause the intervening time to be for nought. Although this complication is uncommon, it does occasionally occur. To prevent this problem it is best to keep the tissue capsule of the expander intact during rotation of the flap. This capsule contains a rich supportive vascular network which provides the expanded skin with its remarkable reliability. Austad [4] also believes it is important to avoid the use of local anesthetics containing epinephrine when transposing expanded flaps, as these caused several flap failures in his experience and have had a similar effect on other delayed flaps reported in the literature. Finally, it is best to avoid closure under tension and traumatic closures, both of which devitalize tissue and increase the likelihood of necrosis.

As mentioned above, the most skilled physician inevitably experiences complications even if all the above actions are followed. The tremendously exciting aspect concerning tissue expansion is that even when complications occur, they usually do not preclude the desired reconstruction or even adversely affect it. In his series of 76 expansions, Antonyshyn reported a 48% overall complication rate but noted that 83% of his intended reconstructions were successfully completed [1]. This experience has been verified by other authors [12, 15]. Further enthusiasm for this reconstructive technique is generated by the relatively rapid improvement in results and decrease in complication rate as an individual physician gains experience with skin expansion. This point was discussed above, but it is interesting to note that experienced reconstructive surgeons may have complication rates as low as 7% [13].

It must be emphasized that reconstruction utilizing the techniques of tissue expansion as outlined above can achieve results which are unattainable or far superior to those attained using other methods [1, 15]. The availability of surplus tissue which matches the desired characteristics of the recipient site allows a high degree of reconstructive sophistication and patient satisfaction. The growing popularity of skin expansion also extends the application of this technique into more difficult and challenging reconstructive dilemmas, such as the treatment of burn deformities and perhaps keloids. Some complications with this technique then are to be expected and can be tolerated; however, hopefully the next decade of tissue expansion will lead to the development of materials that increase its reliability.

Summary

Currently, chronic skin expansion is well suited to the needs of the reconstructive physician. It can be used to reliably correct a local shortage of tissues, particularly those with special qualities such as the scalp and breast, caused by tumor or trauma. It can also be used to increase the amount of donor tissue available from the more sophisticated pedicled and free flaps. The techniques are relatively simple and require no special training or instrumentation, and most of the care can be performed in an outpatient setting.

The growth of skin expansion in the future will center on refinements in materials and techniques, which hopefully will further lower complication rates and identify new applications of this technology. The latter point is exemplified by the recent development of rapid or intraoperative tissue expansion in which skin is expanded within minutes rather than weeks [6]. Unfortunately, little is understood of this latest procedure, and more work is necessary to define its role in future reconstructive efforts. Indeed, more research at the basic science level is also needed concerning chronic tissue expansion, if its current clinical popularity is to be maintained and expanded in the years to come.

References

1. Antonyshyn O, Gruss JS, Mackinnon SE, Zuker R (1988) Complications of soft tissue expansion:,Br J Plast Surg 41:239–250
2. Argenta LC, Marks MW, Pasyk KA (1985) Advances in tissue expansion. Clin Plast Surg 12:159–171
3. Ashail G, Quaba A (1987) A hemorrhagic hazard of tissue expansion. Plast Reconstr Surg 79:627–630
4. Austad ED (1987) Complications in tissue expansion. Clin Plast Surg 14:549–550
5. Austad ED, Rose GL (1982) A self-inflating tissue expander. Plast Reconstr Surg 70:107
6. Baker SR, Swanson NA (1990) Tissue expansion of the head and neck: indications, technique, and complications. Arch Otolaryngol Head Neck Surg 116:1147–1153
7. Cherry GW, Austad ED, Pasyk K et al. (1983) Increased survival and vascularity of random-pattern skin flaps elevated in controlled, expanded skin. Plast Reconstr Surg 72:680–685
8. Cullen KW, Powell B (1989) Tissue expanders in surgery. Br J Clin Pract 43:75–77
9. Elias DL, Baird WL, Zubowicz VN (1991) Applications and complications of tissue expansion in pediatric patients. J Pediatr Surg 26:15–21
10. Hallock GG, Rice DC (1986) Objective monitoring for safe tissue expansion. Plast Reconstr Surg 77:416–420
11. Manders EK, Graham WP, Schenden MJ, Davis TS (1984) Skin expansion to eliminate large scalp defects. Ann Plast Surg 12:305–312
12. Manders EK, Schenden MJ, Furrey JA et al. (1984) Soft-tissue expansion: concepts and complications. Plast Reconstr Surg 74:493–507
13. Marcus J, Horan DB, Robinson JK (1990) Tissue expansion: past, present, and future. J Am Acad Dermatol 23:813–825
14. Masser MR (1990) Tissue expansion: a reconstructive revolution or a cornucopia of complications? Br J Plast Surg 43:344–348
15. Neugan PC, Peters WJ (1989) Advances in burn scar reconstruction: the use of tissue expansion. Ann Plast Surg 22:203–210
16. Neumann CG (1957) The expansion of an area of skin by progressive distention of a subcutaneous balloon. Plast Reconstr Surg 19:124
17. Paletta CF, Bass J, Shehadi SI (1989) Outer table skull erosion causing rupture of scalp expander. Ann Plast Surg 23:538–542
18. Paletta CF, Campbell E, Shehadi SI (1991) Tissue expanders in children. J Pediatr Surg 26:22–25
19. Pasyk KA, Argenta LC, Austad ED (1987) Histopathology of human expanded tissue. Clin Plast Surg 14:435–445
20. Radovan C (1984) Tissue expansion in soft tissue reconstruction. Plast Reconstr Surg 74:482–492
21. Sullivan MJ, Rubinstein MI (1984) Skin expansion. Adv Otolaryngol Head Neck Surg 3:27–38
22. Van Rappard JHAA, Molenaar J, Van Doorn K et al. (1988) Surface area increase in tissue expansion. Plast Reconstr Surg 82:833–837